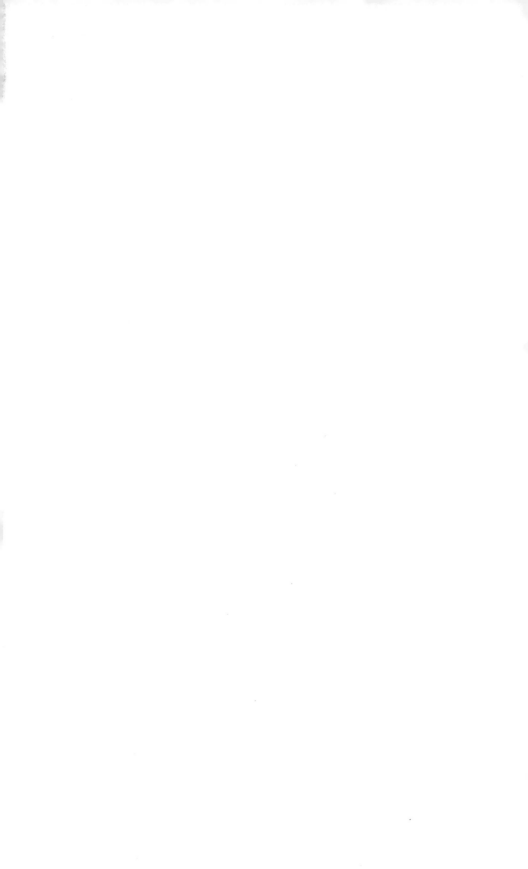

Anesthetic Care for Abdominal Surgery

Editors

TIMOTHY E. MILLER
MICHAEL J. SCOTT

ANESTHESIOLOGY CLINICS

www.anesthesiology.theclinics.com

Consulting Editor
LEE A. FLEISHER

March 2015 • Volume 33 • Number 1

ELSEVIER

1600 John F. Kennedy Boulevard ● Suite 1800 ● Philadelphia, Pennsylvania, 19103-2899

http://www.theclinics.com

ANESTHESIOLOGY CLINICS Volume 33, Number 1
March 2015 ISSN 1932-2275, ISBN-13: 978-0-323-35649-7

Editor: Jennifer Flynn-Briggs
Developmental Editor: Susan Showalter

Anesthesiology Clinics (ISSN 1932-2275) is published quarterly by Elsevier Inc., 360 Park Avenue South, New York, NY 10010-1710. Months of issue are March, June, September, and December. Periodicals postage paid at New York, NY and at additional mailing offices. Subscription prices are $160.00 per year (US student/resident), $330.00 per year (US individuals), $400.00 per year (Canadian individuals), $533.00 per year (US institutions), $674.00 per year (Canadian institutions), $225.00 per year (Canadian and foreign student/resident), $455.00 per year (foreign individuals), and $674.00 per year (foreign institutions). To receive student and resident rate, orders must be accompanied by name of affiliated institution, date of term, and the *signature* of program/residency coordinator on institutions letterhead. Orders will be billed at individual rate until proof of status is received. Foreign air speed delivery is included in all *Clinics'* subscription prices. All prices are subject to change without notice. POSTMASTER: Send address changes to *Anesthesiology Clinics,* Elsevier Health Sciences Division, Subscription Customer Service, 3251 Riverport Lane, Maryland Heights, MO 63043. Customer Service (orders, claims, online, change of address): Elsevier Health Sciences Division, Subscription Customer Service, 3251 Riverport Lane, Maryland Heights, MO 63043. Tel:1-800-654-2452 (U.S. and Canada); 314-447-8871 (outside U.S. and Canada). Fax: 314-447-8029. E-mail: journalscustomerservice-usa@elsevier.com (for print support); journalsonlinesupport-usa@elsevier.com (for online support).

Reprints. For copies of 100 or more of articles in this publication, please contact the Commercial Reprints Department, Elsevier Inc., 360 Park Avenue South, New York, NY 10010-1710. Tel.: 212-633-3874; Fax: 212-633-3820; E-mail: reprints@elsevier.com.

Anesthesiology Clinics, is also published in Spanish by McGraw-Hill Inter-americana Editores S. A., P.O. Box 5-237, 06500 Mexico D. F., Mexico.

Anesthesiology Clinics, is covered in *MEDLINE/PubMed (Index Medicus), Current Contents/Clinical Medicine, Excerpta Medica, ISI/BIOMED,* and *Chemical Abstracts.*

Contributors

CONSULTING EDITOR

LEE A. FLEISHER, MD, FACC, FAHA,
Robert D. Dripps Professor and Chair of Anesthesiology and Critical Care, Professor of Medicine, Perelman School of Medicine, University of Pennsylvania School of Medicine, Philadelphia, Pennsylvania

EDITORS

TIMOTHY E. MILLER, MB ChB, FRCA
Assistant Professor, Department of Anesthesiology, Duke University Medical Center, Durham, North Carolina

MICHAEL J. SCOTT, MB ChB, MRCP, FRCA, FFICM
Consultant in Anesthesia and Intensive Care Medicine, Department of Anesthesia and Perioperative Medicine, Royal Surrey County Hospital NHS Foundation Trust; Senior Fellow, Surrey Peri-operative Anesthesia Critical care Research Group (SPACeR), Faculty of Health and Medical Sciences, University of Surrey, Guildford, Surrey, United Kingdom

AUTHORS

GABRIELE BALDINI, MD, MSc
Anesthesiologist, Assistant Professor, Department of Anesthesia, Montreal General Hospital, McGill University Health Centre, Montreal, Quebec, Canada

JEANETTE R. BAUCHAT, MD
Assistant Professor of Anesthesiology, Northwestern University, Feinberg School of Medicine, Chicago, Illinois

COLIN B. BERRY, MBBS, FRCA
Consultant in Anaesthesia, Exeter, United Kingdom; Lead, Royal College of Anaesthetists Perioperative Medicine Standards and Service Design Group, London, United Kingdom

FRANCESCO CARLI, MD, MPhil, FRCA, FRCPC
Department of Anesthesia, McGill University, Montreal, Quebec, Canada

ADAM CARNEY, MA, MB BChir, MRCP, FRCA
Consultant Anaesthetist, Department of Anaesthesia, Nottingham University Hospitals NHS Trust, Nottingham, United Kingdom

JAMES O.B. COCKCROFT, MB ChB, FRCA
Registrar in Anaesthesia, Royal Devon & Exeter Hospital, Exeter, United Kingdom

MARK O. DAUGHERTY, MBBCh, FRCA
Lead Anaesthetist for Enhanced Recovery and Robotic Surgery in Urology; Consultant in Anaesthesia, Exeter, United Kingdom

MATT DICKINSON, MBBS, MSc, FRCA, FFICM
Consultant Anaesthetist, Department of Anaesthesia, Perioperative Medicine and Pain,
Royal Surrey County Hospital NHS Foundation Trust, Guildford, Surrey, United Kingdom

WILLIAM J. FAWCETT, MB BS, FRCA, FFPMRCA
Consultant in Anesthesia and Pain Medicine, Royal Surrey County Hospital; Senior
Fellow, Postgraduate School, University of Surrey, Guildford, United Kingdom

MICHAEL P.W. GROCOTT, MB BS, MD, FRCA, FRCP, FFICM
Professor, Integrative Physiology and Critical Illness Group, Clinical and Experimental
Sciences, Faculty of Medicine, University of Southampton; Critical Care Research Area,
Southampton NIHR Respiratory Biomedical Research Unit; Anaesthesia and Critical Care
Research Unit, University Hospital Southampton NHS Foundation Trust, Southampton,
United Kingdom

ASHRAF S. HABIB, MBBCh, MSc, MHSc, FRCA
Associate Professor of Anesthesiology, Duke University Medical Center, Durham, North
Carolina

DENNY Z.H. LEVETT, BM, BCh, PhD, MRCP, FRCA
Integrative Physiology and Critical Illness Group, Clinical and Experimental Sciences,
Faculty of Medicine, University of Southampton; Critical Care Research Area,
Southampton NIHR Respiratory Biomedical Research Unit; Anaesthesia and Critical Care
Research Unit, University Hospital Southampton NHS Foundation Trust, Southampton,
United Kingdom

DILEEP N. LOBO, MS, DM, FRCS, FACS, FRCPE
Professor of Gastrointestinal Surgery, Nottingham Digestive Diseases Centre National
Institute for Health Research Biomedical Research Unit, Nottingham University Hospitals,
Queen's Medical Centre, Nottingham, United Kingdom

JOHN S. McGRATH, BMBS, FRCS, MD
National Adviser to NHS England for Enhanced Recovery; Consultant in Urology, Exeter
Health Services Research Unit, Exeter, United Kingdom

TIMOTHY E. MILLER, MB ChB, FRCA
Assistant Professor, Department of Anesthesiology, Duke University Medical Center,
Durham, North Carolina

GARY MINTO, MB ChB, FRCA
Consultant, Department of Anaesthesia & Perioperative Medicine, Plymouth Hospitals
NHS Trust, Honorary Senior Lecturer, Plymouth University Peninsula School of Medicine,
Plymouth, United Kingdom

CAROL PEDEN, MB ChB, MD, FRCA, FFICM, MPH
Consultant in Anaesthesia & Intensive Care Medicine, Royal United Hospital, Bath, United
Kingdom

JAMES PRENTIS, MBBS, FRCA
Consultant Anaesthetist, Department of Perioperative and Critical Care Medicine,
Freeman Hospital, Newcastle upon Tyne, United Kingdom

KARTHIK RAGHUNATHAN, MD MPH
Assistant Professor, Anesthesiology Service, Durham VA Medical Center, Duke University
Medical Center, Durham, North Carolina

CELENA SCHEEDE-BERGDAHL, MSc, PhD
Department of Anesthesia, McGill University; Department of Kinesiology and Physical Education, McGill University, Montreal, Quebec, Canada

MICHAEL J. SCOTT, MB ChB, MRCP, FRCA, FFICM
Consultant in Anesthesia and Intensive Care Medicine, Department of Anesthesia and Perioperative Medicine, Royal Surrey County Hospital NHS Foundation Trust; Senior Fellow, Surrey Peri-operative Anesthesia Critical care Research Group (SPACeR), Faculty of Health and Medical Sciences, University of Surrey, Guildford, Surrey, United Kingdom

MANDEEP SINGH, MD
Division of Anesthesiology and Critical Care Medicine, Duke University Medical Center, Durham, North Carolina

CHRIS SNOWDEN, BMedSci (Hons), MBBS, FRCA, MD
Consultant Anaesthetist, Department of Perioperative and Critical Care Medicine, Freeman Hospital; Honorary Senior Lecturer, Institute of Cellular Medicine, The Medical School, University of Newcastle upon Tyne, Newcastle upon Tyne, United Kingdom

Contents

Reduced exercise capacity is associated with increased postoperative morbidity and mortality. Variables derived from cardiopulmonary exercise testing (CPET) can be used to risk stratify patients and in the future may be combined with other risk predictors to improve outcome prediction. CPET results can be used to improve the process of informed consent and thus contribute to collaborative decision making. CPET can be used to guide the choice of surgical procedure and decide on the most appropriate postoperative care environment. In the future, CPET may also be used to guide prehabilitation training programs, improving fitness and thereby reducing perioperative risk.

Patients who are elderly, malnourished, anxious, and have a low physical function before surgery are likely to have suboptimal recovery from cancer surgery. A multimodal prehabilitation program is proposed, consisting of exercise training and nutritional and psychological support, which increases physiologic reserve before the stress of surgery. This interventional approach seems to improve ability to undergo the stress of surgery and faster recovery. The integration of exercise, adequate nutrition, and psychosocial components, with medical and pharmacologic optimization in the presurgical period, deserves to receive more attention by clinicians to elucidate the most effective interventions.

Patients having major abdominal surgery need perioperative fluid supplementation; however, enhanced recovery principles mitigate against many of the factors that traditionally led to relative hypovolemia in the perioperative period. An estimate of fluid requirements for abdominal surgery can be made but individualization of fluid prescription requires consideration of clinical signs and hemodynamic variables. The literature supports goal-directed fluid therapy. Application of this evidence to justify stroke volume optimization in the setting of major surgery within an enhanced recovery

in perioperative care and more aware of the impact of anesthetic techniques on surgical outcomes and recovery. Key to achieving success is strict adherence to the principle of aggregation of marginal gains. This article reviews anesthetic and analgesic care of patients undergoing elective colorectal surgery in the context of an ERAS program, and also discusses anesthesia considerations for emergency colorectal surgery.

Hepatobiliary surgery outcomes have significantly improved since the early 1970s. Surgical and anesthetic advances related to patient selection, alternative surgical management options, and reduction of operative blood loss have been important. Postoperative analgesic regimens are being modified to include intrathecal opiates and to embrace enhanced recovery regimens.

Esophagectomy is a high-risk operation with significant perioperative morbidity and mortality. Attention to detail in many areas of perioperative management should lead to an aggregation of marginal gains and improvement in postoperative outcome. This review addresses preoperative assessment and patient selection, perioperative care (focusing on pulmonary prehabilitation, ventilation strategies, goal-directed fluid therapy, analgesia, and cardiovascular complications), minimally invasive surgery, and current evidence for enhanced recovery in esophagectomy.

This article details the anesthetic management of robot-assisted and laparoscopic urologic surgery. It includes the key concerns for anesthetists and a guide template for those learning this specialist area. The emphasis is on the principles of enhanced recovery, the preoperative and risk assessments, as well as the specific management plans to reduce the incidence of complications arising as a result of the prolonged pneumoperitoneum and steep head-down positions necessary for most of these procedures.

Studies on enhanced recovery after gynecological surgery are limited but seem to report outcome benefits similar to those reported after colorectal surgery. Regional anesthesia is recommended in enhanced recovery protocols. Effective regional anesthetic techniques in gynecologic surgery include spinal anesthesia, epidural analgesia, transversus abdominis plane blocks, local anesthetic wound infusions and intraperitoneal instillation catheters. Non-opioid analgesics including pregabalin, gabapentin, NSAIDs, COX-2 inhibitors, and paracetamol reduce opioid consumption after surgery. This population is at high risk for PONV, thus, a multimodal

ANESTHESIOLOGY CLINICS

FORTHCOMING ISSUES

June 2015
Airway Management
Lynette Mark, Marek A. Mirski, and
Paul W. Flint, *Editors*

September 2015
Geriatric Anesthesia
Mark D. Neuman and Charles Brown,
Editors

December 2015
Value-Based Care
Lee A. Fleisher, *Editor*

RECENT ISSUES

December 2014
Orthopedic Anesthesiology
Nabil M. Elkassabany and
Edward R. Mariano, *Editors*

September 2014
Vascular Anesthesia
Charles Hill, *Editor*

June 2014
Ambulatory Anesthesiology
Jeffrey L. Apfelbaum
and Thomas W. Cutter, *Editors*

March 2014
Pediatric Anesthesiology
Alan Jay Schwartz, Dean B. Andropoulos,
and Andrew Davidson, *Editors*

RELATED INTEREST

Orthopedic Clinics of North America, January 2015 (Vol. 46, Issue 1)

Foreword

Anesthetic Care for Abdominal Surgery

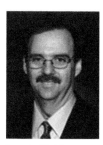

Lee A. Fleisher, MD
Consulting Editor

With the recent interest in providing value in surgical care, enhanced recovery after surgery protocols and the perioperative management of the patient undergoing colorectal surgery has taken on increasing importance. This is particularly true given the recent interest in the Perioperative Surgical Home. In addition, there have been changes in the manner in which anesthesiologists provide care for a group of other abdominal surgeries. In this issue of *Anesthesiology Clinics*, a remarkable group of international experts in the field has written outstanding reviews to help all of us provide state-of-the-art value-based care.

In choosing an editor for an abdominal surgery issue, it was easy to choose two outstanding contributors to this field. Dr. Timothy Miller is currently Assistant Professor of Anesthesiology at Duke University. Dr. Michael Scott is a Consultant in Anaesthesia and Intensive Care Medicine at the Royal Surrey County Hospital NHS Foundation Trust and Senior Fellow at the University of Surrey. Given their expertise, they are well qualified to edit this important issue.

Lee A. Fleisher, MD
Perelman School of Medicine
University of Pennsylvania
Philadelphia, PA 19104, USA

E-mail address:
lee.fleisher@uphs.upenn.edu

Anesthesiology Clin 33 (2015) xiii
http://dx.doi.org/10.1016/j.anclin.2014.12.002   **anesthesiology.theclinics.com**
1932-2275/15/$ – see front matter © 2015 Published by Elsevier Inc.

Preface

Enhanced Recovery and the Changing Landscape of Major Abdominal Surgery

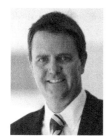   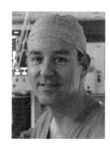

Timothy E. Miller, MB ChB, FRCA

Michael J. Scott, MB ChB, MRCP, FRCA, FFICM

Editors

This issue of *Anesthesiology Clinics* focuses on the anesthetic management and perioperative care pathway for patients undergoing major abdominal surgery. The last decade has seen increasing recognition that a properly planned and managed perioperative care pathway can improve outcomes after major surgery. There has also been widespread adoption of minimally invasive surgical techniques (both laparoscopic and robotic) that when effectively utilized have contributed to accelerated recovery by minimizing surgical injury. When both are done well, it leads to a very short length of stay for surgical procedures that were once performed using open surgical techniques with high morbidity and mortality.

The development of Enhanced Recovery Pathways (ERPs), first in colorectal surgery and now increasingly across all elective surgical specialties, has lead to the development of patient-focused multidisciplinary teams consisting of anesthesiologists, surgeons, physicians, nurses, physiotherapists, and dieticians, all of whom contribute to improving the outcome for patients. ERPs aim to deliver evidence-based practice (and practice-based evidence) across a multitude of treatment elements to reduce the stress response and improve the metabolic response to major surgery. There is increasing evidence this in turn shortens length of stay, reduces complications and costs, and improves long-term outcomes. The ERAS Society has been the first to publish guidelines in a variety of specialties with the aim of reviewing and updating the evidence base in three yearly cycles. Already we have seen significant shifts in evidence base, such as the move away of using epidural anesthesia in laparoscopic colorectal surgery. Medicine moves fast and we must all move with it!

In this issue, we have started with two articles focusing on prehabilitation and assessment for major surgery using cardiopulmonary exercise testing. We then have

Anesthesiology Clin 33 (2015) xv–xvi

http://dx.doi.org/10.1016/j.anclin.2014.12.001

anesthesiology.theclinics.com

1932-2275/15/$ – see front matter © 2015 Published by Elsevier Inc.

an article that outlines the effects an ERP has on the pathophysiology during major surgery, before moving on to articles on abdominal surgical specialties, with the emphasis on surgery within modern ERAS protocols. There are specific articles on fluids and analgesia because they are the two key elements that are delivered by anesthesiologists that, combined with minimally invasive surgery, have a major effect on producing optimal outcomes. We end with an article on Emergency Surgery, which is an area that until recently patients have been very poorly served by, but there are exciting developments with pathways improving care—combining Enhanced Recovery and Surviving Sepsis principles.

All articles in this issue have contributions by experts in their field and eminent anesthesiologists with experience and who have driven changes in the perioperative care pathway. It is now time for anesthesiologists to recognize that they don't just have the best understanding of the perioperative care pathway but are in the perfect position to deliver most of the key factors essential for optimal surgical outcomes. They should embrace their new role as Anesthesiologist and Perioperative Care Physician.

Timothy E. Miller, MB ChB, FRCA
Associate Professor
Department of Anesthesiology
Duke University Medical Center
Durham, NC 27710, USA

Michael J. Scott, MB ChB, MRCP, FRCA, FFICM
Department of Anesthesia and Perioperative Medicine
Royal Surrey County Hospital NHS Foundation Trust
Guildford, Surrey GU1 7XX, UK

Surrey Peri-operative Anesthesia Critical care Research Group (SPACeR)
Faculty of Health and Medical Sciences
University of Surrey
Guildford, Surrey GU2 7XH, UK

E-mail addresses:
timothy.miller2@duke.edu (T.E. Miller)
mjpscott@btinternet.com (M.J. Scott)

Cardiopulmonary Exercise Testing for Risk Prediction in Major Abdominal Surgery

Denny Z.H. Levett, BM, BCh, PhD, MRCP, FRCA[a,b,c],
Michael P.W. Grocott, MB BS, MD, FRCA, FRCP, FFICM[a,b,c],*

KEYWORDS

- Cardiopulmonary exercise testing • Functional capacity • Preoperative
- Incremental exercise test • Anaerobic threshold (AT)
- Peak oxygen consumption ($\dot{V}o_2$ peak) • Risk assessment
- Collaborative decision making

KEY POINTS

- Preoperative exercise capacity is associated with postoperative outcome.
- Lower anaerobic threshold and peak oxygen consumption predict increased postoperative morbidity and mortality.
- Cardiopulmonary exercise testing (CPET) testing may also identify factors limiting exercise capacity.
- CPET-derived variables can be used to guide informed consent, collaborative decision making, and the choice of surgical intervention.
- CPET-derived variables can be used to guide decisions about the most appropriate level of perioperative care, although further studies are required to clarify this role.

THE CHALLENGE FOR PREOPERATIVE RISK STRATIFICATION

It is estimated that globally more than 230 million major surgical procedures are performed each year and that this number is increasing.[1] Surgical interventions are in general cost-effective and thus surgical volume is likely to continue to increase,

Disclosure: See last page of article.
[a] Integrative Physiology and Critical Illness Group, Clinical and Experimental Sciences, Faculty of Medicine, University of Southampton, University Road, Southampton SO17 1BJ, UK; [b] Critical Care Research Area, Southampton NIHR Respiratory Biomedical Research Unit, University Hospital Southampton NHS Foundation Trust, Tremona Road, Southampton SO16 6DY, UK; [c] Anaesthesia and Critical Care Research Unit, University Hospital Southampton NHS Foundation Trust, Tremona Road, Southampton SO16 6DY, UK
* Corresponding author. Anaesthesia and Critical Care Research Unit, Mailpoint 24, E-Level, Centre Block, University Hospital Southampton NHS Foundation Trust, Tremona Road, Southampton SO16 6DY, UK.
E-mail address: mike.grocott@soton.ac.uk

particularly in resource-poor countries.[2] As a consequence the population of patients undergoing elective surgical is expanding. As life expectancy increases, an increasing proportion of these patients are likely to be high-risk elderly patients with multiple comorbidities who present particular challenges to both anesthetists and surgeons. The optimum perioperative management of such patients requires input from a multi-disciplinary team ideally incorporating a process of shared decision making.[3] Accurate preoperative risk stratification is an essential element in such a care pathway, assisting in the process of informed consent, the choice of surgical procedure, and the determination of the appropriate location of postoperative care (critical care or general ward).

Recent cohort studies have reported 3% to 4% mortality associated with surgery in both European[4] and North American[5] patient populations, which was higher than had previously been anticipated. Furthermore, in the prospective European Surgical Outcomes Study (EuSOS) (n = 46,539), wide international variability in mortality was observed, suggesting that there may be the potential to implement measures to improve surgical outcome.[4] In particular, 73% of the patients who died were not admitted to critical care and unplanned critical care admissions were associated with higher mortality than planned admissions. Identifying the subgroup of patients at high risk of mortality preoperatively may allow more appropriate risk counseling and the preemptive focus of personnel, critical care resources, and evidence-based interventions on this needy subgroup. Retrospective studies from the United Kingdom suggest that approximately 12% of patients are in a high-risk group and that these patients account for 80% of perioperative deaths.[6,7]

Postoperative morbidity is more common than mortality (16%–18% in recent case series) and presents significant health care and social burdens.[5,8] Postoperative complications not only increase short-term costs by prolonging hospital length of hospital stay but also have long-term implications for mortality.[5] Furthermore, they may lead to repeated hospital admissions and chronic ill health.[5,9] From the patient perspective this is often associated with a decline in functional capacity and quality of life.[10] The avoidance of postoperative complications is consequently of great importance.[8]

Thus increasing volumes of surgery and an increasingly frail surgical population present perioperative physicians with a significant challenge. Effective shared decision making with patient involvement necessitates accurate individualized perioperative risk prediction, which in turn requires a valid means of stratifying risk.

CARDIOPULMONARY EXERCISE TESTING AND RISK STRATIFICATION

This article explores the utility of cardiopulmonary exercise testing (CPET) in preoperative risk stratification in major abdominal surgery. The hypothesis that preoperative physical fitness predicts surgical outcome is implicit in anesthetic preassessment. The evaluation of functional capacity is included both in clinical practice and perioperative guidelines.[11] However the validity of subjective assessments of functional capacity in a general surgical population is not clear, because patients may not accurately evaluate or report their fitness. Furthermore, the ability of questionnaires such as the Duke Activity Status to discriminate between high-risk and low-risk patients has not been validated.[12] CPET is an objective method of evaluating exercise capacity and is considered to be the gold standard test.[13] It provides a global assessment of the integrated responses of the pulmonary, cardiovascular, hematological, and metabolic systems that are not adequately reflected through the measurement of individual organ system function. Furthermore, as a dynamic assessment it provides greater insights than a resting test into the response to physiologic stress, such as occurs perioperatively, and the physiologic reserve available to respond to such stresses.[14,15]

This article evaluates the evidence supporting the use of CPET for risk stratification in major abdominal surgery. To provide context for this evidence it first summarizes the literature exploring the relationship between health outcomes in general and exercise capacity. It then describes the conduct of CPET and the underlying physiologic rationale, defining the key variables that have been associated with surgical outcome.

PHYSICAL ACTIVITY, EXERCISE, AND HEALTH OUTCOMES

Physical fitness has benefits in almost all contexts of health and disease[16,17] and increasing evidence suggests that physical inactivity is a key public health issue.[18,19] Fitter patients have been shown to have better outcomes in a wide variety of conditions, including diabetes,[20,21] coronary artery disease,[22,23] heart failure,[24–26] hypertension,[27] chronic obstructive pulmonary disease (COPD),[28] chronic kidney disease,[29] cancer,[30] stroke,[31,32] depression,[33] and dementia.[34] Furthermore, physical activity reduces the risk of developing chronic diseases, including type 2 diabetes[35]; cancer of the breast,[36] kidney,[37] and colon[22]; osteoporosis[38]; obesity[39]; and depression.[40] Although there is a transiently increased risk of mortality during physical activity or training,[23,41] this is outweighed by the cumulative benefit of regular physical activity.[22]

Increasing fitness or physical activity also improves clinical outcomes. Supervised and unsupervised training programs have been shown to be beneficial in a variety of conditions, including COPD, stroke, heart failure, and intermittent claudication.[42–46] Furthermore, exercise has been shown to improve the quality of life and the ability to perform the activities of daily living in the frail elderly.[47] Likewise, the public health promotion of physical activity is generally effective.[48]

THE PHYSIOLOGY AND CONDUCT OF CARDIOPULMONARY EXERCISE TESTING

CPET provides an objective method of evaluating exercise capacity (functional capacity or physical fitness). Furthermore, it allows interrogation of the causes of exercise intolerance when exercise capacity is abnormal. CPET integrates expired oxygen and carbon dioxide concentrations with the measurement of ventilatory flow, thus deriving oxygen uptake ($\dot{V}O_2$) and carbon dioxide production ($\dot{V}CO_2$) under conditions of varying physiologic stress imposed by a range of defined external workloads. Heart rate, oxygen saturations, blood pressure, and electrocardiogram are monitored simultaneously.

Two modes of exercise, cycle ergometry and treadmill, are commonly used in CPET, and arm crank ergometry is used occasionally. Cycle ergometry allows accurate determination of the external work rate and thus evaluation of the $\dot{V}O_2$–work rate relationship, which is difficult with a treadmill.[49] In addition, cycle ergometry requires less skill than a treadmill (performance is less affected by practice), it is cheaper, and it takes up less space.[49]

Although a variety of exercise protocols can be used to interrogate different elements of the exercise response, the continuous incremental exercise test (incremental ramp test) to the limit of tolerance (symptom limited) is used most widely to evaluate exercise capacity.[50] The incremental exercise test has several advantages:

- It evaluates the exercise response across the range of exercise capacity.
- The initial work rate is low and the duration of high-intensity exercise is short.
- The test involves only 8 to 12 minutes of exercise.
- It permits assessment of the normalcy or otherwise of the exercise response.

- It allows identification of the site of functional exercise limitation.
- It provides an appropriate frame of reference for training or rehabilitation targets.

A typical test protocol involves 3 minutes of resting measurement, 3 minutes of unloaded cycling (cycling against no resistance), followed by a continuously increasing ramp until exhaustion. The gradient of the ramp is selected by age, gender, and current physical activity levels to achieve a test duration of 8 to 12 minutes. Recovery data are typically collected for 5 minutes or until the heart rate returns to baseline. In early perioperative CPET studies some groups stopped tests above the anaerobic threshold (AT) but before symptom limitation because of safety concerns in this previously unevaluated population.[51,52] Safety studies have subsequently reported very low mortalities of approximately 2 to 5 per 100,000 in patient populations including lung and heart transplant candidates.[13,53] As a result, symptom-limited tests are now most commonly used.

The output from an incremental CPET test is by convention represented graphically in a 9-panel plot.[13,49] The key variables and measurements are summarized in **Table 1**. Exercise capacity can be determined and the causes of exercise limitation can be identified as patterns of abnormality in these plots. CPET can evaluate the severity and physiologic impact of known comorbidities and identify unsuspected disorders such as myocardial ischaemia[54] and pulmonary hypertension[55–57] in preoperative patients.

Peak oxygen consumption ($\dot{V}O_2$ peak) and the AT are indexes of exercise capacity (functional capacity or physical fitness). These variables are metabolic rates expressed in milliliters of $\dot{V}O_2$ per minute absolute, or indexed to bodyweight, or as percentages of predicted values. $\dot{V}O_2$ peak is defined as the highest oxygen uptake recorded during an incremental exercise test at the point of symptom limitation. As such, $\dot{V}O_2$ peak includes a volitional element (the patient may not produce a maximal effort). The AT (also known as the lactate threshold, ventilatory threshold, gas exchange threshold, or lactic acidosis threshold) characterizes the upper limit of

Table 1		
Measurements and variables collected during CPET		
Measurement	**Variables**	**Symbol**
External work	Work rate	WR
Exercise capacity	Peak oxygen uptake	$\dot{V}O_2$ peak
	AT	AT
Metabolic gas exchange	Oxygen uptake	$\dot{V}O_2$
	Carbon dioxide production	$\dot{V}CO_2$
	Respiratory exchange ratio	RER
Ventilatory	Minute ventilation	$\dot{V}E$
	Tidal volume	VT
	Respiratory rate	RR
Pulmonary gas exchange	Ventilatory equivalents for CO_2	$\dot{V}E/\dot{V}CO_2$
	Ventilatory equivalents for O_2	$\dot{V}E/\dot{V}O_2$
	End-tidal oxygen	$PETO_2$
	End-tidal CO_2	$PETCO_2$
	Oxygen saturations	SpO_2
Cardiovascular	Heart rate	HR
	Blood pressure	NIBP
	Oxygen pulse	$\dot{V}O_2/HR$
Symptoms	Dyspnea, fatigue, chest pain, leg pain	—

exercise intensities that can be accomplished almost wholly aerobically.[13] Below the AT, exercise can be sustained indefinitely, whereas above the AT progressive increases in work rate result in progressive reductions in exercise tolerance.[58] The AT is defined as the $\dot{V}O_2$ at which there is a transition from a phase of no increase, or only a small increase in arterial lactate concentration, to a phase of rapidly accelerating increase in arterial lactate concentration associated with a progressive metabolic acidosis.[59] This point can be estimated noninvasively by breath-by-breath expired gas analysis during CPET.[60] The onset of metabolic acidosis at the AT is accompanied by an increase in the pulmonary CO_2 output ($\dot{V}CO_2$) resulting from the intramuscular and blood buffering by bicarbonate of lactate-associated protons.[61,62] This stage can be identified during incremental exercise testing as a change in the gradient of the $\dot{V}CO_2$-$\dot{V}O_2$ relationship (V-slope method[60] or modified V-slope method[63]), typically accompanied by a systematic increase in the ventilatory equivalent for oxygen ($\dot{V}E/\dot{V}O_2$) and in end-tidal PO_2 ($PETO_2$) without a concomitant decrease in end-tidal PCO_2 ($PETCO_2$) or increase in the ventilatory equivalent for CO_2 ($\dot{V}E/\dot{V}CO_2$) (ventilatory equivalents method).[64] Several investigators have shown that these indirect approaches provide a valid estimate of the lactate threshold both in healthy volunteers and in patients with cardiac disease and COPD.[65–68] The AT is independent of patient effort.

The ratio of ventilation ($\dot{V}E$) to $\dot{V}O_2$ is the ventilatory equivalent for oxygen ($\dot{V}E/\dot{V}O_2$) and the ratio of $\dot{V}E$ to $\dot{V}CO_2$ is the ventilatory equivalent for carbon dioxide ($\dot{V}E/\dot{V}CO_2$). The ventilatory equivalents for both O_2 and CO_2 are related to the dead space fraction (dead space volume/tidal volume) and increase as dead space increases (although they also increase with hyperventilation). Abnormally high ventilatory equivalents are thus evident in any pathologic condition with increased dead space; for example, COPD, pulmonary fibrosis, heart failure, and pulmonary embolic disease.

In summary, the incremental exercise test to the limit of tolerance using cycle ergometry (incremental ramp test) has been used extensively as a means of preoperative risk stratification in both clinical practice and clinical trials. It permits the accurate determination of exercise capacity and also allows identification of the site of exercise limitation when this is abnormal. The AT and $\dot{V}O_2$ peak, which are determined from this test, are validated, reliable measures of exercise capacity that can be used to describe physical fitness both in clinical practice and research studies.

CARDIOPULMONARY EXERCISE TESTING AND RISK STRATIFICATION

An association between CPET-derived variables and postoperative outcome is a prerequisite if CPET is to have utility as a preoperative risk stratification tool. The hypothesis that unfit patients are more susceptible to adverse outcomes following major surgery is intuitively appealing. Although CPET had been used for risk stratification in cardiothoracic patients, Older and colleagues[69] were the first group to publish research that used CPET for preoperative assessment in general surgery during the early 1990s. In a cohort study of 184 patients undergoing major elective abdominal surgery, they reported that a lower AT was associated with increased postoperative mortality. Hospital mortality was less than 1% in patients with an AT of more than 11 mL/kg, 18% in patients with an AT of less than 11 mL/kg/min, and 50% in patients with an AT less than 8 mL/kg.[69] Twenty-two cohort studies of preoperative CPET in patients having major intra-abdominal surgery have since been reported (**Table 2** for detailed analysis). These data have been synthesized in several systematic reviews that show a consistent relationship between physical fitness, defined using CPET-derived variables, and postoperative outcome.[77–79] The few studies that

Table 2
Cohort studies evaluating CPET and surgical outcome in major abdominal surgery

Author, Year, Journal	Patients	n	Design	AT Association & Risk Threshold (mls/kg/min)	VO$_2$ Peak Association & Risk Threshold (mls/kg/min)	$\dot{V}E/\dot{V}CO_2$	Outcome
Older et al,[69] 1993	Major Intra Abdominal	187		Y<11	Submaximal tests not measured	Y	CVS Mortality
Older et al,[51] 1999	Major Intra Abdominal	548		Y<11	Submaximal tests not measured	—	Mortality
Wilson et al,[52] 2010	Major Intra Abdominal	847		Y<10.9	Submaximal tests not measured	Y>34	Mortality
Snowden et al,[70] 2010	Major Intra Abdominal	116	Blinded	Y<10.1	Y	N	Morbidity - D7 POMS
Hightower et al,[84] 2010	Major Intra Abdominal	32	Blinded	Y	N	N	Morbidity
West et al,[71] 2014	Colon	136	Blinded	Y<10.1	Y<16.7	Y	Morbidity - D5 POMS
West et al,[85] 2014	Rectal	105	Blinded	Y<10.6	Y<18.6	—	Morbidity - D5 POMS
Prentis et al,[86] 2013	Cystectomy	82	Blinded	Y<12	Y	—	Morbidity - Clavien-Dindo[72], LOS
Nugent et al,[87] 1998	AAA	30		N	N<20 increased morbidity	—	Mortality and complications
Hartley et al,[88] 2012	AAA	415	2 centres	Y<10.2	Y<15	Y	Mortality
Prentis et al,[89] 2012	AAA	185	Blinded	Y<10	Y	—	LOS, Morbidity; ICU LOS
Goodyear et al,[90] 2013	AAA	230		Y<11	—	—	Mortality, LOS, Cost

Study	Surgery	N				Outcome
Carlisle et al,[73] 2007	AAA	130	Y	Y	Y>42	Mortality
Snowden et al,[91] 2013	Major Hepatobiliary	389 *Blinded*	Y	Y	Y	Mortality; LOS
Junejo et al,[74] 2012	Hepatic resection	131	Y 9.9 Mortality	Y	Y>34.5	Mortality; Morbidity
Ausania et al,[92] 2012	Whipples	124 *Blinded*	Y<10.1	Y	Y	Morbidity, Mortality, Pancreatic Leak
Nagamatsu et al,[93] 1994	Upper GI	52	—	Y	—	Cardiopulmonary Morbidity
Nagamatsu et al,[94] 2001	Upper GI	91	N	Y	—	Cardiopulmonary Morbidity
Forshaw et al,[95] 2008	Upper GI	78	Y / N	Y / N	—	Cardiopulmonary Morbidity LOS, unplanned ICU
Moyes et al,[96] 2013	Upper GI	108	Y<9	Y	Y	Cardiopulmonary Morbidity
McCullough et al,[75] 2006	Bariatric	109	Y	Y<15.6	N	Morbidity & Mortality composite
Hennis et al,[97] 2012	Bariatric	106	Y<11	Y	Y	Morbidity POMS D5

Abbreviations: AAA, abdominal aortic aneurysm; CVS, cardiovascular; D, day; GI, gastrointestinal; ICU, intensive care unit; LOS, hospital length of stay; N, no significant association between variable and outcome; NR, association between variable and outcome not reported; POMS, postoperative morbidity score[76]; Y, significant association between variable and postoperative outcome.
Data from Refs.[52,69–71,73–75]

did not find a statistically significant relationship included fewer than 100 patients and are likely to have had inadequate sample size to have sufficient statistical power to identify a clinically important difference. In most studies, both AT and $\dot{V}O_2$ peak were associated with outcome, although this association was statistically stronger for the AT in most cases (see **Table 2**). Abnormal ventilatory equivalents for carbon dioxide reflecting increased dead space were also associated with both mortality and morbidity in some case series,[52,73,74] but not in others.[70,75]

The AT threshold of 11 mL/kg/min to identify high-risk patients initially proposed by Older[69] was based on criteria used for the diagnosis of heart failure. Analysis of area under the receiver operating curve has since been used in several case series to identify predictive cutoffs for discriminating between low-risk and high-risk patient groups. As is evident from **Table 2**, more recent case series in general have reported a lower AT threshold, in the region of 9 to 10 mL/kg/min, which may reflect different patient populations, changes in surgical technique with greater laparoscopic surgery (and a reduced surgical stress response), or improvements in perioperative care with more critical care provision. It may be that some types of surgery present a greater physiologic challenge (open Whipple procedure compared with laparoscopic colectomy), or that the process of care is different for different subspecialties. For example, in the United Kingdom, some populations are routinely admitted to a critical care environment postoperatively (eg, esophagectomy, liver resection), whereas others are routinely cared for on general wards (eg, colorectal surgery). Thus perioperative care in a critical care environment may compensate for a reduced physiologic reserve. Further studies are required to explore this variability.

The strength of the association between AT and postoperative morbidity and mortality may be underestimated in many of these case series because clinicians were not blinded to the CPET results and used them to make clinical decisions. A high-risk test is likely to result in the institution of management to reduce risk such as changing the choice of surgical procedure, electively admitting the patient to critical care, or optimizing comorbidities preoperatively. The effect of this confounding by indication would be to dilute the strength of the association between risk and outcome.[80]

CARDIOPULMONARY EXERCISE TESTING AND OTHER RISK STRATIFICATION TOOLS

The ability of CPET-derived variables to predict outcome has also been evaluated compared with and in combination with other candidate risk predictors. Carlisle and colleagues[73] showed improved prediction of mortality following abdominal aortic aneurysm surgery when CPET-derived variables were used in combination with a clinical risk score (Revised Cardiac Risk Index; Lee score). Snowdon and colleagues[70] similarly reported better prediction of postoperative morbidity when AT was combined with the Veterans Activity Questionnaire Index (VASI). James and colleagues[81] recently reported that CPET-derived variables were better able to predict major adverse cardiac events and complications than plasma biomarkers (B natriuretic peptide). They did not evaluate the predictive ability of the two used in combination. In the future, increasingly sophisticated risk prediction may be achieved by combining CPET data, clinical risk scores, and plasma biomarkers. The limited available data suggest that unrelated but effective tests would give additive predictive ability.[70,73] In the future, a hierarchy of tests may be used to describe risk: simple clinical risk scores and screening biomarkers may be used to screen out low-risk patients at low cost, whereas patients at high or uncertain risk could be evaluated by a more complex battery of tests, including CPET.

USING CARDIOPULMONARY EXERCISE TESTING–DERIVED RISK INFORMATION
Informed Consent and Collaborative Decision Making

Risk data derived from CPET can be used to contribute to the discussion between patients and clinicians about the best course of action for an individual patient. The aim of collaborative decision making is to provide patients with sufficient information to allow them to decide on the most appropriate course of treatment in their particular circumstances. CPET is of value in this process because it provides risk information in a way that is intuitively easy to understand: the idea of fitness for surgery provides the starting point for a discussion about the specific risks and benefits of a particular procedure for a particular patient, and the CPET-derived data can inform clinician estimates of risk. Thus CPET allows patients to make more informed decisions about surgical intervention.

Cardiopulmonary Exercise Testing Guided Perioperative Care

CPET has also been used to guide clinicians' decision making when deciding on the appropriate choice of operative procedure and perioperative care environment. Patients defined as high risk for adverse outcome may be scheduled for less physiologically challenging procedures or for nonsurgical management. For example, a defunctioning colostomy may be chosen instead of a more definitive tumor resection. More commonly, CPET data have been used to guide the choice of postoperative care with less fit patients being allocated to a critical care environment postoperatively. Older and colleagues,[51] in a prospective study, used CPET-derived variables (AT, ventilatory equivalents for oxygen, myocardial ischemia), along with magnitude of surgery to allocate patients to intensive care, high-dependency care, and ward care. There was no cardiovascular mortality in the patients allocated to ward care and the mortalities on the high-dependency unit and intensive care unit were lower than historical control data from the same institution. This study is limited by the nonrandomized design and historical control data and by the risk of bias in the attribution of the criteria for cardiovascular death (all-cause mortality was not reported). Although it does not meet criteria for the demonstration of a causal link between the intervention (postoperative care allocated by CPET-derived variables) and outcome (mortality), the results merit further investigation. A case-controlled study of outcome in colorectal patients with an AT of less than 11 mL/kg/min who were randomly assigned to either ward care or critical care subsequently reported increased cardiac events in those allocated to the ward, again suggesting that intervening because of AT may improve outcomes.[82] A pilot double-blind, randomized controlled trial evaluating the usefulness of CPET for directing perioperative care has recently been completed in the United Kingdom. The study enrolled 228 patients undergoing elective colorectal cancer surgery within an enhanced recovery after surgery program and results are expected early in 2015.[83] Further studies exploring the impact of CPET-guided direction of postoperative care on outcome are needed, but the difficulty of evaluating such a complex intervention has so far limited the available data. In general in these studies, the critical care unit is treated as a so-called black box that provides benefit. Increased focus on the elements of critical care that might offer benefit will also be important if this approach is to be effectively evaluated. An alternative perspective on CPET is that it can identify low-risk patients who are safe to triage to the general ward postoperatively and should have high chance of following an enhanced recovery–type pathway without deviation. CPET can thus be used to target resources to those patients whose need is greatest, which is vital in a resource-constrained health care environment.

Prehabilitation: Exercise Training Before a Physiologic Challenge

CPET risk stratification can also be used to identify patients who may benefit from preoperative exercise training to increase fitness and thereby improve outcomes; this is known as prehabilitation. Preliminary data have confirmed the feasibility of this approach in patients having intra-abdominal surgery and has produced encouraging pilot data.[71] Furthermore, there are more than 20 ongoing clinical trials evaluating exercise training programs in surgical patients registered with the clinical trials database (ClinicalTrials.Gov, #2795). The advent of neoadjuvant therapies has created the opportunity to train patients before major cancer operations for which previously the pressure of reducing the time between diagnosis and surgery precluded such an intervention. Improved understanding of the optimal duration, pattern, intensity, and qualities of such interventions are needed to maximize efficacy.

SUMMARY

Reduced exercise capacity defined by a low AT or $\dot{V}o_2$ peak is associated with increased postoperative morbidity and mortality. CPET-derived variables can be used to risk stratify patients and in the future may be combined with other risk predictors (clinical scores and biomarkers) to improve the precision of outcome prediction. CPET results can be used to improve the process of informed consent and thus contribute to collaborative decision making. Furthermore, CPET can be used to guide the choice of surgical procedure and decide on the most appropriate postoperative care environment, although further clinical trial evidence is required in this area. In this way scarce resources can be concentrated on the patients at highest risk. In the future, CPET may also be used to guide prehabilitation training programs, improving fitness and thereby reducing perioperative risk.

DISCLOSURE

Dr D.Z.H. Levett is course director for the UK Perioperative Cardiopulmonary Exercise Course and is an executive board member of the Xtreme-Everest oxygen research consortium, which have received unrestricted research grant funding from (among others) BOC Medical (Linde Group) and Smiths Medical. Professor M.P.W. Grocott is a cochair of the annual UK National Perioperative Cardiopulmonary Exercise Testing Meeting and a board member of CPX International. He has received honoraria for speaking for and/or travel expenses from BOC Medical (Linde Group) and Cortex GmBH. He leads the Fit-4-Surgery research collaboration and also leads the Xtreme-Everest oxygen research consortium, which has received unrestricted research grant funding from (among others) BOC Medical (Linde Group) and Smiths Medical. Professor M.P.W. Grocott is also funded in part from the British Oxygen Company Chair of the Royal College of Anaesthetists, awarded by the National Institute of Academic Anesthesia. Some of this work was undertaken at University Southampton NHS Foundation Trust – University of Southampton NIHR Respiratory Biomedical Research Unit, which received a portion of funding from the UK Department of Health Research Biomedical Research Units funding scheme. All funding was unrestricted. The funders had no role in study design, data collection and analysis, decision to publish, or preparation of the article.

REFERENCES

1. Weiser TG, Regenbogen SE, Thompson KD, et al. An estimation of the global volume of surgery: a modelling strategy based on available data. Lancet 2008; 372(9633):139–44.
2. Chao TE, Sharma K, Mandigo M, et al. Cost-effectiveness of surgery and its policy implications for global health: a systematic review and analysis. Lancet Glob Health 2014;2(6):e334–45.
3. Glance LG, Osler TM, Neuman MD, et al. Redesigning surgical decision making for high-risk patients. N Engl J Med 2014;370(15):1379–81.
4. Pearse RM, Moreno RP, Bauer P, et al. Mortality after surgery in Europe: a 7 day cohort study. Lancet 2012;380(9847):1059–65.
5. Khuri S, Henderson W, DePalma R, et al. Determinants of long-term survival after major surgery and the adverse effect of postoperative complications. Ann Surg 2005;242(3):326–41 [discussion: 341–3].
6. Findlay GP, Goodwin APL, Protopapa K, et al. Knowing the risk: a review of the peri-operative care of surgical patients. London: National Confidential Enquiry into Patient Outcome and Death; 2011.
7. Pearse R, Harrison D, Protopapa K, et al. Identification and characterisation of the high-risk surgical population in the United Kingdom. Crit Care 2006;10(3):R81.
8. Ghaferi AA, Birkmeyer JD, Dimick JB. Variation in hospital mortality associated with inpatient surgery. N Engl J Med 2009;361(14):1368–75.
9. Rhodes A, Cecconi M, Hamilton M, et al. Goal-directed therapy in high-risk surgical patients: a 15-year follow-up study. Intensive Care Med 2010;36(8):1327–32.
10. Finlayson E, Zhao S, Boscardin WJ, et al. Functional status after colon cancer surgery in elderly nursing home residents. J Am Geriatr Soc 2012;60(5):967–73.
11. Fleisher LA, Fleischmann KE, Auerbach AD, et al. 2014 ACC/AHA guideline on perioperative cardiovascular evaluation and management of patients undergoing noncardiac surgery: executive summary: a report of the American College of Cardiology/American Heart Association Task Force on Practice Guidelines. Circulation 2014;130:2215–45.
12. Struthers R, Erasmus P, Holmes K, et al. Assessing fitness for surgery: a comparison of questionnaire, incremental shuttle walk, and cardiopulmonary exercise testing in general surgical patients. Br J Anaesth 2008;101(6):774–80.
13. American Thoracic Society, American College of Chest Physicians. American Thoracic Society and American College of Chest Physicians Statement on cardiopulmonary exercise testing. Am J Respir Crit Care Med 2003;167(2):211–77.
14. Desborough JP. The stress response to trauma and surgery. Br J Anaesth 2000; 85(1):109–17.
15. Older P, Smith R. Experience with the preoperative invasive measurement of haemodynamic, respiratory and renal function in 100 elderly patients scheduled for major abdominal surgery. Anaesth Intensive Care 1988;16(4):389–95.
16. Fiuza-Luces C, Garatachea N, Berger NA, et al. Exercise is the real polypill. Physiology (Bethesda) 2013;28(5):330–58.
17. Sallis RE. Exercise is medicine and physicians need to prescribe it! Br J Sports Med 2009;43(1):3–4.
18. Kohl HW 3rd, Craig CL, Lambert EV, et al. The pandemic of physical inactivity: global action for public health. Lancet 2012;380(9838):294–305.
19. Lee IM, Shiroma EJ, Lobelo F, et al. Effect of physical inactivity on major noncommunicable diseases worldwide: an analysis of burden of disease and life expectancy. Lancet 2012;380(9838):219–29.

20. Hayashino Y, Jackson JL, Fukumori N, et al. Effects of supervised exercise on lipid profiles and blood pressure control in people with type 2 diabetes mellitus: a meta-analysis of randomized controlled trials. Diabetes Res Clin Pract 2012; 98(3):349–60.

21. Thomas DE, Elliott EJ, Naughton GA. Exercise for type 2 diabetes mellitus. Cochrane Database Syst Rev 2006;(3):CD002968.

22. Thompson PD, Buchner D, Pina IL, et al. Exercise and physical activity in the prevention and treatment of atherosclerotic cardiovascular disease: a statement from the Council on Clinical Cardiology (Subcommittee on Exercise, Rehabilitation, and Prevention) and the Council on Nutrition, Physical Activity, and Metabolism (Subcommittee on Physical Activity). Circulation 2003;107(24):3109–16.

23. Thompson PD, Franklin BA, Balady GJ, et al. Exercise and acute cardiovascular events placing the risks into perspective: a scientific statement from the American Heart Association Council on Nutrition, Physical Activity, and Metabolism and the Council on Clinical Cardiology. Circulation 2007;115(17):2358–68.

24. Belardinelli R, Georgiou D, Cianci G, et al. Randomized, controlled trial of long-term moderate exercise training in chronic heart failure: effects on functional capacity, quality of life, and clinical outcome. Circulation 1999;99(9):1173–82.

25. Mandic S, Myers J, Selig SE, et al. Resistance versus aerobic exercise training in chronic heart failure. Curr Heart Fail Rep 2012;9(1):57–64.

26. O'Connor CM, Whellan DJ, Lee KL, et al. Efficacy and safety of exercise training in patients with chronic heart failure: HF-ACTION randomized controlled trial. JAMA 2009;301(14):1439–50.

27. Cornelissen VA, Smart NA. Exercise training for blood pressure: a systematic review and meta-analysis. J Am Heart Assoc 2013;2(1):e004473.

28. Waschki B, Kirsten A, Holz O, et al. Physical activity is the strongest predictor of all-cause mortality in patients with COPD: a prospective cohort study. Chest 2011;140(2):331–42.

29. Heiwe S, Jacobson SH. Exercise training for adults with chronic kidney disease. Cochrane Database Syst Rev 2011;(10):CD003236.

30. Des Guetz G, Uzzan B, Bouillet T, et al. Impact of physical activity on cancer-specific and overall survival of patients with colorectal cancer. Gastroenterol Res Pract 2013;2013:340851.

31. Austin MW, Ploughman M, Glynn L, et al. Aerobic exercise effects on neuroprotection and brain repair following stroke: A systematic review and perspective. Neurosci Res 2014;87C:8–15.

32. Saunders DH, Sanderson M, Brazzelli M, et al. Physical fitness training for stroke patients. Cochrane Database Syst Rev 2013;(10):CD003316.

33. Cooney GM, Dwan K, Greig CA, et al. Exercise for depression. Cochrane Database Syst Rev 2013;(9):CD004366.

34. Forbes D, Thiessen EJ, Blake CM, et al. Exercise programs for people with dementia. Cochrane Database Syst Rev 2013;(12):CD006489.

35. Hopper I, Billah B, Skiba M, et al. Prevention of diabetes and reduction in major cardiovascular events in studies of subjects with prediabetes: meta-analysis of randomised controlled clinical trials. Eur J Cardiovasc Prev Rehabil 2011;18(6): 813–23.

36. Friedenreich CM. Physical activity and breast cancer: review of the epidemiologic evidence and biologic mechanisms. Recent Results Cancer Res 2011;188: 125–39.

37. Behrens G, Leitzmann MF. The association between physical activity and renal cancer: systematic review and meta-analysis. Br J Cancer 2013;108(4):798–811.

38. Howe TE, Shea B, Dawson LJ, et al. Exercise for preventing and treating osteoporosis in postmenopausal women. Cochrane Database Syst Rev 2011;(7):CD000333.
39. Tate DF, Jeffery RW, Sherwood NE, et al. Long-term weight losses associated with prescription of higher physical activity goals. Are higher levels of physical activity protective against weight regain? Am J Clin Nutr 2007;85(4):954–9.
40. Mammen G, Faulkner G. Physical activity and the prevention of depression: a systematic review of prospective studies. Am J Prev Med 2013;45(5):649–57.
41. De Backer G, Ambrosioni E, Borch-Johnsen K, et al. European guidelines on cardiovascular disease prevention in clinical practice: third joint task force of European and other societies on cardiovascular disease prevention in clinical practice (constituted by representatives of eight societies and by invited experts). Eur J Cardiovasc Prev Rehabil 2003;10(4):S1–10.
42. Carson KV, Chandratilleke MG, Picot J, et al. Physical training for asthma. Cochrane Database Syst Rev 2013;(9):CD001116.
43. Lane R, Ellis B, Watson L, et al. Exercise for intermittent claudication. Cochrane Database Syst Rev 2014;(7):CD000990.
44. Mehrholz J, Pohl M, et al. Treadmill training and body weight support for walking after stroke. Cochrane Database Syst Rev 2014;(1):CD002840.
45. Puhan MA, Gimeno-Santos E, Scharplatz M, et al. Pulmonary rehabilitation following exacerbations of chronic obstructive pulmonary disease. Cochrane Database Syst Rev 2011;(10):CD005305.
46. Taylor RS, Sagar VA, Davies EJ, et al. Exercise-based rehabilitation for heart failure. Cochrane Database Syst Rev 2014;(4):CD003331.
47. Chou CH, Hwang CL, et al. Effect of exercise on physical function, daily living activities, and quality of life in the frail older adults: a meta-analysis. Arch Phys Med Rehabil 2012;93(2):237–44.
48. Heath GW, Parra DC, Sarmiento OL, et al. Evidence-based intervention in physical activity: lessons from around the world. Lancet 2012;380(9838):272–81.
49. Porszasz J, Stringer W, Casaburi R. Equipment, measurements and quality control. In: Ward SA, Palange P, editors. Clinical exercise testing, vol. 12. European Respiratory Monograph; 2007. p. 108–28.
50. Whipp BJ, Davis JA, Torres F, et al. A test to determine parameters of aerobic function during exercise. J Appl Physiol Respir Environ Exerc Physiol 1981;50(1):217–21.
51. Older P, Hall A, Hader R. Cardiopulmonary exercise testing as a screening test for perioperative management of major surgery in the elderly. Chest 1999;116(2):355–62.
52. Wilson RJ, Davies S, Yates D, et al. Impaired functional capacity is associated with all-cause mortality after major elective intra-abdominal surgery. Br J Anaesth 2010;105(3):297–303.
53. Myers J, Voodi L, Umann T, et al. A survey of exercise testing: methods, utilization, interpretation, and safety in the VAHCS. J Cardiopulm Rehabil 2000;20(4):251–8.
54. Belardinelli R, Lacalaprice F, Carle F, et al. Exercise-induced myocardial ischaemia detected by cardiopulmonary exercise testing. Eur Heart J 2003;24(14):1304–13.
55. Glaser S, Obst A, Koch B, et al. Pulmonary hypertension in patients with idiopathic pulmonary fibrosis - the predictive value of exercise capacity and gas exchange efficiency. PLoS One 2013;8(6):e65643.

56. Guazzi M, Cahalin LP, et al. Cardiopulmonary exercise testing as a diagnostic tool for the detection of left-sided pulmonary hypertension in heart failure. J Card Fail 2013;19(7):461–7.
57. Held M, Grun M, Holl R, et al. Cardiopulmonary exercise testing to detect chronic thromboembolic pulmonary hypertension in patients with normal echocardiography. Respiration 2014;87(5):379–87.
58. Sullivan CS, Casaburi R, Storer TW, et al. Non-invasive prediction of blood lactate response to constant power outputs from incremental exercise tests. Eur J Appl Physiol Occup Physiol 1995;71(4):349–54.
59. Beaver WL, Wasserman K, Whipp BJ. Improved detection of lactate threshold during exercise using a log-log transformation. J Appl Physiol (1985) 1985; 59(6):1936–40.
60. Beaver WL, Wasserman K, Whipp BJ. A new method for detecting anaerobic threshold by gas exchange. J Appl Physiol (1985) 1986;60(6):2020–7.
61. Wasserman K. The anaerobic threshold: definition, physiological significance and identification. Adv Cardiol 1986;35:1–23.
62. Wasserman K, Beaver WL, Whipp BJ. Gas exchange theory and the lactic acidosis (anaerobic) threshold. Circulation 1990;81(1 Suppl):II14–30.
63. Sue DY, Wasserman K, Moricca RB, et al. Metabolic acidosis during exercise in patients with chronic obstructive pulmonary disease. Use of the V-slope method for anaerobic threshold determination. Chest 1988;94(5):931–8.
64. Whipp BJ, Ward SA, Wasserman K. Respiratory markers of the anaerobic threshold. Adv Cardiol 1986;35:47–64.
65. Dickstein K, Barvik S, Aarsland T, et al. A comparison of methodologies in detection of the anaerobic threshold. Circulation 1990;81(1 Suppl):II38–46.
66. Matsumura N, Nishijima H, Kojima S, et al. Determination of anaerobic threshold for assessment of functional state in patients with chronic heart failure. Circulation 1983;68(2):360–7.
67. Patessio A, Casaburi R, Carone M, et al. Comparison of gas exchange, lactate, and lactic acidosis thresholds in patients with chronic obstructive pulmonary disease. Am Rev Respir Dis 1993;148(3):622–6.
68. Simonton C, Higginbotham M, Cobb F. The ventilatory threshold: quantitative analysis of reproducibility and relation to arterial lactate concentration in normal subjects and in patients with chronic congestive heart failure. Am J Cardiol 1988;62(1):100–7.
69. Older P, Smith R, Courtney P, et al. Preoperative evaluation of cardiac failure and ischemia in elderly patients by cardiopulmonary exercise testing. Chest 1993; 104(3):701–4.
70. Snowden CP, Prentis JM, Anderson HL, et al. Submaximal cardiopulmonary exercise testing predicts complications and hospital length of stay in patients undergoing major elective surgery. Ann Surg 2010;251(3):535–41.
71. West MA, Lythgoe D, Barben CP, et al. Cardiopulmonary exercise variables are associated with postoperative morbidity after major colonic surgery: a prospective blinded observational study. Br J Anaesth 2014;112(4):665–71.
72. Dindo D, Demartines N, Clavien PA. Classification of surgical complications: a new proposal with evaluation in a cohort of 6336 patients and results of a survey. Ann Surg 2004;240(2):205–13.
73. Carlisle J, Swart M. Mid-term survival after abdominal aortic aneurysm surgery predicted by cardiopulmonary exercise testing. Br J Surg 2007;94(8):966–9.
74. Junejo MA, Mason JM, Sheen AJ, et al. Cardiopulmonary exercise testing for preoperative risk assessment before hepatic resection. Br J Surg 2012;99(8):1097–104.

75. McCullough P, Gallagher M, Dejong A, et al. Cardiorespiratory fitness and short-term complications after bariatric surgery. Chest 2006;130(2):517–25.
76. Grocott M, Browne J, Van der Meulen J, et al. The Postoperative Morbidity Survey was validated and used to describe morbidity after major surgery. J Clin Epidemiol 2007;60(9):919–28.
77. Hennis PJ, Meale PM, Grocott MP. Cardiopulmonary exercise testing for the evaluation of perioperative risk in non-cardiopulmonary surgery. Postgrad Med J 2011;87(1030):550–7.
78. Smith TB, Stonell C, Purkayastha S, et al. Cardiopulmonary exercise testing as a risk assessment method in non cardio-pulmonary surgery: a systematic review. Anaesthesia 2009;64(8):883–93.
79. West M, Jack S, Grocott MP. Perioperative cardiopulmonary exercise testing in the elderly. Best Pract Res Clin Anaesthesiol 2011;25(3):427–37.
80. Grocott MP, Pearse RM. Prognostic studies of perioperative risk: robust methodology is needed. Br J Anaesth 2010;105(3):243–5.
81. James S, Jhanji S, Smith A, et al. Comparison of the prognostic accuracy of scoring systems, cardiopulmonary exercise testing, and plasma biomarkers: a single-centre observational pilot study. Br J Anaesth 2014;112(3):491–7.
82. Swart M, Carlisle J. Case-controlled study of critical care or surgical ward care after elective open colorectal surgery. Br J Surg 2012;99(2):295–9.
83. ClinicalTrials.Gov. Cardiopulmonary exercise testing and preoperative risk stratification. Available at: https://clinicaltrials.gov/ct2/show/NCT00737828?term=grocott&rank=3. Accessed January 12, 2015.
84. Hightower CE, Riedel BJ, Feig BW, et al. A pilot study evaluating predictors of postoperative outcomes after major abdominal surgery: physiological capacity compared with the ASA physical status classification system. Br J Anaesth 2010;104(4):465–71.
85. West MA, Parry MG, Lythgoe D, et al. Cardiopulmonary exercise testing for the prediction of morbidity risk after rectal cancer surgery. Br J Surg 2014;101: 1166–72.
86. Prentis JM, Trenell MI, Vasdev N, et al. Impaired cardiopulmonary reserve in an elderly population is related to postoperative morbidity and length of hospital stay after radical cystectomy. BJU Int 2013;112(2):E13–9.
87. Nugent A, Riley M, Megarry J, et al. Cardiopulmonary exercise testing in the preoperative assessment of patients for repair of abdominal aortic aneurysm. Ir J Med Sci 1998;167(4):238–41.
88. Hartley RA, Pichel AC, Grant SW, et al. Preoperative cardiopulmonary exercise testing and risk of early mortality following abdominal aortic aneurysm repair. Br J Surg 2012;99(11):1539–46.
89. Prentis JM, Trenell MI, Jones DJ, et al. Submaximal exercise testing predicts perioperative hospitalization after aortic aneurysm repair. J Vasc Surg 2012;56(6): 1564–70.
90. Goodyear SJ, Yow H, Saedon M, et al. Risk stratification by pre-operative cardiopulmonary exercise testing improves outcomes following elective abdominal aortic aneurysm surgery: a cohort study. Perioper Med (Lond) 2013;2(1):10.
91. Snowden CP, Prentis J, Jacques B, et al. Cardiorespiratory fitness predicts mortality and hospital length of stay after major elective surgery in older people. Ann Surg 2013;257(6):999–1004.
92. Ausania F, Snowden CP, Prentis JM, et al. Effects of low cardiopulmonary reserve on pancreatic leak following pancreaticoduodenectomy. Br J Surg 2012;99(9): 1290–4.

93. Nagamatsu Y, Yamana H, Fujita H. The simultaneous evaluation of preoperative cardiopulmonary funcitons of esophageal cancer patients in the analysis of expired gas with exercise testing (In Japanese). Nihon Kyobu Geka Gakkai Zasshi 1994;42:2037–40.

94. Nagamatsu Y, Shima I, Yamana H, et al. Preoperative evaluation of cardiopulmonary reserve with the use of expired gas analysis during exercise testing in patients with squamous cell carcinoma of the thoracic esophagus. J Thorac Cardiovasc Surg 2001;121(6):1064–8.

95. Forshaw M, Strauss D, Davies A, et al. Is cardiopulmonary exercise testing a useful test before esophagectomy? Ann Thorac Surg 2008;85(1):294–9.

96. Moyes LH, McCaffer CJ, Carter RC, et al. Cardiopulmonary exercise testing as a predictor of complications in oesophagogastric cancer surgery. Ann R Coll Surg Engl 2013;95(2):125–30.

97. Hennis PJ, Meale PM, Hurst RA, et al. Cardiopulmonary exercise testing predicts postoperative outcome in patients undergoing gastric bypass surgery. Br J Anaesth 2012;109(4):566–71.

Prehabilitation to Enhance Perioperative Care

Francesco Carli, MD, MPhil, FRCA, FRCPC[a],*, Celena Scheede-Bergdahl, MSc, PhD[a,b]

KEYWORDS

- Surgery • Elderly • Cancer • Prehabilitation • Exercise • Nutrition

KEY POINTS

- Despite advances in surgical care, there remain patients with suboptimal recovery; elderly patients, especially those with cancer and limited protein reserve are at highest risk for negative postsurgical outcomes.
- Although more traditional approaches have targeted the postoperative period for rehabilitation, it has been shown that the preoperative period is most effective for intervention.
- Surgical prehabilitation is an emerging concept, deriving from the realization that effective perioperative care must include in addition to the clinical and pharmacological preparation of the surgical preparation, preoperative physical, nutritional and psychological optimization.

THE STRESS OF SURGERY AND TRAJECTORY OF RECOVERY

Tissue trauma, physical inactivity, quasi-starvation and psychological distress represent major stresses to the body. In turn, immediate systemic changes are initiated, resulting in both short- and long-term effects on the capacity to perform activities of daily living and on overall quality of life.

Despite advances in surgical technology, anesthesia and perioperative care, which have made surgery safer and more accessible to a variety of patients potentially at risk, there remains a group of patients who still have suboptimal recovery. Almost 30% of patients undergoing major abdominal surgery have postoperative complications,[1] and, even in absence of morbid events, major surgery is associated with a 40% reduction in functional capacity.[2] After surgery, patients experience physical fatigue, disturbed sleep, and a decreased capacity to concentrate for up to 9 weeks after discharge.[3] Long periods of physical inactivity induce loss of muscle mass, deconditioning, pulmonary complications, and decubitus. Postoperative fatigue and

[a] Department of Anesthesia, McGill University, Montreal, Quebec, Canada; [b] Department of Kinesiology and Physical Education, McGill University, Montreal, Quebec, Canada
* Corresponding author. Department of Anesthesia, McGill University Health Centre, 1650 Cedar Avenue, Room D10.144, Montreal, Quebec H3H 2R4, Canada.
E-mail address: franco.carli@mcgill.ca

Anesthesiology Clin 33 (2015) 17–33
http://dx.doi.org/10.1016/j.anclin.2014.11.002   anesthesiology.theclinics.com
1932-2275/15/$ – see front matter © 2015 Elsevier Inc. All rights reserved.

complications have been found to be correlated with preoperative health status, functional capacity, and muscle strength.[4] The elderly, persons with cancer, and persons with limited protein reserve are the most susceptible to the negative effects of surgery.

There is mounting evidence that many of the negative immediate effects of surgery such as pain, fatigue, and weakness, are potentially amenable to intervention. If proper interventions are carried out, these symptoms may be readily controlled, allowing for a faster recovery and early hospital discharge. However, the effects of surgery are felt far beyond the immediate convalescent period and patients can feel fatigued for many weeks; fatigue delays return to usual function and reduces quality of life. Thus, it would be of practical benefit if ways of improving postsurgery physical function and quality of life could be identified.

Traditionally, efforts have been made to improve the recovery process by intervening in the postoperative period. However, the postoperative period may not be the most opportune time to introduce interventions to accelerate recovery. Many of these surgical patients are concerned about perturbing the healing process as well as being depressed and anxious as they await extra treatment of the tumor and, therefore, are unwilling to be engaged in the process.

The preoperative period may be, then, a more emotionally opportune time to intervene in the factors that contribute to recovery. Patients are often scheduled for extra tests, anxiously waiting for surgery, and searching for explanation and reassurance. In the face of the powerlessness and diminished self-esteem that often follow a health threat, active engagement of the individual in the preparation process may have benefits beyond the physical and alleviate some of the emotional distress surrounding the anticipation of surgery and the recovery process.

SURGICAL PREHABILITATION AND THE PUBLISHED EVIDENCE

The process of enhancing functional capacity of the individual to enable them to withstand an incoming stressor has been termed prehabilitation.[5] Although several programs have attempted to prepare patients for the postoperative recovery through education and positive reinforcement, little has been developed to systematically enhance functional capacity before surgery.

The theory of prehabilitation was initially supported in animal models. To investigate the effect of voluntary exercise on the tolerance to trauma, female rats, kept in cages with running wheels for periods of 3 to 7 weeks (exercise group), were subjected to trauma and compared with rats kept in cages without running wheels for the same period (sedentary group).[6] Mortality was significantly decreased in rats kept in cages with running wheels for 5 weeks or 7 weeks, but not those in the 3-week group. These results indicated that voluntarily exercising rats showed increased resistance to trauma compared with rats kept under sedentary conditions.

Although the benefits of physical activity have been shown in many disabling conditions, there are limited clinical data on the role of exercise before surgery. However, the evidence of the role of exercise in disease prevention is overwhelming. In medicine, regular exercise has been shown to decrease the incidence of ischemic heart disease, diabetes, stroke, and fractures in the elderly as a result of improved balance and strength. As a result of exercise, there is an increase in aerobic capacity, decreased sympathetic overreactivity, increased antioxidant capacity, improved insulin sensitivity, and increasing ratio of lean body mass to body fat.[7] Exercise training, particularly in sports medicine, has been used as a method of preventing a specific injury or facilitating recuperation. Thus, one would assume that by increasing the patient's aerobic and muscle strength capacity through increased physical activity before surgery, physiologic reserve would be enhanced and postoperative recuperation would be facilitated.

In 2002, Topp and colleagues[5] proposed that, by applying an exercise program before the stress of surgery, postoperative recovery would occur more rapidly compared with patients who remained sedentary. Since then, several studies have been undertaken, using different types of exercise programs.

The first systematic review of fair to good methodological quality was published in 2011 and included 12 studies.[8] The effect of preoperative exercise therapy on postoperative complication rate and length of hospital stay was studied, and it showed that preoperative exercise therapy can be effective for reducing postoperative complication rates and accelerate discharge from hospital in patients undergoing cardiac and abdominal surgery. Conversely, the outcome after joint arthroplasty was not significantly affected by preoperative exercise therapy.

All 4 studies that investigated cardiac and abdominal surgery included inspiratory muscle training as an intervention. The results showed that the risk of developing postoperative pulmonary complications was significantly higher in the group not receiving inspiratory muscle training. The interventions included in the review varied with respect to the type of exercise, frequency, duration, and intensity and lacked detailed about the precise implementation of the programs. In the orthopedic groups, the prehabilitation lasted up to 6 weeks, whereas in the cardiac and abdominal group, the average was 3 to 4 weeks. Also, some interventions were home based, whereas others were partly supervised or fully supervised by a physiotherapist. Functional measures such as exercise capacity and muscle strength were not included as outcome measures. In the studies involving joint replacement surgery, there was a large variety of physical exercises, with different emphasis on either joint mobility or muscle strength. The results of these studies indicated that preoperative exercise therapy does not affect length of hospital stay or complication rate after surgery.

Santa Mina and colleagues[9] reviewed 15 studies and concluded that total-body prehabilitation improved postoperative pain, length of stay, and physical function, but it was not consistently effective in improving health-related quality of life or aerobic fitness in the studies that examined these outcomes.

More recently, another systematic review of 8 studies[10] reported that exercise confers some physiologic improvement with limited clinical benefit. However, the data analyzed were limited, with great heterogeneity between the studies because of the differences in surgery type. Also, the exercise regimens were not uniformly reported with regard to the individual components of exercise (eg, the duration and the intensity), and the lack of adherence to high-intensity exercise. Although some physiologic improvement during the preoperative period was reported by most of the studies, this change did not translate into improved clinical outcomes.

A previous randomized controlled trial (RCT), conducted by our group,[11] in patients undergoing colorectal surgery compared the effects of a home-based program, which included a sham intervention (basic recommendation to walk daily and do breathing exercises), and a high-intensity training program, which consisted of both aerobic and resistance exercise. We found that, unexpectedly, a third of the patients in the intense exercise group deteriorated in their functional walking capacity (a measure of functional exercise capacity) during the presurgical period. Their compliance was recorded at a mere 16%, thus indicating that the prescribed exercise regimen could not be maintained. Only 33% improved during prehabilitation, and 29% deteriorated despite the intervention. Predictors of poor surgical outcome included deterioration while waiting for surgery, age greater than 75 years, and high anxiety, thus supporting the need to better identify which factors, such as disease progression, catabolic state, poor compliance, and psychological stress, in addition to exercise, contributed to functional deterioration before surgery. These results suggest that an intervention based on exercise alone may not have been sufficient to enhance functional capacity if factors such as nutrition, anxiety, and perioperative care were not taken into consideration during the program. Also, the intensity of the exercise program should be carefully considered as well. Although physical activity has undoubtedly several benefits in restoring physiologic reserve in preparation for abdominal surgery, the role played by other modalities cannot be excluded, such as pharmacologic optimization, smoking cessation, alcohol reduction, dietetic counseling, nutritional supplementation, cognitive enhancement, and psychosocial support beside education.

In a recent pilot study[12] followed by an RCT,[13] a multimodal prehabilitation program composed of moderate-intensity physical exercise and complemented by nutritional counseling and protein supplementation, and anxiety and reduction strategies within the context of the ERAS (enhanced recovery after surgery) protocol, showed that more than 80% of patients with cancer undergoing colorectal resection were able to return to preoperative functional capacity by 8 weeks, compared with 40% of a control group who did not receive the prehabilitation program.

Although some components of a prehabilitation program are common to all types of surgery, specific interventions need to be tailored on a personal basis to improve definite body functions. For instance, the requirement of prehabilitation for someone going for lung surgery concentrates on the aerobic component, whereas peripheral and core muscle strengthening are needed for those undergoing hip and knee surgery. In addition, the timing of prehabilitation in relationship to the time of surgical intervention needs to be appropriately evaluated. In most studies, the time interval for prehabilitation has been proposed to be between 4 and 8 weeks, with short periods for patients with lung or abdominal cancer, and long periods for more chronic conditions, such as spine surgery or arthroplasty.

INCREASING PHYSIOLOGIC RESERVE WITH PHYSICAL EXERCISE: HOW DOES EXERCISE BENEFIT?

The participation in an acute bout of strenuous exercise is met with the need for the body to compensate for potentially major systemic perturbations. For example, blood volume can be quickly recruited and flow redirected to active muscle groups from less metabolically active tissue. Depending on the intensity and duration of exercise performed, cardiac output and systolic blood pressure increase to adequately perfuse blood to the working tissue. Breathing rate and the depth of each breath also increase, to ensure adequate oxygenation of the blood. Metabolism increases and shift nutrient source to reflect the availability of oxygen to the mitochondria and need for adenosine triphosphate, the primary energy source of the human body. Motor units that control skeletal muscle fiber recruitment become activated, and neural pathways fire to reflect the work undertaken. Many other body systems also adjust to minimize the stress of physical activity. As with other events that disrupt homeostasis, the body attempts to compensate for these perturbations to reestablish its natural environment.[14,15]

When exercise is undertaken on a regular basis, the body becomes more efficient in its adaptation to the stress of exercise. Physiologic systems, such as cardiovascular, respiratory, muscular, neural, and endocrine, all become more adept at both the anticipation and the compensation for each individual bout of exercise. As the body is exposed to repeated bouts of exercise, the systems become trained to adapt to the stress of work, and the body resets what is considered to be in its normal range for daily living. Trained individuals are able to tax a greater percentage of their functional range, or maximal physiologic capacity, during periods of physical stress.[15] For example, if a sedentary person is required to run for a bus, their body is not accustomed to performing the acute bout of activity. They are able to use only a smaller portion of their potential functional capacity, thus resulting in a limited ability for adaptation to that particular stress. Heart racing, sweating, feeling slightly ill, with shaky legs, and out of breath, they might be unable to speak with a bus driver or have difficulty climbing stairs. In the case of someone who performs regular exercise, they encounter a similar situation and are better able to adapt to the stress by means of their ability to tap into a greater percentage of their physiologic reserve. Although they run the same amount to catch up with a bus, their bodies are better able to cope with the bout of activity undertaken.

Physiologic reserve is the overall range of functional capacity in an individual, defined by genetics, and including all organ systems in the human body. The aging process is associated with some degree of diminishment, which starts in early adulthood.[16] Depending on the degree of loss of physiologic reserve, there may be negative consequences on the ability to perform activities of daily living, and, in more severe cases, frailty and increased morbidity/mortality may ensue. Although the aging process itself compromises physiologic reserve, the effects are compounded by sedentary behavior. Regular physical exercise can attenuate the degree of physical decline associated with aging.[17] Despite the known benefits of active living, only 30% of individuals older than 65 years participate in some form of daily exercise.[18] Despite increasing efforts to promote physical activity in this population, the figures remain consistent.[19]

The ability to adapt to physical stress and the preservation of physiologic reserve are both relevant concepts for prehabilitation. Functional capacity, as determined by cardiopulmonary exercise testing, has been associated with surgical outcomes in noncardiopulmonary procedures: patients who are less fit have been shown to have a higher incidence of postsurgical morbidity and mortality.[20] In addition, impaired handgrip strength before surgery, as assessed by dynamometry, also seems to be related to poorer postoperative outcomes in patients undergoing nonemergency, cardiac and noncardiac procedures.[21] The goal of prehabilitation is to improve these fitness parameters, among others such as flexibility, to optimize postsurgical recovery and maintain physical function.

A critical aspect of improving physiologic reserve lies in the postsurgical healing process. There is a decrease in functional decline in the period after surgery (**Fig. 1**).[22] Although the functional decline is primarily caused by surgical trauma, inflammation, or the cancer itself, it can be further amplified by the effects of bed rest or a need to take it easy. The health of physiologic systems quickly diminish as a result of inactivity, with the process beginning in as little as the first week after cessation of activity.[23] This factor is also important during the presurgical time frame, where diminished physical activity can directly affect surgical outcomes. Bed rest, in as little as 7 days, has been shown to decrease insulin-mediated glucose extraction.[24] The vasodilator effects of insulin diminish with 10 days of bed rest, even in healthy populations.[25] Those at risk for developing type 2 diabetes are subject to a disproportionate aggravation of existing systemic low-grade inflammation during periods of physical inactivity.[26] These effects of physical inactivity are critical for the surgical process, when inflammation is already of concern.

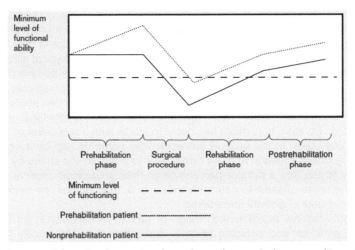

Fig. 1. Trajectory of functional capacity throughout the surgical process. (*From* Sultan P, Hamilton MA, Ackland GL. Preoperative muscle weakness as defined by handgrip strength and postoperative outcomes: a systematic review. BMC Anesthesiol 2012;12:1.)

As rapid as the physiologic decline caused by sedentary behaviors, the effects of training also occur quickly. For example, cardiovascular improvements can be seen within 3 weeks on commencement of physical training, even in older individuals.[27] The effective use of strength training programs is also not exclusive to younger populations: regular resistance training can reverse the age-related declines in skeletal muscle strength and function, even in frail, elderly individuals.[28] The limited time between diagnosis and surgery also seems to be an adequate time frame to obtain objectively measurable training effects.[29]

In 2007, the American College of Sports Medicine and the American Heart Association issued exercise recommendations specifically for the older adult, taking into consideration their heterogeneous health status and individual needs/goals for performing physical activity.[19] Other organizations have also released similar guidelines (eg, 2008 Physical Activity Guidelines for Americans, Canadian Society for Exercise Physiology, World Health Organization). A summary of the comprehensive guidelines published by the US Department of Health and Human Services (2008 Physical Activity Guidelines for Americans) has been presented in **Box 1**. Considering that the older adult is the least likely to regularly exercise,[19] it is important that their physical activity be meaningful, feasible, and something that they enjoy to maximize adherence. The main message is that the elderly should be encouraged to maintain a lifestyle as active as possible to promote and maintain good health practices.[30]

EXERCISE: WHAT TO DO?

Current recommendations include a combination of moderate and vigorous exercise, if deemed appropriate for the individual (see **Box 1**). What does moderate and vigorous represent for the patient? On a scale of 1 to 10 (1 representing a resting activity with no effort and 10 representing all-out, exhaustive exercise), moderate activity can be thought of as being a 5 to 6. Vigorous exercise falls within the range of 7 to 8. This scale, otherwise known as Rating of Perceived Exertion (RPE) or Borg Scale, is

Box 1
Physical activity guidelines for older adults.

Key Guidelines for Older Adults (2008 Physical Activity Guidelines for Americans)

The following Guidelines are the same for adults and older adults:

- All older adults should avoid inactivity. Some physical activity is better than none, and older adults who participate in any amount of physical activity gain some health benefits.

- For substantial health benefits, older adults should do at least 150 minutes (2 hours and 30 minutes) a week of moderate-intensity, or 75 minutes (1 hour and 15 minutes) a week of vigorous-intensity aerobic physical activity, or an equivalent combination of moderate- and vigorous-intensity aerobic activity. Aerobic activity should be performed in episodes of at least 10 minutes, and preferably, it should be spread throughout the week.

- For additional and more extensive health benefits, older adults should increase their aerobic physical activity to 300 minutes (5 hours) a week of moderate-intensity, or 150 minutes a week of vigorous-intensity aerobic physical activity, or an equivalent combination of moderate- and vigorous-intensity activity. Additional health benefits are gained by engaging in physical activity beyond this amount.

- Older adults should also do muscle-strengthening activities that are moderate or high intensity and involve all major muscle groups on 2 or more days a week, as these activities provide additional health benefits.

The following Guidelines are just for older adults:

- When older adults cannot do 150 minutes of moderate-intensity aerobic activity a week because of chronic conditions, they should be as physically active as their abilities and conditions allow.

- Older adults should do exercises that maintain or improve balance if they are at risk of falling.

- Older adults should determine their level of effort for physical activity relative to their level of fitness.

- Older adults with chronic conditions should understand whether and how their conditions affect their ability to do regular physical activity safely.

From US Department of Health and Human Services. Physical Activity Guidelines for Americans. Available at: http://www.health.gov/paguidelines/guidelines/. Accessed November 5, 2014.

easy to use and gives a rough indication of the intensity of activity performed (**Fig. 2**). It can easily be transferred onto an easy to read poster (large print) and hung up within view of the patients while exercising. This strategy allows for a common reference point for both the tester and testee. Although it does not represent a perfect representation of exercise intensity, it is commonly used in many populations of patients chronic disease (eg, American Thoracic Society). There are other scales, such as the Modified Borg Scale, which work on the same concept but use different numbers to represent perceived exertion. The use of a simple RPE scale is especially relevant for patients who have been prescribed medications that affect the heart rate response to exercise (eg, β-blockers), therefore limiting the use of heart rate as an indication of intensity. The benefit of the RPE scale is that it reflects the perceived intensity of the activity on a given day, taking into consideration any fatigue, illness, or other condition that negatively affects the individual's health status at a given moment. Conversely, it also takes into consideration positive adaptations caused by training, and the patient must increase their work intensity to maintain the same range of RPE values.

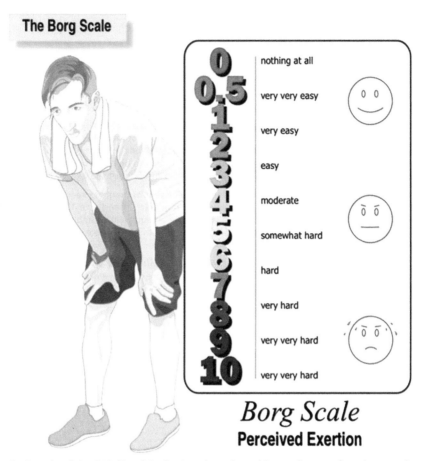

Fig. 2. Sample of the RPE (Borg) Scale. A scale such as this may be transferred onto a large poster board and mounted within view of the exercising patient. Often the RPE is color coded (from *green* or *blue* at rest to *red* at maximal efforts) or has cartoons representing effort. Key words represent exercise intensity.

Another important point raised in the more recent guidelines is that aerobic exercise does not have to take place in continuous bouts but has been shown to be of benefit in smaller sessions of at least 10 minutes. In patients with type 2 diabetes, 3 x 10 minutes of aerobic exercise during the day had more desirable effects on glycemic control than performing a single session of 30 minutes. The multiple short daily sessions may be associated with a higher energy expenditure than occurs during a single bout.[31] Besides possible physiologic benefits, the 10-minute sessions may be more feasible in this patient population, because of perceived time restraints, fatigue, or motivational factors.

Regarding exercise in general, it can be said that more is better but something is better than nothing.[32] In terms of exercise prescription, there is a clear dose response, with more health benefits occurring with higher amounts of physical activity.[30] However, when considering the prehabilitation patient, there are 2 issues to keep in mind: first, there is a clearly defined period between diagnosis and surgery, which depends on individual health care programs and, second, the presurgical patient may have a host of health conditions, including anxiety, depression, malnutrition, concurrent conditions, and the cancer itself, which might affect how they perform physical activity. For these reasons, encouraging the patient to do as much as they can in the period that is available may be the most efficient and effective approach. This strategy is especially important for the patient who has been previously sedentary or who has engaged in very low levels of physical activity. Programming for prehabilitation should introduce exercise that is more than what the individual already partakes in, so that the body experiences the stress of additional work, but avoiding an exercise protocol that is too intense, which may result in fatigue, injury, or (in our previous experience) poor adherence.[11] Prehabilitation in a 4-week period (diagnosis to surgery) has been shown to be sufficient to improve distance in the 6-minute walk test, decrease heart rate/oxygen consumption at submaximal workloads, and improve peak power output.[33] In addition, the program should be varied, touching on the various components outlined in **Box 1** (ie, aerobic and muscle strengthening exercises) and reflecting the needs of the individual. A sample exercise program from our laboratory is presented in **Box 2**. Allowing adequate rest between bouts of exercise is also important, both for physical recovery and to reap the physiologic benefits from the previous activity bout.[34] To continue physical improvements, the program must progress by slowly increasing the challenge of the exercise intensity. The concept of specificity should also be addressed when designing an exercise program for prehabilitation: an individual improves their functional capacity according to the type of stress delivered.[15] For instance, someone who trains on a bicycle may not achieve a higher peak oxygen consumption if evaluated on a treadmill. For that reason, the method of evaluation should reflect the type of training prescribed. Specificity may also be evident when the exercise testing occurs at intensities higher than training values (ie, measuring peak oxygen consumption [Vo_2peak] after training at values 50%–60% of Vo_2peak). In this instance, submaximal evaluation may be reflective of training and more appropriate to detect improvements in the elderly population.[35]

In general, individuals who have been the least fit and the most sedentary show the most improvements when they commence an exercise program.[32] Since the ratio of actual physiologic reserve to total physiologic reserve is small, even small amounts of physical training are remarkable. Patients following simple walking and breathing exercise guidelines have made marked improvements in walking capacity, as measured by the 6-minute walk test.[11] Older adults are particular susceptible to bed rest and physical inactivity, because of their already low functional capacity, this is a patient population who particularly benefit from targeted intervention.[22] In addition, prehabilitation programs that are multimodal (including physical, nutritional, and psychological components) seem to be more effective than programs that are unimodal.[36] As indicated by systemic reviews, preoperative exercise intervention before cardiac or abdominal surgery has been shown to reduce postoperative complications.[8] For these reasons, a multimodal prehabilitation program, with the aim of improving physical capacity before cancer surgery, seems to be an efficient and cost-effective method to ameliorate patient outcome after surgery.[22]

OPTIMIZING NUTRITION FOR PREHABILITATION

The nutritional status of patients scheduled for abdominal surgery is directly influenced by the presence of cancer or other chronic conditions, such as inflammatory bowel disease, which have an impact on all aspects of intermediary (protein,

Box 2
Example of 4-week prehabilitation program including physical activity and nutrition and relaxation exercises

Aerobic exercise

- Start a slow walk to adequately warm up
- 30 minutes minimum of aerobic activity (walking/biking) 3 times per week at moderate intensity (4–6 on the Borg Scale). If the participant finds the activity to be easier (2–3 on the Borg Scale), then, the walking pace or duration should be gradually increased. It is recommended not to surpass 7 to 8 on the Borg Scale. Example: walk at a normal pace for 5 minutes and then walk at a quicker pace for 2 minutes and repeat for the duration of time.

Resistance exercise

- All exercises are to be performed starting with 1 set of about 10 to 12 repetitions. Number of sets and repetitions gradually increase to 2 sets and 12 to 15 repetitions.
  - Use of a resistance band/handheld weights and some body weight exercises
  - Body weight exercise involve the following:
    - Push-ups (wall, modified, or full)
    - Squats with the use of a chair
    - Hamstring curls
    - Calf raises
    - Abdominal crunches (chair or floor)
  - Theraband/handheld weight exercises involve the following
    - Chest exercise
    - Deltoid lifts
    - Bicep curls
    - Triceps extension

Flexibility

- Flexibility exercises are given for the following muscles (each exercise should be performed twice and held for a minimum of 20 seconds).
  - Chest
  - Biceps
  - Triceps
  - Quadriceps
  - Hamstring
  - Calf

Breathing Relaxation Exercise

- Abdominal breathing (15 minutes twice daily)
- Use of relaxation CD (nature sounds and breathing instructions)

It is instructed to take protein within 30 minutes on completion of the exercise regimen.

carbohydrate, lipid, trace element, vitamin) metabolism, and by other factors, such as age, adjuvant cancer therapy, and stage of the disease. In addition, a patient who is undernourished before surgery has a greater risk of morbidity and mortality.[37] The primary goal of nutrition therapy is to optimize nutrient stores preoperatively and provide adequate nutrition to compensate for the catabolic response of surgery postoperatively.[38,39]

The purpose of nutritional prehabilitation is therefore to prepare (or optimize) the patient for surgery, not necessarily to replace nutritional deficits. To be successful, nutrition intervention requires a timeline that needs to start with preoperative assessment and extend into the postoperative period. The shift to preemptive preoperative nutritional therapy (which is focused on prevention) is strongly considered if the patient meets risk criteria.[40]

The greater sensitivity of protein catabolism to nutritional support, in particular to amino acids, could have important implications for the nutritional management of these patients during periods of catabolic stress, with particular emphasis on substrate utilization and energy requirement during the healing process. The European Society for Clinical Nutrition and Metabolism recommends 1.2 to 1.5 g protein/kg, for surgical patients. Protein intake is calculated as 20% of total energy expenditure, determined individually, using a stress factor of 1.3 for major surgery and an appropriate activity factor.[41]

The benefits of an interaction between nutrition and physical exercise have been studied in elderly patients, in whom it been shown that a minimum of 140 g of carbohydrate taken 3 hours before exercise increases liver and muscle glycogen and facilitates the completion of the exercise session.[42] Also, the time of ingesting a protein meal after surgery is of importance; elderly individuals who consume 10 g proteins immediately after weight training have their mean quadriceps fiber area increased by 24% as well as their dynamic muscular strength.[43,44]

With regard to the type of nutrients, administration of a pharmaconutrition formula containing arginine, fish oil, and nucleotides has been shown to reduce infection, other complications, and hospital length of stay in patients undergoing major upper or lower gastrointestinal surgeries, regardless of preexisting nutritional status.[45,46] A synergistic effect may exist between arginine and fish oils, and therefore, a combination of the 2 agents should be used. Timing of delivery is optimized by starting 5 to 7 days preoperatively (500–1000 mL per day) and continuing postoperatively. No prehabilitation studies have been performed with administration of immunonutrition coupled with physical activity/exercise.

Whey protein is another nutritional component that has attracted the interest of exercise physiologists, because it is a protein that is highly bioavailable, is rapidly digested, and contains all the indispensable amino acids.[47,48] Compared with casein, whey protein is also associated with an increase in protein synthesis.[49] In addition, when whey protein is compared with other sources of complete proteins, whey is found to score highest on the quality assessments used to assess protein quality, such as net protein utilization, biological value, and the protein digestibility corrected amino acid score (a measure of how well a particular protein provides indispensable amino acids).[50] Whey protein plays a role in oxidative stress defense, by increasing the content of intracellular stores of the antioxidant glutathione (GSH). The mechanism of GSH is believed to be related to the in vivo synthesis of GSH being limited by the availability of the amino acid cysteine, found in rich supply in whey protein. GSH is a major intracellular antioxidant that neutralizes reactive oxygen species (ROS) by donating its sulfridryl proton.[51] Because ROS is involved in cytokine signaling during the acute phase response, the consumption of whey protein and resultant increase in GSH levels, which neutralize ROS, may aid in blunting the inflammatory processes characteristic of the stress induced by surgery. In a recent prehabilitation nutrition (no physical exercise) RCT, patients who had undergone colorectal cancer surgery were given a daily whey protein supplement (10–20 g) for 4 weeks before surgery and the functional walking capacity (assessed by the 6-minute walk test) increased more than 20 m (minimal clinically important difference for the measure of surgical recovery) in more than 50% of the subjects (C Gillis, personal communication, 2014).

STRATEGIES TO MINIMIZE THE EMOTIONAL BURDEN OF SURGERY

The physical burden of surgery is closely linked to the emotional one. Increased levels of psychosocial distress seen in patients undergoing abdominal surgery are related to the diagnosis (eg, cancer), the treatment (chemotherapy), and most often to the disability (stoma siting). Several studies have identified that anxiety and depression can affect postoperative outcome (eg, those who were more stressed on the third day after surgery stayed longer in hospital, and those who were more optimistic were not often hospitalized).[52] Depression was associated with more infection-related complication and poor wound healing.[53–55] In a recent prehabilitation study conducted in patients who underwent colorectal resections,[56] those who improved in functional capacity showed also positive changes in mental health and some aspects of the Short Form 36 subscale vitality. Anxiety at baseline was also associated with poorer recovery. The belief that fitness aided recovery was a strong predictor of improvement. Stress management before prostate surgery has been shown to affect immune function.[57]

These observations indicate that there is a need to address the importance of incorporating mental strategies to attenuate the stress response and enhance the effect of prehabilitation. Interventional studies that improve healing outcomes by reducing psychological stress provide further evidence of the impact of psychological and behavioral factors in wound repair.

Physical exercise can reduce psychological distress in addition to improving cardiovascular function. Older adults were randomized to an exercise intervention (1-hour aerobic exercise session, 3 times per week) or a nonintervention control group. One month after the beginning of the intervention, participants received a 3.5-mm punch biopsy on the back of their nondominant upper arm. Older adults who exercised healed their wounds on average 18 days earlier than those in the control group.[58]

Another aspect inherent to prehabilitation is related to the benefits of informing patients of all aspects of the perioperative process. The benefits of giving preoperative information to patients include decreased length of stay, less demand for analgesia postoperatively, and increased patient satisfaction.[59] The use of information booklets and tailored messages on how to promote personal health help to empower patients in the control of their own health and become more involved in the healing process. The prehabilitation program can provide adequate information that is made to suit individual-level psychological characteristics, such as motivational orientation or cognitive processing style. This process can elicit motivation and participation.

Although there has been great effort in studying the impact of physical exercise on postoperative outcome, little has been done to address patient and caregiver's emotional burden of surgery. There is a growing interest in mind-body interventions, with the intent to attenuate the stress of anxiety and sleep deprivation. Therefore, it makes sense that a multimodal prehabilitation program includes all these aspects of care in a multidisciplinary fashion.

WHO BENEFITS FROM PREHABILITATION?

Because people are living well in their late 70s, they are more likely to undergo surgery. Morbidity and mortality associated with surgery increase with advancing age once individuals are older than 75 years. There is a large heterogeneity in this population, with frail and cognitively impaired on one side and highly functional and robust on the other side. There has also been a shift in the comorbidity of this population, with an increase in cancer, obesity, diabetes, cognitive impairment, and osteoarthritis.[36,60]

Comprehensive preoperative assessments that take into consideration functionality, comorbidity, cognition, social support, nutrition, and medical assessment could help identify those who are at risk of adverse events and formulate a treatment plan before surgery.

Although there have been several studies emphasizing the benefit of long-term endurance training in patients with chronic heart failure and the positive effect of rehabilitation physical exercise after reconstructive surgery, few studies have focused on surgical prehabilitation in the elderly and patients with cancer with the intent to increase physiologic reserve and enhance functional capacity in preparation for surgery. It is assumed that elderly, frail patients with medical comorbidities, poor functional and social status, at risk of malnutrition need some attention.[61–63]

The appropriate time for the development of a prehabilitation program is during the preoperative assessment period for elective operations. At this time, the multidisciplinary team, which should include internal medicine, geriatrics, anesthesia, surgery, dietetics, kinesiology/physiotherapy, and nursing, would devise a risk stratification model and identify the type and duration of prehabilitation needed to balance the potential benefit of such intervention versus the potential harms of delaying surgery.

RECOVERY AND EVALUATION OF PREHABILITATION

Traditionally, successful recovery from surgery has been identified with the patient leaving the hospital and without complications during the first 30 postoperative days. However, length of hospital stay may be affected by external elements, such as socioeconomic, cultural, and institutional factors, and complications and mortality are uncommon and often inconsistently measured.[64] These measures are important to clinicians and administrators but may not be relevant to the patient, who wants to go back to baseline activities and to be able to function socially. This situation implies that recovery is a more complex construct, because it includes physiologic, social, functional, and economic domains.[65] For example, with the trend of declining 30-day morbidity and mortality as a result of better perisurgical and anesthesia care, advances in cancer therapy, and pharmacologic optimization, patients who have cancer live longer, and, therefore, emphasis has shifted to cancer survivorship and community reintegration.[36]

This situation shifts the paradigm from addressing short-term health issues to considering long-term functional and psychosocial capacity and improving patient-centered longitudinal outcome. The measures used to assess the impact of prehabilitation intervention on recovery need to be relevant in the context of the time chosen. For example, in the first 3 weeks after surgery, the recovery trajectory focuses on mobility, pain relief, and coping with side effects of medications, whereas at 6 to 8 weeks, the focus is more on quality of life and reintegration in the community and the workplace.[66]

Outcome measures to evaluate the impact of prehabilitation need to take into consideration 2 aspects of this program: the preoperative period, during which the prehabilitation program is implemented, and the postoperative period, during which the impact of the prehabilitation program is evaluated. The scope of the preoperative period is to increase physiologic, physical, nutritional, and mental reserve. It is during this time that the multidisciplinary interventions aimed at making patients stronger for surgery are chosen, taking into consideration the type of surgery and the patient's physiologic and metabolic conditions. In the second period, after surgery, the increased reserve obtained during the prehabilitation phase is available to provide sufficient energy and sustain the recovery process, which, in cases of cancer, might facilitate earlier administration of adjuvant therapy.

Because recovery is a complex phenomenon to assess, it is clear that a single outcome measure is not able to capture the evolution of the healing trajectory. Preferably, a composite of objective performance measures together with self-reported measures assessing functional status, independence, and feelings would help the clinician to follow the progress.[67]

SUMMARY

Surgical prehabilitation is an emerging concept that derives from the realization that perioperative care must include, beside clinical and pharmacologic preparation of the surgical patient, preoperative physical, nutritional, and mental optimization. As the population ages and mortality decreases, additional concerns in patients who undergo surgery and other treatment include quality of life, community reintegration, and physical and mental performance after surgery and cancer treatment. Multidisciplinary prehabilitation programs that incorporate innovative comprehensive preoperative risk evaluation need to be developed, tested, implemented, and directed to patients, especially those at risk. The integrated role of physical exercise, adequate nutrition, and psychosocial balance, together with medical and pharmacologic optimization, deserves to receive more attention by clinicians.

REFERENCES

1. Schilling PL, Dimick JB, Birkmeyer JD. Prioritizing quality improvement in general surgery. J Am Coll Surg 2008;207:698–704.
2. Christensen T, Kehlet H. Postoperative fatigue. World J Surg 1993;17(2):220–5.
3. Salmon P, Hall GM. A theory of postoperative fatigue: an interaction of biological, psychological, and social processes. Pharmacol Biochem Behav 1997;56(4): 623–8.
4. Schroeder D, Hill GL. Predicting postoperative fatigue: importance of preoperative factors. World J Surg 1993;17(2):226–31.
5. Topp R, Ditmyer M, King K, et al. The effect of bed rest and potential of prehabilitation on patients in intensive care unit. AACN Clin Issues 2002;13:263–76.
6. Asoh T, Takeuchi Y, Tsuji H. Effect of voluntary exercise on resistance to trauma in rats. Circ Shock 1986;20:259–67.
7. Pierson LM, Herbert WG, Norton HJ, et al. Effects of combined aerobic and resistance training versus aerobic training alone in cardiac rehabilitation. J Cardiopulm Rehabil 2001;21(2):101–10.
8. Valkenet K, Van de port IG, Dronkers JJ, et al. The effects of preoperative exercise therapy on postoperative outcome: a systematic review. Clin Rehabil 2011; 25:99–111.
9. Santa Mina D, Clarke D, Ritvo P, et al. Effect of total-body prehabilitation on postoperative outcomes: a systematic review and meta-analysis. Physiotherapy 2014; 100(3):196–207.
10. Lemanu DP, Singh PP, MacCormick AD, et al. Effect of preoperative exercise on cardiorespiratory function and recovery after surgery: a systematic review. World J Surg 2013;37:711–20.

11. Carli F, Charlebois P, Stein B, et al. Prehabilitation to improve recovery of physical function following colorectal surgery: a randomized trial. Br J Surg 2010;97: 1187–97.
12. Li C, Carli F, Lee L, et al. Impact of trimodal prehabilitation programme on functional recovery after colorectal cancer surgery. Surg Endosc 2013;27(4):1072–82.
13. Gillis C, Li C, Lee L, et al. Prehabilitation vs rehabilitation, a randomized control trial in patients undergoing colorectal resection for cancer. Anesthesiology 2014;121(5):937–47.
14. Fletcher GF, Balady GJ, Amsterdam EA, et al. Exercise standards for testing and training: a statement for healthcare professionals from the American Heart Association. Circulation 2001;104(14):1694–740.
15. Astrand P, Rodahl K, Dahl HA, et al. Textbook of work physiology: physiological bases of exercise. 4th edition. Champaign (IL): Human Kinetics; 2003.
16. Hawkins S, Wiswell R. Rate and mechanism of maximal oxygen consumption decline with aging: implications for exercise training. Sports Med 2003;33(12): 877–88.
17. Cadore EL, Pinto RS, Bottaro M, et al. Strength and endurance training prescription in healthy and frail elderly. Aging Dis 2014;5(3):183–95.
18. Heath JM, Stuart MR. Prescribing exercise for frail elders. J Am Board Fam Pract 2002;15(3):218–28.
19. Haskell WL, Lee IM, Pate RR, et al. Physical activity and public health: updated recommendation for adults from the American College of Sports Medicine and the American Heart Association. Med Sci Sports Exerc 2007;39(8):1423–34.
20. Hennis PJ, Meale PM, Grocott MP. Cardiopulmonary exercise testing for the evaluation of perioperative risk in non-cardiopulmonary surgery. Postgrad Med J 2011;87:550–7.
21. Sultan P, Hamilton MA, Ackland GL. Preoperative muscle weakness as defined by handgrip strength and postoperative outcomes: a systematic review. BMC Anesthesiol 2012;17(12):1.
22. Carli F, Zavorsky GS. Optimizing functional exercise capacity in the elderly surgical population. Curr Opin Clin Nutr Metab Care 2005;8(1):23–32.
23. Mujika I, Padilla S. Cardiorespiratory and metabolic characteristics of detraining in humans. Med Sci Sports Exerc 2001;33(3):413–21.
24. Biensø RS, Ringholm S, Kiilerich K, et al. GLUT4 and glycogen synthase are key players in bed rest-induced insulin resistance. Diabetes 2012;61(5):1090–9.
25. Sonne MP, Højbjerre L, Alibegovic AC, et al. Endothelial function after 10 days of bed rest in individuals at risk for type 2 diabetes and cardiovascular disease. Exp Physiol 2011;96(10):1000–9.
26. Højbjerre L, Sonne MP, Alibegovic AC, et al. Impact of physical inactivity on adipose tissue low-grade inflammation in first-degree relatives of type 2 diabetic patients. Diabetes Care 2011;34(10):2265–72.
27. Murias JM, Kowalchuk JM, Paterson DH. Time course and mechanisms of adaptations in cardiorespiratory fitness with endurance training in older and young men. J Appl Physiol (1985) 2010;108(3):621–7.
28. Fielding RA. The role of progressive resistance training and nutrition in the preservation of lean body mass in the elderly. J Am Coll Nutr 1995;14(6):587–94.
29. Jack S, West M, Grocott MP. Perioperative exercise training in elderly subjects. Best Pract Res Clin Anaesthesiol 2011;25(3):461–72.
30. Nelson ME, Rejeski WJ, Blair SN, et al. Physical activity and public health in older adults: recommendation from the American College of Sports Medicine and the American Heart Association. Med Sci Sports Exerc 2007;39(8):1435–45.

31. Eriksen L, Dahl-Petersen I, Haugaard SB, et al. Comparison of the effect of multiple short-duration with single long-duration exercise sessions on glucose homeostasis in type 2 diabetes mellitus. Diabetologia 2007;50(11):2245–53.

32. Haskell WL. J.B. Wolffe Memorial Lecture. Health consequences of physical activity: understanding and challenges regarding dose-response. Med Sci Sports Exerc 1994;26(6):649–60.

33. Kim do J, Mayo NE, Carli F, et al. Responsive measures to prehabilitation in patients undergoing bowel resection surgery. Tohoku J Exp Med 2009;217(2): 109–15.

34. Brentano MA, Martins Kruel LF. A review on strength exercise-induced muscle damage: applications, adaptation mechanisms and limitations. J Sports Med Phys Fitness 2011;51(1):1–10.

35. De Vito G, Hernandez R, Gonzalez V, et al. Low intensity physical training in older subjects. J Sports Med Phys Fitness 1997;37(1):72–7.

36. Silver JK, Baima J. Cancer prehabilitation: an opportunity to decrease treatment-related morbidity, increase cancer treatment options, and improve physical and psychological health outcomes. Am J Phys Med Rehabil 2013;92(8):715–27.

37. Schwegler I, von Holzen A, Gutzwiller JP, et al. Nutritional risk is a clinical predictor of postoperative mortality and morbidity in surgery for colorectal cancer. Br J Surg 2010;97(1):92–7.

38. Howard L, Ashley C. Nutrition in the perioperative patient. Annu Rev Nutr 2003; 23:263–82.

39. Weimann A, Braga M, Harsanyi L, et al. ESPEN guidelines on enteral nutrition: surgery including organ transplantation. Clin Nutr 2006;25:224–44.

40. McClave SA, Kozar R, Martindale RG, et al. Summary points and consensus recommendation from the North American Surgical Nutrition Summit. JPEN J Parenter Enteral Nutr 2013;37(suppl):99S–105S.

41. Braga M, Ljungqvist O, Soeters P, et al. ESPEN Guidelines on Parenteral Nutrition: surgery. Clin Nutr 2009;28:378–86.

42. Hargreaves M. Pre-exercise nutritional strategies: effects on metabolism and performance. Can J Appl Physiol 2001;26(Suppl):S64–70.

43. Esmarck B, Andersen JL, Olsen S, et al. Timing of postexercise protein intake is important for muscle hypertrophy with resistance training in elderly humans. J Physiol 2001;535:301–11.

44. Burke LM, Hawley JA, Ross ML, et al. Preexercise aminoacidemia and muscle protein synthesis after resistance exercise. Med Sci Sports Exerc 2012;44: 1968–77.

45. Jie B, Jiang ZM, Nolan MT, et al. Impact of preoperative nutritional support on clinical outcome in abdominal surgical patients at nutritional risk. Nutrition 2012;29:420–33.

46. Drover JW, Dhaliweal R, Weitzel L, et al. Perioperative use of arginine-supplemented diets: a systematic review of the evidence. J Am Coll Surg 2011;212:385–99.

47. Marshall K. Therapeutic applications of whey protein. Altern Med Rev 2004;9: 136–56.

48. Walzem RL, Dillard CJ, German JB. Whey components: millennia of evolution create functionalities for mammalian nutrition: what we know and what we may be overlooking. Crit Rev Food Sci Nutr 2002;42:353–75.

49. Campbell WW, Leidy HJ. Dietary protein and resistance training effects on muscle and body composition in older persons. J Am Coll Nutr 2007;26:696S–703S.

50. Yalcin AS. Emerging therapeutic potential of whey proteins and peptides. Curr Pharm Des 2006;12:1637–43.

51. Grey V, Mohammed SR, Smountas AA, et al. Improved glutathione status in young adult patients with cystic fibrosis supplemented with whey protein. J Cyst Fibros 2003;2:195–8.
52. Munafo M, Stevenson J. Anxiety and surgical recovery. Reinterpreting the literature. J Psychosom Res 2001;51:589–96.
53. Singh NA, Clements KM, Fiatarone MA. A randomized controlled trial of progressive resistance training in depressed elders. J Gerontol 1997;52:M27–35.
54. Gouin JP, Kiecolt-Glasera JK. The impact of psychological stress on wound healing: methods and mechanisms. Immunol Allergy Clin North Am 2011;31:81–93.
55. Walburn J, Vedhara K, Hankins M, et al. Psychological stress and wound healing in humans: a systematic review and meta-analysis. J Psychosom Res 2009;67(3):253–71.
56. Mayo NE, Feldman L, Scott S, et al. Impact of preoperative change in physical function on postoperative recovery: arguments supporting prehabilitation for colorectal surgery. Surgery 2011;150:504.
57. Cohen L, Parker PA, Vence L, et al. Presurgical stress management improves postoperative immune function in men with prostate cancer undergoing radical prostatectomy. Psychosom Med 2011;73:18–25.
58. Emery CF, Kiecolt-Glaser JK, Glaser R, et al. Exercise accelerates wound healing among healthy older adults: a preliminary investigation. J Gerontol 2005;60:1432–6.
59. Sjoling M, Nordahl G, Olofsso N, et al. The impact of preoperative information on state anxiety, postoperative pain and satisfaction with pain management. Patient Educ Couns 2003;51:169–76.
60. Cheema FN, Abraham NS, Berger DH, et al. Novel approaches to perioperative assessment and intervention may improve long-term outcomes after colorectal cancer resection in older adults. Ann Surg 2011;253:867–74.
61. Dronkers JJ, Chorus AM, van Meeteren NL, et al. The association of preoperative physical fitness and physical activity with outcome after scheduled major abdominal surgery. Anaesthesia 2013;68:67–73.
62. Fearon KC, Jenkins JT, Carli F, et al. Patient optimization for gastrointestinal cancer surgery. Br J Surg 2013;100(1):15–27.
63. Carli F, Brown S, Kennepohl S. Prehabilitation to enhance postoperative recovery of an octogenarian following robotic-assisted hysterectomy with endometrial cancer. Can J Anaesth 2012;59:779–84.
64. Carli F, Mayo N. Measuring the outcome of surgical procedures: what are the challenges? Br J Anaesth 2001;87(4):531–3.
65. Allvin R, Berg K, Idvall E, et al. Postoperative recovery: a concept analysis. J Adv Nurs 2007;57(5):552–8.
66. Lee L, Tran T, Mayo NE, et al. What does it really mean to "recover" from an operation? Surgery 2014;155(2):211–6.
67. Amtmann D, Cook KF, Johnson KL, et al. The PROMIS initiative: involvement of rehabilitation stakeholders in development and examples of applications in rehabilitation research. Arch Phys Med Rehabil 2011;92:S12–9.

Monitoring Needs and Goal-directed Fluid Therapy Within an Enhanced Recovery Program

 CrossMark

Gary Minto, MB ChB, FRCA[a],*, Michael J. Scott, MB ChB, MRCP, FRCA, FFICM[b],
Timothy E. Miller, MB ChB, FRCA[c]

KEYWORDS

- Fluid therapy • Colorectal surgery • Cardiac output monitoring • Enhanced recovery

KEY POINTS

- Enhanced recovery principles mitigate against many of the factors that traditionally led to relative hypovolemia in the perioperative period.
- Individualization of fluid prescription requires consideration of clinical signs and hemodynamic variables.
- A large literature spanning 4 decades supports goal-directed fluid therapy.
- Application of this evidence to justify stroke volume optimization in the setting of major surgery within an enhanced recovery program is controversial.

Individuals having major abdominal surgery need perioperative fluid supplementation. This requirement is caused by:

- A physiologic stress response to the surgery. Incision and tissue handling trigger endocrine and inflammatory changes that lead to:
  - Redistribution of water from body fluid compartments
  - Endothelial changes promoting leakage of fluid out of capillaries
  - Redistribution of blood flow
  - Activation of sodium and water retention mechanisms
- The magnitude of the stress response varies between individuals, and even within the same individual, depending on the condition in which they present

Conflicts of interest: G. Minto declares he has no conflicts of interest.
[a] Department of Anaesthesia & Perioperative Medicine, Plymouth Hospitals NHS Trust, Plymouth University Peninsula School of Medicine, Plymouth PL6 8DH, UK; [b] Department of Anaesthesia and Intensive Care Medicine, Royal Surrey County Hospital, University of Surrey, Guildford GU1 7XX, UK; [c] Department of Anesthesiology, Duke University Medical Center, Durham, NC 27710, USA
* Corresponding author.
E-mail address: gary.minto@nhs.net

for surgery. Patients who are acutely ill tend to have a greater inflammatory response; this may be modified by preoperative factors such as nutritional status, neoadjuvant chemotherapy and radiotherapy, antibiotics, and steroids.

- Replacement of losses:
  - Preoperative dehydration if oral fluids are withheld
  - These effects may be magnified by bowel preparation
  - Losses caused by the underlying disorder (eg, preoperative vomiting, diarrhea, or evaporative losses)
  - Blood loss, although major hemorrhage is rare during elective bowel surgery
- Hemodynamic changes induced by anesthesia:
  - Vasoparesis and venodilatation in response to neuraxial blockade[1]
  - Drug effects on vasomotor tone and cardiac contractility; in general, anesthesia promotes vasodilatation
  - Vasoconstriction in response to pressor agents
- Hemodynamic changes induced by surgical conditions:
  - Positioning (eg, head up or down, prone[2])
  - Pneumoperitoneum to facilitate laparoscopic surgery
- Reduced oral intake in the postoperative period, which may be complicated by intestinal ileus, excessive use of opioids, gastric tubes, nausea, vomiting.

Many of these mechanisms promote hypovolemia, which is a deficit in intravascular fluid volume.

PERIOPERATIVE FLUID REQUIREMENTS IN THE CONTEXT OF ENHANCED RECOVERY

In contrast with the emergency setting, in which many of the pathophysiologic perturbations discussed earlier are already in place at the time of surgery, enhanced recovery mitigates against most of these factors.

- Patients are brought to theater in a well-hydrated state, having also been provided with preoperative carbohydrate drinks.
- Routine bowel preparation is avoided for most colonic resections.
- Laparoscopic or small-incision surgery seeks to minimize physiologic disturbance.
- Long-acting opioids, which may cause ileus, are avoided.
- In many enhanced recovery (ER) programs, epidural blockade is also avoided, minimizing hemodynamic changes caused by regional anesthesia.[3]
- ERs incorporate a general fluid therapy philosophy of avoidance of sodium and water overload (discussed later).
- Early resumption of enteral feeding, early mobilization, and reduced tubes and drains are intended to allow patients to self-regulate their fluid and nutritional intake from soon after surgery.[4]

For these reasons perioperative fluid management may be different within ER pathways than in other settings.

GENERAL APPROACHES TO INTRAOPERATIVE FLUID THERAPY
Fixed-volume Strategies

During surgery, intravenous fluid administration is necessary. In the past, a simplistic fixed-volume approach has been used, whereby an estimated baseline fluid regimen is commenced, and then modified based on measurement of preoperative and ongoing losses, and on information from conventional hemodynamic monitoring.

Whether this baseline fluid regimen should be liberal or restrictive has been the source of much debate. A key factor here is so-called third-space loss, which is the concept that a large amount of fluid (perhaps 10 mL/kg/h) shifts from the intravascular into the peritoneal space and evaporates when the abdomen is open during surgery, and that a degree of fluid redistribution and capillary leak persists for a time after surgery, creating a risk of relative hypovolemia. A liberal intraoperative fluid regimen is variably defined, but typically involves a bolus of 500 to 1000 mL of intravenous crystalloid before the commencement of surgery, around 10 mL/kg/h during surgery, and a further 2 to 3 L intravenous fluid after surgery, totaling more than 5 L in the first postoperative day.[5]

Although deeply entrenched in clinical teaching and practice for decades, there is minimal evidence that third-space loss occurs.[6]

There is a paucity of large-scale perioperative studies to date, but many small trials, systematic reviews, and meta-analyses consistently favor a restrictive approach.[5,7–9] It is relevant that a recent randomized controlled trial (RCT) of resuscitation strategies for gastroenteritis in sub-Saharan African children linked liberal fluid prescription with an increased mortality.[10]

What constitutes restrictive is also variably defined; avoidance of fluid excess is perhaps a more appropriate terminology.[11] The summary from meta-analysis is that patients in the restrictive arms of studies received around 1500 mL less intraoperative crystalloid (95% confidence interval [CI], 986–2154 mL) than those in the liberal group[5] and that this was associated with a lower rate of complications and a shorter hospital stay.

A problem with fixed-volume strategies is that they disregard interindividual variation. The ideal is to individualize fluid therapy so as to avoid harmful effects of either hypovolemia or fluid overload (**Fig. 1**).

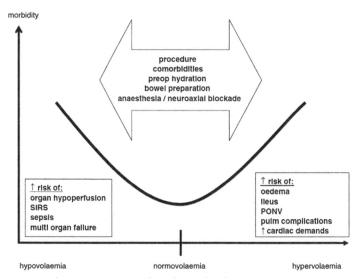

Fig. 1. A conceptual curve portraying the relationship between perioperative administered fluid volume and postoperative morbidity, and factors influencing shift of the curve (*arrow*). Boxes indicate the risk of complications associated with deviation from normovolemia. PONV, postoperative nausea and vomiting; SIRS, systemic inflammatory response syndrome. (*From* Bundgaard-Nielsen M, Secher N, Kehlet H. 'Liberal' vs. 'restrictive' perioperative fluid therapy – a critical assessment of the evidence. Acta Anaesthesiol Scand 2009;53:850; with permission.)

Conventional Hemodynamic Monitoring

Individualization of fluid prescription needs to take into account gender, age, compli-cating illnesses, body composition, and preoperative hydration.[12] In clinical practice, regimens are not fixed doses; fluid administration is modified at the discretion of attending clinicians, based on consideration of various clinical signs, hemodynamic variables, and biomarkers.

- Heart rate, systolic and diastolic blood pressure, and pulse pressure are real-time hemodynamic measurements that are readily available during and after sur-gery; however, these are not a good reflection of central blood volume, because they are also affected by anesthesia and surgical stress. Moreover, compensa-tory changes, particularly splanchnic vasoconstriction, can mask hypovolemia. In a healthy volunteer study, heart rate and BP remained stable despite venesec-tion of 25% of blood volume.[13]
- Peripheral perfusion and temperature may similarly be influenced by other peri-operative factors.
- Urine output is an inaccurate reflection of central blood volume: pressure diuresis may occur even if there is relative hypovolemia; conversely, the surgical stress response promotes water and salt retention, and pneumoperitoneum may cause oliguria.
- Central venous pressure measurements do not correlate well with intravascular volume because a multitude of factors (muscle relaxation, remifentanil infusions, epidural and spinal anesthesia, and pneumoperitoneum) affect venous tone. In general, central venous pressure does not predict fluid responsiveness (unless very low) so cannot be used to identify when patients need more fluid,[14] although it may serve as an indicator of venous capacitance to avoid overinfusion.
- Biomarkers, such as arterial lactate, and a comparison of central venous and arterial oxygen saturations to characterize tissue oxygen extraction have some potential,[15] but are not highly responsive to real-time hemodynamic changes. Global measurements may not reflect perfusion in particular tissues, especially the intestines, and algorithms incorporating their use are complex. The situation is further complicated because central venous sampling is from the superior vena cava and therefore a true mixed venous saturation is not obtained. Trending and response to fluid boluses may be useful in the immediate postoperative period (4–6 hours); however, in most surgical patients, perturbations in measured tissue oxygenation during surgery are minimal in contrast with the oxygen delivery changes seen in critically ill patients.[16–18]

Advanced Hemodynamic Monitoring

The ability to use extra hemodynamic information to judge fluid administration during surgery is an attractive concept. This technique was previously difficult because it generally required insertion of a pulmonary artery catheter and thermodilution tech-niques to measure cardiac stroke volume and other variables. However, minimally invasive technology is now readily available in the form of cardiac output or flow-based monitors, which seem to provide reasonably accurate estimations of functional circulating volume and can be used continuously throughout surgery to monitor for any deficit or excess. Prominent techniques are:

- Arterial waveform analysis; converting the pulse pressure signal into a nominal stroke volume

- Esophageal Doppler; deriving stroke volume from blood flow in the descending thoracic aorta
- Plethysmography; in effect, using the fullness of the fingertip with each heartbeat to estimate circulating blood volume
- Finger cuffs; using the volume clamp method to continuously measure blood pressure and stroke volume from a finger cuff
- Partial carbon dioxide rebreathing; using the reverse Fick principle to calculate cardiac output
- Transthoracic bioimpedance and bioreactance; exploiting the variation in electrical resistance with intrathoracic blood volume during the cardiac cycle

In practice, a monitor's ability to display a nominal cardiac output is of questionable value. To be of practical use for perioperative fluid therapy, measured variables need to be incorporated into a dynamic algorithm, so that the user can direct fluid therapy toward specific hemodynamic targets; so-called goal-directed fluid therapy (GDFT). Most perioperative algorithms are based on stroke volume optimization (SVO) (**Box 1**).

A perioperative fluid therapy strategy based on detection and treatment of occult hypovolemia with small fluid challenges should reduce adverse effects related to

---

Box 1
Cardiac output monitors in practice: the SVO concept

Although the new generation of advanced hemodynamic monitors are commonly referred to as cardiac output monitors, their main clinical application is to characterize fluid responsiveness; that is, a measurable increase in stroke volume in response to a fluid challenge. Fluid responsiveness is taken as being synonymous with hypovolemia. It is thought that individuals are normovolemic when their stroke volume is at the shoulder of the Frank-Starling curve in the supine position. According to this model, patients are hypovolemic when the stroke volume is on the steep, ascending leftward part of the Frank-Starling curve, whereas an increase in preload does not translate to an increase in stroke volume when stroke volume is on the plateau. It is possible to exploit this clinically with a fluid challenge: a minimal response suggests that stroke volume is on the plateau. If the stroke volume increases 10% or more within 5 minutes, then the patient is assumed be on the steep upward part of the curve and to have been fluid responsive (as opposed to no increase, which would place the patient on the flat normovolemic portion of the curve).

Most stroke volume monitors use this concept in their suggested algorithms for fluid therapy. Some monitors in addition are able to continuously display so-called dynamic flow indicators: stroke volume variability, pulse pressure variation, and systolic pressure variability, all derived from the arterial pressure waveform. These indicators are essentially mini fluid challenges provided by swings in intrathoracic pressure induced by intermittent positive pressure mechanical ventilation. The stroke volume (or pulse pressure or systolic pressure) response during each respiratory cycle is inversely related to circulating volume. When the stroke volume is on the plateau of the Starling curve, arterial pressure swings are minimized; when hypovolemia is present, variability increases. Certain conditions are essential when using dynamic flow indices: a regular pulse (so that variability in diastolic filling time is not a factor), a sufficiently large tidal volume to cause a swing in intrathoracic pressure with mechanical ventilation, and an absence of spontaneous breathing efforts (which would interfere with intrathoracic pressure) (**Fig. 2**).

In clinical practice, the SVO algorithm is used, and other information, such as conventional hemodynamic signals to maintain the ideal stroke volume, is also considered. In effect, the additional advanced monitoring gives the user confidence to administer or withhold fluid at certain stages of the operation at which they otherwise might not (ie, bespoke individualized fluid therapy).

Intraoperative conditions such as pain, position, and pneumoperitoneum may have an effect on stroke volume (or stroke volume variation) at a particular moment, but the ultimate aim is to have each patient euvolemic at the end of surgery.

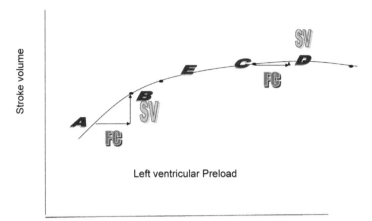

Fig. 2. Response of stroke volume (SV) to a fluid challenge (FC) is a marker of position on the Frank-Starling curve. Where SV increases more than 10% in response to 200 mL of isotonic fluid (*A to B*), patients are described as fluid responsive. Where SV does not increase to this extent (*C to D*), then no further FC is given. In the case of SV variation and other dynamic flow indices, the SV (or other variable such as systolic pressure) varies in response to preload changes induced by mechanical ventilation rather than an FC per se, but the concept is similar. Where SV variation is greater than 12% patients are likely to be fluid responsive, and where SV variation is less than 10% they are not likely to be. SVO refers to using fluid (either colloid or isotonic crystalloid) to keep the SV at the shoulder of the curve (*E*), which is similar to keeping SV variation less than 10%.

inadequate circulating volume, and, overall, this is what the literature shows. Compared with a fixed-dose fluid regimen modified by conventional static measurements, GDFT is associated with better clinical outcomes.

The definitive 2013 Cochrane Systematic Review on the subject, "Perioperative Increase in Global Blood Flow to Explicit Defined Goals and Outcomes after Surgery," includes 31 studies comprising 5292 participants and shows a clear reduction in complications, particularly renal and respiratory failure and wound infections.[19]

There is also biological plausibility. In early studies, patients in the GDFT group had significantly higher end-operative stroke volume[20–23] compared with conventional practice, suggesting that occult hypovolemia was being avoided. The amounts of fluid were not very different; the GDFT group on average received a larger amount of intraoperative colloid (467 mL; 95% CI, 331–603) than the non–goal-directed group.[5] The hypothesis is that the effect is caused by timing; not only is tissue ischemia avoided but patients are also saved from fluid loading at inappropriate times. Excess fluid given at the wrong time is not neutral, it results in edema[24] and can damage the endothelial glycocalyx,[25] promoting further edema.

In 2011, from the available evidence, the UK National Institute for Healthcare and Clinical Excellence strongly endorsed cardiac output monitoring to guide perioperative fluid administration in appropriate cases,[26] and GDFT has been enthusiastically adopted as a pillar of enhanced recovery care.[27]

TERMINOLOGY: GOAL DIRECTED OR GOAL MISDIRECTED?

On a cautionary note, although systematic reviews of the literature may consistently support goal-directed therapy (GDT),[19,28–31] all of these meta-analyses combine evidence from many settings. GDT is a vague term, meaning different things to different people and, depending on the clinical environment, sometimes even different things to the same person.[11] It can refer to perioperative fluid management, clinicians driving oxygen delivery to supramaximal levels in critical care patients, or early treatment of sepsis in the emergency department.

Even when considered just in surgical patients, fluid therapy can be delivered with or without inotropes, preoperatively, intraoperatively, and postoperatively, and to patients who may or may not be critically ill. GDFT, in whatever guise, is designed to optimize global tissue oxygen delivery and oxygen consumption. For most elective perioperative patients it seems that this can be achieved by optimization of preload alone (ie, provision of fluid).

Therefore when interpreting the extensive available literature on GDFT, it is important to appreciate the distinction between these 3 clinical questions:

- In high-risk patients, do interventions to increase global oxygen delivery during the perioperative period produce clinical benefit?
- For all patients having major surgery, is the use of additional monitoring to measure fluid responsiveness beneficial? – Does SVO work?
- Is it necessary to optimize patients all the way through surgery or does a period of postoperative optimization of oxygen delivery and reperfusion restore oxygen, nutrients, and blood pressure after a period of cellular injury?

Perhaps clinicians should be cautious in extrapolating evidence from one setting to the other. Stroke volume is a surrogate; in the theater environment, it is hoped that hemodynamic interventions will optimize oxygen delivery but there is currently no useful monitor of tissue well-being to verify that interventions are working in real time.

GOAL-DIRECTED FLUID THERAPY SPECIFICALLY IN THE ENHANCED RECOVERY SETTING

The ER is viewed as a package to be applied, bringing such an improvement in quality of care that there is little need to unpick the particular element of the package that affords the most benefits. There is a clear association between compliance with all the elements and a better clinical outcome.[32] Perioperative GDFT is such a cornerstone of enhanced recovery that the 20 or so steps that constitute recognizable ER programs have been simplified into a trimodal system of:

- GDFT
- Good analgesia
- Everything else[33]

GDFT is successfully incorporated into 23-hour-stay laparoscopic colorectal[34] and short-stay liver resection pathways.[35] Even this evidence is conflicting because patients in colorectal surgery were stroke volume optimized throughout, whereas patients having liver resection were rendered hypovolemic with low-pulse-pressure anesthesia during surgery and resuscitated to restore stroke volume as rapidly as possible after the end of the liver resection. This raises the question of whether there are key periods to aim for SVO and whether it is necessary throughout the operative period. It may be more beneficial to reduce stroke volume and blood pressure to reduce blood loss as long as hypoperfusion is limited and parameters are restored at the end of surgery.

So much of the evidence for GDFT is from an era when perioperative surgical practice was different; it is probable that many control patients in those trials were hypovolemic during surgery. As overall perioperative care changes, so apparently does the measurable impact of any particular intervention, including a complex intervention like

GDFT.[28] If clinicians confine their analysis to RCTs of GDFT versus conventional management within a defined ER program, it is apparent that there is a paucity of them. A systematic review published in 2014 found only 4 in elective colorectal surgery.[36–40] Two of these[37,38] were not included in the Cochrane Review of perioperative increase in global blood flow to the explicit defined goals cited earlier. The largest multicentre study of perioperative GDFT to date, OPTIMISE, contains a meta-analysis of all relevant trials up to early 2014, including those two, and indicates an overall benefit for GDFT, but the overall result is still influenced by all the early studies.[31]

Current evidence suggests no effect of SVO guided by esophageal Doppler monitoring on complication rates (**Table 1**) or length of stay after colorectal surgery conducted within ER pathways.

This lack of effect may be a result of newer trials being conducted within an environment of optimized perioperative care. As a result, patients are more likely to be fluid replete during surgery and may not have benefitted from targeted fluid administration (**Fig. 3**). Even among these 4 trials, there is some statistical heterogeneity, reflecting different conditions of the included studies. In 2 of the RCTs,[37,38] GDFT was tested against fluid restriction, whereby meticulous attention was paid to fluid balance. Patients came to theater in a euvolemic state, a conservative baseline infusion of intraoperative crystalloid was advocated, intraoperative losses were carefully monitored and replaced volume for volume with colloid, and response was monitored with conventional hemodynamic signals. Around two-thirds of the participants in 1 study had laparoscopic surgery, minimizing blood loss and physiologic fluid shifts.[38] An average of 900 to 1300 mL of crystalloid and 300 to 500 mL of colloid were given during surgery lasting around 2 hours. Esophageal Doppler–guided GDFT had no benefit compared with this regimen in either study.

In contrast, in a third study, although perioperative care was provided within an ER pathway, control patients had a considerably more liberal perioperative fluid regimen.[39] In addition, intervention patients were given an additional 1.3 L of intraoperative colloid by an investigator; apparently to their detriment because they remained in hospital for 2 days longer than controls. Our interpretation is that the GDFT algorithm that was used failed to guard against fluid overload in patients who were receiving a liberal baseline fluid regimen (discussed later).

Table 1
Forest plot comparing overall complication rates in esophageal Doppler monitor (ODM) and control groups after colorectal surgery within an enhanced recovery protocol. A Mantel-Haenszel random-effects model was used for meta-analysis. Odds ratios are shown with 95% confidence intervals

References	Complications ODM	Restriction	Weight (%)	Odds Ratio	Odds Ratio
Brandstrup et al[38]	23 of 71	24 of 79	37.5	1.10 (0.55, 2.19)	
Challand et al[39]	63 of 89	60 of 90	44.6	1.21 (0.64, 2.28)	
Srinivasa et al[37]	26 of 37	26 of 37	18.0	1.00 (0.37, 2.71)	
Total	112 of 197	110 of 206	100.0	1.13 (0.74, 1.72)	

0·1   0·2   0·5   1   2   5   10
Favours ODM   Favours control

Heterogeneity: $\tau^2 = 0.00$; $\chi^2 = 0.11$, 2 degrees of freedom, $P = .95$; $I^2 = 0\%$.
Test for overall effect: $Z = 0.56$, $P = .58$.
From Srinivasa S, Lemanu D, Singh P, et al. Systematic review and meta-analysis of oesophageal Doppler-guided fluid management in colorectal surgery. Br J Surg 2013;100:1705; with permission.

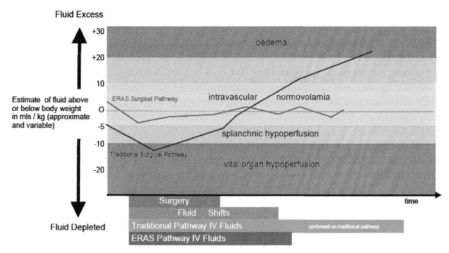

Fig. 3. Conceptual model contrasting perioperative fluid status changes and fluid therapy in the settings of enhanced recovery after surgery (ERAS) and traditional surgery. Surgery and physiologic shifts tend to reduce intravascular volume during the early stages of the perioperative period, whereas intravenous (IV) fluid may promote a relative fluid excess in the hours to days afterward. In general, ERAS minimizes these physiologic changes.

Perioperative fluid therapy may be restrictive, liberal, goal directed, or a combination thereof. Overall, there is evidence that, within an ER setting, a carefully monitored restrictive regimen is equivalent to intraoperative GDFT for patients having elective colorectal surgery, and that both of these are better than liberal fluid therapy supplemented by SVO.

Note that, in a small study of 32 patients having 2-hour colonic resections within a multimodal ER regimen, a regimen of restrictive fluids (median 1640 mL of intravenous fluid on the day of surgery) compared with liberal fluids (median 5050 mL) was associated with more complications (18 in 6 patients vs 1),[41] suggesting that it is possible to be overly restrictive. In contrast, in a study examining compliance with components of ER, avoidance of fluid overload was the most important factor in avoiding complications: for every liter of fluid administered, postoperative complications (mainly cardiorespiratory) increased by 32%.[32] Every liter of postoperative fluid excess is associated with an additional day in hospital stay.[3] For colorectal surgery within ER, euvolemia is desirable, but the best way to achieve this has not been resolved.

In other major abdominal surgical settings evidence is more limited. A study of esophageal Doppler monitor (ODM)–guided GDFT in cystectomy[42] suggests benefit, although the study is not specified as being within ER, and an RCT of GDFT for major gynecology[43] showed no difference in complication rates, although it had an overall length of stay of 11 days. Single studies constitute insufficient evidence to make conclusions.

CONTROVERSIES: VALIDITY OF THE STROKE VOLUME OPTIMIZATION CONCEPT

A valid question is whether novel hemodynamic devices and indices provide a false sense of security. As discussed, the monitors are claimed to be effective to characterize fluid responsiveness, which is taken as a sign of hypovolemia (see **Box 1**). A problem with this approach is that the scientific foundations are not well established. Guidance that clinicians should give 200 mL of fluid (until recently colloid was advocated) and wait 5 minutes for a 10% increase in stroke volume seems arbitrary.

The association of dynamic flow indices with fluid responsiveness has a more sound methodological basis. A receiver operator curve comparing the variable in question (eg, stroke volume variation) with a gold standard method of assessing volume status (eg, LV volume measured by transesophageal echo) is used to establish thresholds for prediction of fluid responsiveness.[44] A further degree of sophistication is introduced by identifying 2 thresholds; one that prioritizes specificity (not giving fluid to patients who do not need it) and the other that prioritizes sensitivity (ie, making sure that all cases of hypovolemia are detected). The interval between them is a zone of uncertainty (clinicians cannot be certain whether patients are– fluid responsive or not) in which around 25% of readings from typical perioperative cohorts occur.[45]

Sophisticated as they may be, clear evidence of benefit using dynamic flow indices to guide GDFT during contemporary surgery is scarce. The variables require certain conditions: a delivered tidal volume more than 7 mL/kg, absence of spontaneous breathing activity, absence of cardiac rhythm abnormalities (which make diastolic filling inconsistent), and ideally a responsive breath-by-breath calculation method, many of which are lacking in a high proportion of intraoperative patients.[46] The possibility exists that an open abdomen attenuates pressure swings, whereas a pneumoperitoneum accentuates it.

Moreover, comparisons of monitors to predict fluid responsiveness in the same patients often do not agree closely with one another.[47] In addition, even the assertion that fluid responsiveness indicates hypovolemia is questionable. In a recent study around half of the well-hydrated volunteer subjects showed a stroke volume increase of more than 10% in response to a passive leg raise (in effect, a fluid challenge).[48]

Further, in contrast with the more sequentially evolving environment of critical care, the intraoperative setting is characterized by rapid changes in stimuli, endogenous catecholamine levels, effects of drugs, and hemorrhage, all of which may affect stroke volume. Rather than having a single Frank-Starling curve, depending on these factors, individuals move serially between a family of ventricular function curves (depending on cardiac contractility and afterload), so it is difficult to be sure what the optimum stroke volume is at a particular moment.[49]

It has been implied with SVO that advanced hemodynamic monitoring protects against a fluid overload, but perhaps this is not the case. The distinction between SVO and stroke volume maximization is more than semantic[50]: any excess fluid could be detrimental.[24] As well as signals about relative hypovolemia, GDFT algorithms require clear stopping thresholds (ie, signs that the circulating volume is full) and it is possible that this aspect of the algorithm has been found wanting when SVO has been tested under ER conditions.

REQUIRED RESEARCH
Effectiveness Trial Within an Enhanced Recovery Environment

Translation of a complex intervention into clinical benefit requires that the intervention is shown to work when clinicians apply it to patients in routine hospital practice. There are as yet no large RCTs investigating the clinical effectiveness of GDFT to improve outcomes within an ER context. It seems unlikely that additional hemodynamic information can lead to harm[39] but, in a cost-constrained environment, in order to be cost-effective GDFT has to be shown to be better.

Adequate blinding of GDFT is difficult, so several trials are biased in that perioperative clinicians knew which group patients were allocated to,[21,23,40] which may systematically affect their overall care or the determination of outcomes. In contrast, attempts to blind delivery of the intervention[22,37–39] render the study protocol different from real-life use.

Any literature that comprises many single-center efficacy studies is open to the possibility of publication bias (ie, that only studies with a positive result are published); the Cochrane meta-analysis suggests that this is the case with the GDFT literature.[19]

Definitive sufficiently powered effectiveness trials are difficult to conduct: they require a cooperative network of centers capable of delivering an intervention (in this case GDFT) consistently within an ER program that is broadly similar across all the centers. Within an effectiveness trial, prospectively defined subgroup analysis (eg, types of surgery, levels of comorbidity, or aerobic fitness) may be analyzed to identify particular settings in which GDFT may be useful.[51] An RCT of restrictive versus liberal fluid therapy for contemporary major abdominal surgery intending to recruit more than 2800 patients is underway[52] in which there is a planned statistical interaction analysis to investigate the effect of GDFT superimposed on the basal fluid regimens, although this is no substitute for a prospective large head-to-head trial.

DO PERIOPERATIVE INOTROPES CONVEY ADDITIONAL BENEFIT?

A large proportion of trials included in meta-analyses allow for the use of inotropes as well as fluid challenges. OPTIMISE, the largest perioperative GDFT study to date, showed a strong but nonsignificant trend toward benefit for an arterial wave form–derived SVO algorithm in 730 surgical patients; however, the intervention group in addition received a fixed-dose regimen of dopexamine during surgery and for 6 hours afterward.[31] Positive outcomes may be caused by beta-agonist drugs having beneficial antiinflammatory and other metabolic effects.[53] A much larger multicentre RCT investigating this premise further is currently being set up by the OPTIMISE investigating group, but this will take at least 5 years to produce answers. Another interpretation of the results is that it is 6 postoperative hours of close attention that pays dividends. This interpretation has echoes in the evolution of the literature[17] on early GDT in patients presenting to the emergency department with septic shock. In a single-center efficacy trial, dramatic benefits were shown for GDFT compared with usual care. The protocol-based care for early septic shock (ProCESS) study recently tested the same GDFT regimen against 2 other fluid therapy strategies applied for 6 hours in 1341 patients across 31 centers and showed no difference in 60-day mortality from septic shock.[54] It may be that what affects clinical outcomes is care being closely applied and monitored by diligent personnel, rather than monitors and algorithms per se.

ER focuses on simple steps of care delivered consistently and meticulously.

SUBGROUPS OF BENEFIT?

Laparoscopic colorectal surgery, involving a long period of pneumoperitoneum in a head-down position, has been described as minimally invasive surgery with maximal cardiovascular stress. This hemodynamic model of cardiac failure is in contrast with the compensated hypovolemia model of supine open abdominal surgery. Several observational and quality-improvement studies have been published by the Guildford group, for example, describing a Do_2 target of 400 mL/min-1/m-2 to be a useful threshold in reducing complications,[55] and several prominent GDFT studies include a large proportion of laparoscopic patients,[38–40] with some attempt to adapt a generic

SVO algorithm during pneumoperitoneum.[38] However, prospective subgroup analysis (or ideally a GDFT RCT with a bespoke algorithm confined to laparoscopic resection patients) is lacking.

Some patients, by dint of comorbidities, underlying functional capacity, neoadjuvant chemoradiotherapy, or magnitude of surgical resection, are at higher risk than others of complications, but possible differential effects of GDFT in subgroups have not been adequately investigated in studies to date.

CURRENT BEST PRACTICE

Meticulous adherence to perioperative fluid administration is effective.[27]

GDT does not seem to cause harm (if done correctly) and although there is no evidence it seems sensible to match monitoring to surgical and patient risk.

Current consensus is that, for patients who arrive in theater in a euvolemic state, a crystalloid infusion of around 1.5 mL/kg/h during surgery is a reasonable baseline; additional fluid challenges can be used in response to measured losses and hemodynamic signals. It is perhaps easier to achieve individualized fluid therapy with a stroke volume–targeted approach guided by an advanced hemodynamic monitor, as long as particular attention is paid to stopping thresholds so as to avoid fluid excess. Because of a lack of specific evidence of benefit for GDFT when the physiologic disturbance attributable to the surgery is minimized, as in enhanced recovery, the point is not proved.

All fluid therapy and vasopressors should be administered according to the hemodynamic model at the particular stage of the operation; for example, steep head-up or head-down positions present different hemodynamic conditions. The aim is to have sufficient circulating volume and blood flow to avoid tissue hypoxia at all stages of the operation, and ultimately to have each patient euvolemic in the awake, supine state at the end of surgery, so that minimal postoperative intravenous fluid is required, and then only in response to clear clinical evidence of hypovolemia.

REFERENCES

1. Gould TH, Grace K, Thorne G, et al. Effect of thoracic epidural anaesthesia on colonic blood flow. Br J Anaesth 2002;89:446–51.
2. Biais M, Bernard O, Ha JC, et al. Abilities of pulse pressure variations and stroke volume variations to predict fluid responsiveness in prone position during scoliosis surgery. Br J Anaesth 2010;104(4):407–13.
3. Levy BF, Scott MJ, Fawcett WJ, et al. Randomized clinical trial of epidural, spinal or patient-controlled analgesia for patients undergoing laparoscopic colorectal surgery. Br J Surg 2011;98:1068–78.
4. Fearon KC, Ljungqvist O, Von Meyenfeldt M, et al. Enhanced recovery after surgery: a consensus review of clinical care for patients undergoing colonic resection. Clin Nutr 2005;24:466–77.
5. Corcoran T, Clarke S, Myles P, et al. Perioperative fluid management strategies in major surgery: a stratified meta-analysis. Anesth Analg 2012;114:640–51.
6. Brandstrup B, Svendsen C, Engquist A. Hemorrhage and operation cause a contraction of the extra cellular space needing replacement—evidence and implications? A systematic review. Surgery 2006;139:419–32.
7. Brandstrup B, Tønnesen H, Beier-Holgersen R, et al, Danish Study Group on Perioperative Fluid Therapy. Effects of intravenous fluid restriction on postoperative complications: comparison of two perioperative fluid regimens: a randomized assessor-blinded multicenter trial. Ann Surg 2003;238:641–8.

8. Lobo DN, Bostock KA, Neal KR, et al. Effect of salt and water balance on recovery of gastrointestinal function after elective colonic resection: a randomised controlled trial. Lancet 2002;359:1812–8.

9. Nisanevich V, Felsenstein I, Almogy G, et al. Effect of intraoperative fluid management on outcome after intraabdominal surgery. Anesthesiology 2005;103:25–32.

10. Maitland K, Kiguli S, Opoka RO, et al, for FEAST Trial Group. Mortality after fluid bolus in African children with severe infection. N Engl J Med 2011;364(26):2483–95.

11. Roche A, Miller T. Goal-directed or goal-misdirected–how should we interpret the literature? Crit Care 2010;14:129.

12. Bundgaard-Nielsen M, Secher N, Kehlet H. 'Liberal' vs. 'restrictive' perioperative fluid therapy – a critical assessment of the evidence. Acta Anaesthesiol Scand 2009;53:843–51.

13. Hamilton-Davies C, Mythen M, Salmon J, et al. Comparison of commonly used clinical indicators of hypovolaemia with gastrointestinal tonometry. Intensive Care Med 1997;23:276–81.

14. Marik P, Baram M, Vahid B. Does central venous pressure predict fluid responsiveness? Chest 2008;134:172–8.

15. Donati A, Loggi S, Preiser JC, et al. Goal-directed intraoperative therapy reduces morbidity and length of hospital stay in high-risk surgical patients. Chest 2007; 132:1817–24.

16. Cohn S, Pearl R, Acosta S, et al. A prospective randomized pilot study of near-infrared spectroscopy-directed restricted fluid therapy versus standard fluid therapy in patients undergoing elective colorectal surgery. Am Surg 2010;76: 1384–92.

17. Rivers E, Nguyen B, Havstad S, et al, Early Goal-Directed Therapy Collaborative Group. Early goal-directed therapy in the treatment of severe sepsis and septic shock. N Engl J Med 2001;345(19):1368–77.

18. Shoemaker W, Appel P, Kram H, et al. Prospective trial of supranormal values of survivors as therapeutic goals in high-risk surgical patients. Chest 1988;94: 1176–86.

19. Grocott M, Dushianthan A, Hamilton M, et al, Optimisation Systematic Review Steering Group. Perioperative increase in global blood flow to explicit defined goals and outcomes following surgery. Cochrane Database Syst Rev 2012;(11):CD004082.

20. Conway DH, Mayall R, Abdul-Latif MS, et al. Randomised controlled trial investigating the influence of intravenous fluid titration using oesophageal Doppler monitoring during bowel surgery. Anaesthesia 2002;57:845–9.

21. Gan T, Soppitt A, Maroof M, et al. Goal-directed intraoperative fluid administration reduces length of hospital stay after major surgery. Anesthesiology 2002;97: 820–6.

22. Noblett SE, Snowden CP, Shenton BK, et al. Randomized clinical trial assessing the effect of Doppler-optimized fluid management on outcome after elective colorectal resection. Br J Surg 2006;93:1069–76.

23. Wakeling H, McFall M, Jenkins C, et al. Intraoperative oesophageal Doppler guided fluid management shortens postoperative hospital stay after major bowel surgery. Br J Anaesth 2005;95:634–42.

24. Jacob M, Chappell D, Rehm M. Clinical update: perioperative fluid management. Lancet 2007;369:1984–6.

25. Woodcock TE, Woodcock TM. Revised Starling equation and the glycocalyx model of transvascular fluid exchange: an improved paradigm for prescribing intravenous fluid therapy. Br J Anaesth 2012;108(3):384–94.

26. National Institute for Health and Clinical Excellence. CardioQ-ODM oesophageal Doppler monitor. Medical Technology Guide 3, March 2011. Available at: http://www.nice.org.uk/nicemedia/live/13312/52624/52624.pdf. Accessed August 18, 2014.

27. Fawcett W, Mythen M, Scott M. Enhanced recovery: more than just reducing length of stay? Br J Anaesth 2012;109:671–4.

28. Hamilton MA, Cecconi M, Rhodes A. A systematic review and meta-analysis on the use of preemptive hemodynamic intervention to improve postoperative outcomes in moderate and high-risk surgical patients. Anesth Analg 2011;112:1392–402.

29. Gurgel ST, do Nascimento P. Maintaining tissue perfusion in high-risk surgical patients: a systematic review of randomized clinical trials. Anesth Analg 2011; 112:1384–91.

30. Lees N, Hamilton M, Rhodes A. Clinical review: goal-directed therapy in high risk surgical patients. Crit Care 2009;13:231.

31. Pearse RM, Harrison DA, MacDonald N, et al. Effect of a perioperative, cardiac output-guided hemodynamic therapy algorithm on outcomes following major gastrointestinal surgery: a randomized clinical trial and systematic review. JAMA 2014. http://dx.doi.org/10.1001/jama.2014.5305.

32. Gustafsson UO, Hausel J, Thorell A, et al. Adherence to enhanced recovery after surgery protocol and outcomes after colorectal cancer surgery. Arch Surg 2011; 46:571–7.

33. Mythen MG, Scott MJ. Anaesthetic considerations for enhanced recovery. In: Francis N, Kennedy RH, Ljungqvist O, et al, editors. Manual of fast track recovery for colorectal surgery. London: Springer; 2012. p. 49–72.

34. Levy BF, Scott MJP, Fawcett WJ, et al. 23-hour stay laparoscopic colectomy. Dis Colon Rectum 2009;52:1239–43.

35. Jones C, Kelliher L, Dickinson M, et al. Randomized clinical trial on enhanced recovery versus standard care following open liver resection. Br J Surg 2013; 100:1015–24.

36. Srinivasa S, Lemanu D, Singh P, et al. Systematic review and meta-analysis of oesophageal Doppler-guided fluid management in colorectal surgery. Br J Surg 2013;100:1701–8.

37. Srinivasa S, Taylor M, Singh P, et al. Randomized clinical trial of goal- directed fluid therapy within an enhanced recovery protocol for elective colectomy. Br J Surg 2012;100:66–74.

38. Brandstrup B, Svendsen P, Rasmussen M, et al. Which goal for fluid therapy during colorectal surgery is followed by the best outcome: near maximal stroke volume or zero fluid balance? Br J Anaesth 2012;109:191–9.

39. Challand C, Struthers R, Sneyd JR, et al. Randomized controlled trial of intraoperative goal-directed fluid therapy in aerobically fit and unfit patients having major colorectal surgery. Br J Anaesth 2012;108:53–62.

40. Senagore AJ, Emery T, Luchtefeld M, et al. Fluid management for laparoscopic colectomy: a prospective, randomized assessment of goal-directed administration of balanced salt solution or hetastarch coupled with an enhanced recovery program. Dis Colon Rectum 2009;52:1935–40.

41. Holte K, Foss N, Andersen J, et al. Liberal or restrictive fluid administration in fast-track colonic surgery: a randomized, double-blind study. Br J Anaesth 2007;99:500–8.

42. Pillai P, McEleavy I, Gaughan M, et al. A double-blind randomized controlled clinical trial to assess the effect of Doppler optimized intraoperative fluid management on outcome following radical cystectomy. J Urol 2011;186(6):2201–6.

43. McKenny M, Conroy P, Wong A, et al. A randomised prospective trial of intra-operative oesophageal Doppler-guided fluid administration in major gynaecological surgery. Anaesthesia 2013;68:1224–31.
44. Michard F. Stroke volume variation: from applied physiology to improved outcomes. Crit Care Med 2011;39:402–3.
45. Cannesson M, Le Manach Y, Hofer CK, et al. Assessing the diagnostic accuracy of pulse pressure variations for the prediction of fluid responsiveness: a "gray zone" approach. Anesthesiology 2011;115:231–41.
46. Lansdorp B, Lemson J, van Putten M, et al. Dynamic indices do not predict volume responsiveness in routine clinical practice. Br J Anaesth 2012;108(3): 395–401.
47. Nordstrom J, Hallsjo-Sander C, Shore R, et al. Stroke volume optimization in elective bowel surgery: a comparison between pulse power wave analysis (LiDCOrapid) and oesophageal Doppler (CardioQ). Br J Anaesth 2013;110: 374–80.
48. Godfrey G, Dubrey S, Handy J. A prospective observational study of stroke volume responsiveness to passive leg raise in healthy non-starved volunteers as assessed by trans-thoracic echocardiography. Anaesthesia 2014;69:306–13.
49. Minto G, Struthers R. Stroke volume optimisation: is the fairy tale over? Anaesthesia 2014;69(4):291–6.
50. Bouwman RA, Boer C. Minimal invasive cardiac output monitoring: get the dose of fluid right. Br J Anaesth 2012;109(3):299–302.
51. Miller T, Roche A, Gan T. Poor adoption of hemodynamic optimization during major surgery: are we practicing substandard care? Anesth Analg 2011;112: 1274–6.
52. Myles PS, Bellomo R. A pivotal trial of fluid therapy for major abdominal surgery: need and equipoise. Crit Care Resusc 2011;13(4):278–80.
53. Bangash MN, Patel NS, Benetti E, et al. Dopexamine can attenuate the inflammatory response and protect against organ injury in the absence of significant effects on hemodynamics or regional microvascular flow. Crit Care 2013;17(2): R57. http://dx.doi.org/10.1186/cc12585.
54. ProCESS Investigators. A randomized trial of protocol-based care for early septic shock. N Engl J Med 2014;370(18):1683–93.
55. Levy BF, Fawcett WJ, Scott MJP, et al. Intra-operative oxygen delivery in infusion volume optimized patients undergoing laparoscopic colorectal surgery within an enhanced recovery programme: effect of different analgesic modalities. Colorectal Dis 2012;14:887–92.

Fluid Management in Abdominal Surgery

What, When, and When Not to Administer

Karthik Raghunathan, MD, MPH[a],*, Mandeep Singh, MD[b],
Dileep N. Lobo, MS, DM, FRCS, FACS, FRCPE[c]

KEYWORDS

- Intravenous fluids • Crystalloids • Colloids • Balanced fluids • Fluid responsiveness
- Noninvasive monitoring

KEY POINTS

- Intravenous fluids are drugs with predominantly cardiovascular and renal effects, potentially significant gastrointestinal effects, and possible immune effects.
- Distribution of administered fluid volume across compartments (such as the intravascular, interstitial, and intracellular spaces) depends on several factors, including the integrity of the endothelial glycocalyx and intravascular volume context.
- Before the administration of fluid therapy, determination of volume responsiveness and volume status is recommended.
- Balanced crystalloids, with a physiologic strong ion difference and chloride content, may avoid the potentially deleterious effects of chloride-rich isotonic fluids like normal (0.9%) saline.
- Intravascular volume status may be assessed with variable accuracy using minimally invasive or noninvasive technologies.

INTRODUCTION

Intravenous fluid therapy is a key part of perioperative care, and surgical outcomes have been shown to be affected by the type and volume of fluid used. This review

Funding sources: None.
Conflicts of interest: K. Raghunathan has received funding from Baxter for an Investigator-initiated trial. D.N. Lobo has received unrestricted research grants and speaker's honoraria from B. Braun Melsungen, Baxter, and Fresenius Kabi.
[a] Anesthesiology Service, Durham VA Medical Center, Duke University Medical Center, Box 3094, Durham, NC 27710, USA; [b] Division of Anesthesiology and Critical Care Medicine, Duke University Medical Center, 2301 Erwin Road, Durham, NC 27710, USA; [c] Division of Gastrointestinal Surgery, Nottingham Digestive Diseases Centre National Institute for Health Research Biomedical Research Unit, Nottingham University Hospitals, Queen's Medical Centre, Nottingham NG7 2UH, UK
* Corresponding author.
E-mail address: Karthik.Raghunathan@duke.edu

presents an overview of the basic principles that underlie fluid management in the perioperative setting, includes evidence-based recommendations (where tenable), and suggests a rational approach to the timing and choice of fluids for administration.

TYPE OF FLUID

A variety of fluid types are available, including different types of crystalloids, colloids, blood products, and even hemoglobin-based oxygen-carrying solutions. The use of normal or isotonic (0.9%) saline solution dates to the work of a Dutch chemist named Hartog Hamburger in 1896.[1] In an in vitro study of red blood cell (RBC) lysis in response to changes in tonicity, human RBCs were found to be most stable in a preparation of 0.92% saline. More recently, studies have reported an association between resuscitation with isotonic saline and several undesirable effects when compared with resuscitation with physiologically balanced crystalloids (eg, lactated Ringer solution, Plasma-Lyte, Hartmann solution).[2] Administration of 0.9% saline results in hyperchloremia and a decrease in the plasma strong ion difference with consequent metabolic acidosis.[3] This condition, in turn, has been associated with reduced cardiac contractility, decreased renal perfusion, reduced gastric blood flow, and impaired gastric motility.[4-7] Elevated serum chloride concentrations have been associated with renal vasoconstriction and renal parenchymal swelling in animal studies[8,9] and an increase in postoperative 30-day mortality in large database analyses.[10] The deleterious effects of administration of large volumes of 0.9% saline on the kidney have also been shown in a human study that demonstrated decreased renal blood flow velocity and cortical tissue perfusion.[11] Acknowledging potential clinical implications, the British Consensus Guidelines on Intravenous Fluid Therapy for Adult Surgical Patients recommended the use of balanced crystalloids rather than isotonic saline in most routine clinical settings.[12] The case for balanced crystalloids has also been presented comprehensively in a review.[13] Populations for whom isotonic saline remains a reasonable choice include patients with nausea/vomiting or gastric suction (and thus hypochloremic alkalosis) and neurosurgical patients for whom avoiding other hypotonic crystalloids may be reasonable.

Hadimioglu and colleagues[14] conducted a double-blind study randomizing kidney transplant recipients to receive isotonic saline, lactated Ringer solution, or Plasma-Lyte and compared subsequent changes in acid-base balance and potassium and lactate levels. No significant changes in pH or acid-base measures were seen in patients receiving lactated Ringer solution or Plasma-Lyte as opposed to those who received saline (7.44 ± 0.50 vs 7.36 ± 0.05, and 0.4 ± 3.1 vs −4.3 ± 2.1, respectively). However, there were no subsequent significant differences in postoperative renal function. The best metabolic profile was seen in patients receiving Plasma-Lyte. Shaw and colleagues[15] conducted an observational study evaluating the use of normal saline versus a calcium-free isotonic balanced crystalloid solution in adult patients undergoing major abdominal surgery using the Premier Perspective Comparative Database. A total of 926 patients who received Plasma-Lyte on the day of surgery were propensity-matched (in a 3:1 ratio) with 2778 patients who received saline. Hemodialysis occurred approximately 5 times more often in the matched saline group (1.0% [95% confidence interval (CI) 0.05–1.8] vs 4.8% [95% CI 4.1–5.7], P<.001); the matched saline group also had significantly increased odds of postoperative infection, blood transfusion, and electrolyte disturbance (sodium, potassium, and/or magnesium). In addition, in-hospital mortality was higher for the saline group (5.6%) than for the balanced crystalloid–Plasma-Lyte group (2.9%), although the difference was not significant after correcting for confounders. Further literature has confirmed the association between fluids with high chloride ion content (and a lower strong ion difference) and renal vasoconstriction and decreased glomerular filtration rate.[16]

Clinicians may prefer colloids (such as albumin, starches, and gelatins) based on the theory that intravascular retention is prolonged as compared with crystalloids (a theoretic premise that larger particles are trapped in the vascular space by an intact endothelial barrier). However, large multicenter clinical trials suggest that the advantage in volume expansion is usually only about 30% to 40%.[17,18] In a hypovolemic context, the potency of colloids is perhaps up to twice that of crystalloids.[19] Using a prospective study setup with double-tracer blood volume measurements (to assess volume status before and after crystalloid administration), Jacob and colleagues[20] evaluated the traditional model of replacement of blood loss with 3 times as much crystalloid. The volume effect of lactated Ringer solution was less than 20% (and additional infusions of hypertonic albumin were used to restore blood volume to original value) under these conditions.

The major drawbacks of colloid use include increased cost, potentially limited availability (with albumin, which is a blood product), possibly impaired coagulation (notable with larger quantities of hetastarch), and persistent evidence of renal injury seen with starch solutions.[21] Hetastarch use has been associated with increased bleeding in cardiac and neurologic surgery[22,23] and may increase the incidence of renal failure in septic patients[24] as well as in patients undergoing renal transplantation and cardiac surgery.[25,26] Meta-analyses show no improvement in survival with the use of colloids versus crystalloids among patients with trauma, burns, and following surgery.[27] Specific blood products (packed RBCs, fresh frozen plasma, cryoprecipitate, platelets, specific factor solutions) may be used for selected indications such as anemia or coagulation factor deficiencies in respective subgroups or during resuscitation (eg, hemorrhagic shock). Perioperative cell salvage and hemoglobin-based oxygen-carrying solutions are less commonly used.

AMOUNT OF FLUID

Various volume strategies have been studied including individualized goal-directed therapy (iGDT) and liberal, zero-balance, or restrictive approaches.[28] However, there is no uniform definition for what constitutes a liberal versus restrictive approach. Varadhan and Lobo[28] developed definitions to better compare outcomes: liberal was defined as greater than 2.75 L/day, zero-balance as 1.75 to 2.75 L/day, and restrictive as less than 1.75 L/day in the postoperative period. Brandstrup and colleagues[29] defined fluid management strategies for elective colorectal surgery based on quantities transfused for preloading with epidural analgesia, replacement of so-called third space losses, replacement of fasting deficits (maintenance requirements), and replacement of estimated blood losses. Fluid restriction resulted in fewer complications and earlier return of bowel function. Other studies have used different definitions of liberal versus standard fluid management approaches (incorporating the quantity of electrolytes received in a given day). Lobo and colleagues[5] evaluated the recovery of gastrointestinal function after elective colonic resection with a standard group receiving 3 L of intravenous fluids with 154 mmol sodium daily versus a restricted group receiving no more than 2 L of fluid with 77 mmol sodium. Patients in the standard group gained more weight, suffered delayed recovery of gastrointestinal function, endured increased overall complications, and had an extended hospital length of stay.

Perioperative iGDT aims to optimize circulation in the operating room via real-time individualized hemodynamic monitoring and therapeutic interventions to maximize stroke volume (SV).[30] iGDT may incorporate the use of fluid boluses, inotropic medications directed to maximize specific parameters such as cardiac index, SV, or minimize pulse pressure variation (PPV), or oxygen extraction ratio. A systematic review and meta-analysis of 29 trials involving 4805 moderate- and high-risk surgical patients by Hamilton and colleagues[31] and by Pearse and colleagues[32] showed a significant reduction in morbidity with the use of both fluids and inotropes (as opposed to fluids alone). Other studies evaluating preemptive iGDT have shown earlier return of bowel function, decreased incidence of nausea and vomiting, and reductions in hospital length of stay.[33,34] Although there are no standardized recommendations for the type and amount of fluid or inotrope to administer, therapy should be guided with real-time monitoring of fluid responsiveness so that the administration of fluid to a volume nonresponsive patient is avoided.[35,36]

A review of the literature on iGDT in colorectal surgery[37] drew attention to the fact that comparisons had not been made in the setting of restrictive fluid therapy (near-zero fluid balance) in the postoperative period and patients had not been managed within an enhanced recovery after surgery pathway.[38] This review also noted the heterogeneity in trials involving iGDT. The benefits observed in initial trials may be minimized by advances in surgical techniques and perioperative care.[37] Two trials support this position.[39,40] In a double-blind multicenter trial on 150 patients undergoing elective colorectal surgery, Doppler-guided iGDT to near-maximal SV added no benefit compared with the use of a zero-balance approach (ie, maintenance of near-normal body weight).[39] There were no significant differences in complications or duration of hospital stay. These results were confirmed in another study that randomized 85 patients undergoing elective colectomy within an established enhanced recovery protocol (including fluid restriction) to flow-guided or no flow-guided fluid therapy.[40] Based on these consistent findings, it may not be necessary to use flow-directed fluid volume therapy in all patients undergoing major surgery, particularly in the context of an existing enhanced recovery protocol in which postoperative fluid overload is avoided.[39,40] However, when blood loss is expected to be in excess of 500 mL, or if preoperative volume status is uncertain, Doppler-guided iGDT may remain potentially useful. The current safety warnings on hydroxyethyl starch (HES) add to the uncertainty surrounding iGDT because most trials were conducted with colloid. However, one study has suggested that either crystalloid or HES may be used with equal efficacy for flow-directed fluid therapy.[41]

A fluid challenge may be administered to evaluate hemodynamic response, with the volume administered being delivered rapidly (studies report timing the challenge over 5–10 minutes) and the bolus being large enough to recruit preload (inducing myocardial stretch), thereby increasing end-diastolic volume and SV.[35] In most iGDT protocols, SV maximization continues (with boluses of approximately 3 mL/kg) until SV no longer increases with volume loading (with a 10%–15% increase in SV set as the threshold for responsiveness). This concept differs from liberal strategies whereby the proximate dynamic hemodynamic response is not routinely monitored in real time. The overall goal includes maximization of cardiac output (CO) to preempt the development of an oxygen debt. Most studies support avoiding routine empirical fluid loading. Zero-balance techniques avoid net weight gain due to fluids with the use of volume removal where necessary (eg, with diuretics when there is a weight gain of approximately 2.5–3 kg).[42]

FLUID THERAPY WITHIN ENHANCED RECOVERY AFTER SURGERY

Traditional intravenous fluid regimens for patients undergoing abdominal surgery have incorporated large volumes often exceeding actual/measured fluid losses.[43] Patients may have received 3.5 to 7 L of fluids intraoperatively and up to 3 L per day on the surgical wards with ramifications as discussed earlier.[5,42] For many years, a third space was believed to exist and has been described in textbooks as a fluid compartment that needed to be replete.[38,44,45] Studies have confirmed that damage to the endothelial glycocalyx occurs with such administration of crystalloids and could result in accumulation of fluid in the interstitial space with consequent complications.

Concerns pertinent to patients undergoing elective abdominal surgery may be considered in 3 stages. In the preoperative setting, possible depletion of circulating volume secondary to prolonged fasting, mechanical bowel preparation, nausea/vomiting/diarrhea, or decreased oral intake due to gastrointestinal pathology may occur, resulting in a volume-responsive hypovolemic patient presenting for surgery. Intraoperatively, large incisions (during open laparotomy) resulting in evaporative fluid loss may be compounded by surgical blood loss. Postoperatively, patients may experience additional fluid depletion from a lack of oral intake, drains, fistulae, and/or increased ileostomy output. Hypotension due to hypovolemia is exacerbated by internal redistribution of effective circulating blood volume from thoracic epidural analgesia-induced sympathectomy (ie, there may be an increase in venous pooling of circulating blood volume leading to reduced preload).

In 2012, the Enhanced Recovery after Surgery (ERAS) Society, the European Society of Clinical Nutrition and Metabolism, and the International Association for Surgical Metabolism and Nutrition issued updated consensus recommendations: ERAS in colonic,[46] pelvic/rectal,[47] and pancreatic surgery.[48] The goal was to decrease hospital length of stay and time to resumption of normal activities and improve survival.[38] Preoperative optimization of the patient's fluid status before gastrointestinal surgery is achieved via 2 major initiatives: (1) avoiding excessive starvation by allowing solid food intake up to 6 hours and clear liquids up to 2 hours before anesthetic induction and (2) avoiding routine mechanical bowel preparation. Prolonged starvation (beyond 8 hours) may place patients in a catabolic state, increasing insulin resistance and prolonging hospital length of stay. Preoperative carbohydrate intake has been shown to reduce insulin resistance[49] without increasing the risk of aspiration[50] and may reduce hospital stay by a day in patients undergoing major abdominal surgery.[51] Bowel preparation has been shown to cause significant fluid and electrolyte imbalance, including hypocalcemia and hypophosphatemia.[52] Bucher and colleagues[53] performed a meta-analysis of 4 randomized controlled trials with a total of 1297 patients undergoing elective colorectal surgery. Anastomotic leakage was significantly more common in the bowel preparation group (5.6% vs 2.8%) in addition to general morbidity and mortality rates. Thus, the guidelines recommend bowel preparation solely for those patients undergoing low rectal resection with a diverting stoma.

Intraoperatively, the ERAS guidelines recommend the use of warmed intravenous fluids, preferring boluses with colloid and crystalloids for background maintenance. Thus, iGDT is recommended to optimize intravascular volume status and ensure an optimized SV while minimizing fluid overload. Targeting supranormal global oxygen delivery was demonstrated to have a significant survival benefit (by Shoemaker and colleagues[54] who conducted a prospective, longitudinal study analyzing hemodynamic and oxygen transport variables in 708 high-risk surgical patients). Cardiac index, oxygen delivery, and oxygen consumption were found to increase in the immediate postoperative setting, more dramatically in survivors as compared with nonsurvivors. Shoemaker and colleagues hypothesized that the need for increased CO may be due to increased metabolic demands after surgical trauma in the setting of previously low and maldistributed intraoperative blood flow due to neural and hormonal mechanisms. The combined use of fluids and inotropes (as opposed to fluids alone) has been shown to better facilitate achievement of supranormal oxygen delivery and reduce mortality (odds ratio, 0.41; 95% CI 0.23–0.73), although the exact doses of ino-tropes used were not evaluated. In addition, vasopressors should be administered to normovolemic hypotensive patients to avoid complications associated with using fluids alone (such as bowel edema and increased extravascular lung water).[46] Large-volume blood loss should prompt replacement (1:1) with allogeneic packed RBCs and fresh frozen plasma, with platelets administered as needed.

Postoperatively, no more than 2 to 2.5 L of water and 70 to 100 mmol sodium should be administered per day for most patients who require only maintenance fluid replace-ment (ie, without volume deficits or ongoing fluid and electrolyte losses). The ERAS guidelines advocate avoiding nasogastric tubes and the aggressive treatment of post-operative nausea and vomiting to enhance oral intake and wean intravenous fluids (ideally within 48 hours after colonic surgery). Optimal management thus includes the combination of iGDT with an overall aim to achieve a state of zero-balance in terms of weight gain. Patients undergoing laparotomy have fluid requirements different from those undergoing laparoscopic surgery. Increased fluid requirements in open laparot-omy may result from a greater systemic inflammatory response syndrome (with greater loss of the endothelial glycocalyx), increased evaporative losses, and increased bowel handling/manipulation.[46] Patients undergoing laparotomy are more likely to have thoracic epidural analgesia and require intravenous fluids to counteract the sympathectomy-induced hypotension (from increased venous capacitance and relative hypovolemia), further exacerbated by the increased release of inflammatory mediators. Abdominal insufflation and Trendelenburg positioning during laparoscopic surgery have been shown to reduce tissue oxygen delivery.[55] Thus, appropriate deci-sions regarding fluid therapy must be made to augment SV during laparoscopy based on individualized assessments of hemodynamic variables.

CLINICAL ASSESSMENT AND MONITORING TO GUIDE FLUID THERAPY

Assessment of fluid status can be difficult in the operative setting where a formal phys-ical examination cannot always be conducted. Traditional evaluation has focused on assessment of the heart rate, blood pressure, and urine output.[56] Volume deficits may not become apparent until they exceed 10% of body weight.[57] As noted by Vincent and Weil,[57] hypotension can be a nonspecific sign due to vascular inflow obstruction, heart failure, or a vasodilatory process. Changes in heart rate to maintain CO may be skewed by medications such as β-blockers and vasopressors. Other common intra-operative events such as surgical stimulatory actions activating nociceptive pathways and changes in body temperature may distort an anesthesiologist's interpretation of the patient's real-time volume status. Static measurements such as end-diastolic pressure and central venous pressure can also be influenced by a myriad of factors including patient comorbid cardiovascular pathologies and, thus, may not accurately reflect volume responsiveness.

Assessment of volume responsiveness may be performed with dynamic methods such as the administration of a rapid fluid bolus (3 mL/kg as earlier in the context of iGDT) or by a passive leg raise maneuver. Stroke volume variation (SVV) and/or PPV (with pulse pressure equal to the difference between systolic and diastolic pressure) can also be formally assessed. Analysis of various systems that quantify SVV, including the PiCCO plus system (Pulsion Medical Systems, Munich, Germany), Flo-Trac/Vigileo (Edwards Lifesciences, Irvine, CA, USA), and LiDCO plus technique (LiDCO Ltd, London, UK), revealed fluid responsiveness with SVV threshold values be-tween 10% and 13%.[56,58–66] Marik and colleagues[67] conducted a meta-analysis of 29 studies encompassing a total of 685 patients to compare the accuracy of SVV, PPV, and systolic pressure variation (SPV) in predicting change in SV index or cardiac index after a fluid challenge during controlled mechanical ventilation. Roughly 56% of patients showed a demonstrable response to a fluid bolus. Pooled correlation coefficients between baseline SVV, PPV, and SPV and change in stroke/cardiac index were 0.72, 0.78, and 0.72, respectively. Areas under the receiver operating characteristic curves were 0.84, 0.94, and 0.86, respectively. This result favored PPV in comparison with SVV.

Monitors can help distinguish between hypovolemia and other causes of hypotension (such as cardiogenic, neurogenic or distributive, and obstructive). Pulmonary artery catheters (PACs), although frequently used in the past, have been associated with conflicting data.[68,69] Esophageal Doppler-based monitoring (EDM, Deltex Medical Inc, Chichester, West Sussex, United Kingdom) directly measures blood flow velocity in the descending thoracic aorta. Then, using a nomogram-based estimate of aortic cross-sectional area, CO and SV are estimated. Fluid boluses may be titrated to target an increase of at least 10% in the SV and CO. Dynamic arterial pressure–based computations such as SPV, PPV, and SVV may also help in defining fluid responsiveness (as described earlier). Noblett and colleagues[70] conducted a double-blind prospective randomized controlled trial with 108 patients randomized to either receive perioperative fluid at the discretion of the anesthetist (control group) or EDM-based optimization of SV. The intervention group had overall higher average SV, had shorter hospital length of stay (7 vs 9 days), tolerated enteral nutrition earlier, had a reduced increase in interleukin 6 level, and had decreased morbidity. Abbas and Hill[71] conducted a systematic review of EDM-guided therapy in major abdominal surgery and reported reduced hospital length of stay, faster return of gastrointestinal function, and reduced requirement for inotropes postoperatively. These studies were conducted before ERAS guidelines and fluid-restrictive strategies were commonplace.

The bioreactance-based noninvasive cardiac output monitor (NICOM, Cheetah Medical, Vancouver, WA, USA) uses 4 surface electrodes across the chest to compute an approximation of the CO, SV, and SVV. Waldron and colleagues[72] compared 100 adult patients undergoing elective colorectal surgery with goal-directed fluid therapy (using 250-mL colloid boluses) guided by either EDM or NICOM. Both monitors were used to assess monitor discrepancies in both patient groups. A 10% increase in SV was used for the fluid challenge. There was no statistically significant difference between monitor readings and no clinically significant differences in outcomes including postoperative pain, nausea, return of bowel function, organ dysfunction, and hospital length of stay. Critchley and Critchley[73] conducted a meta-analysis using Bland-Altman statistics (bias and precision) to compare novel CO measurement technology against gold standard techniques. They determined that a lack of precision of up to 30% was acceptable for routine clinical purposes. Peyton and Chong[74] conducted a meta-analysis reviewing data on EDM, NICOM, pulse contour techniques, and partial carbon dioxide rebreathing to assess percentage error versus PAC-based thermodilution. None of the techniques had less than 30% error (most were only about 45% precise).

New noninvasive systems display continuous noninvasive arterial pressures (CNAPs) recreating a beat-to-beat waveform. This technology is based on arterial tonometry and the volume clamp method. Current devices include Nexfin (BMEYE B.V., Amsterdam, The Netherlands), CNAP (CNSystems, Graz, Austria), and T-line (Tensys Medical, Inc, San Diego, CA, USA). Kim and colleagues[75] conducted a systematic review and meta-analysis of 28 studies (919 patients) reporting pooled random-effects bias and standard deviation (SD) measures of systolic arterial pressure, diastolic arterial pressure, and mean arterial pressure. Acceptable standards

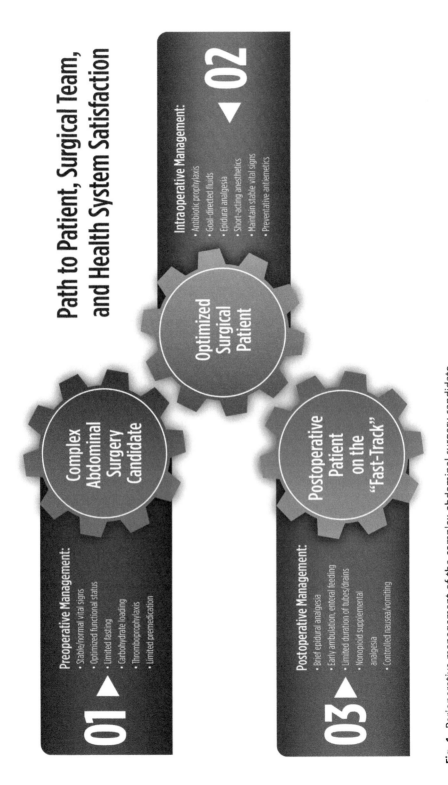

Path to Patient, Surgical Team, and Health System Satisfaction

01 ▲

Preoperative Management:
- Stable/normal vital signs
- Optimized functional status
- Limited fasting
- Carbohydrate loading
- Thromboprophylaxis
- Limited premedication

Complex Abdominal Surgery Candidate

Optimized Surgical Patient

02 ▼

Intraoperative Management:
- Antibiotic prophylaxis
- Goal-directed fluids
- Epidural analgesia
- Short-acting anesthetics
- Maintain stable vital signs
- Preventative antiemetics

Postoperative Patient on the "Fast-Track"

03 ▶

Postoperative Management:
- Brief epidural analgesia
- Early ambulation, enteral feeding
- Limited duration of tubes/drains
- Nonopioid supplemental analgesia
- Controlled nausea/vomiting

Fig. 1. Perioperative management of the complex abdominal surgery candidate.

for bias and SD were less than 5 and 8 mm Hg, respectively. The overall pooled bias and SD were -1.6 ± 12.2 mm Hg (95% limits of agreement -25.5 to 22.2 mm Hg) for systolic arterial pressure, 5.3 ± 8.3 mm Hg (-11.0 to 21.6 mm Hg) for diastolic arterial pressure, and 3.2 ± 8.4 mm Hg (-13.4 to 19.7 mm Hg) for mean arterial pressure. Kim and colleagues stressed the importance of this finding, noting that a patient with an invasive systolic arterial pressure reading of 100 mm Hg could have a CNAP reading of systolic arterial pressure anywhere from 74 to 123 mm Hg. These devices thus do not comply with standards created by the Arlington Association for the Advancement of Medical Instrumentation but are nevertheless clinically useful to monitor trends in certain settings.

In the late 1990s, physicians began analyzing the pulse oximetry waveform to obtain noninvasive data regarding volume status in mechanically ventilated patients in normal sinus rhythm.[76] Indices of fluid responsiveness include respiratory variation in pulse oximetric plethysmographic (POP) waveform amplitude (delta POP; manually calculated) and pleth variability index (PVI; continuous/automated calculation; measure of dynamic change in perfusion index occurring during the respiratory cycle where perfusion index is defined as the ratio of nonpulsatile to pulsatile blood flow through the peripheral capillary bed). Sandroni and colleagues[77] reported results of a meta-analysis of 10 studies with 233 patients that evaluated the accuracy of delta POP and/or PVI in predicting the hemodynamic response to a large or small fluid bolus (approximately 500 mL vs 250 mL, respectively). There was no major difference in change in the cardiac index, SV, or SV index found within studies incorporating the same-size fluid bolus. There was also no significant difference found between studies using delta POP and those using PVI. Sensitivity and specificity of the diagnostic techniques were more accurate with studies incorporating larger boluses, which likely indicates inaccuracy with poor capillary perfusion (eg, low CO, peripheral vasoconstriction, hypothermia). Analysis by Sandroni and colleagues suggests that plethysmographic indices are adequate for detecting fluid responsiveness, but less accurate in quantifying the magnitude of change in CO after fluid administration.

Fluid and electrolyte overload may result from liberal fluid replacement strategies or from moderate strategies in patients with comorbidities (such as congestive heart failure or end-stage renal disease). Patients may present with hypertension and significant weight gain (>2.5 kg), display jugular venous distention, develop pitting/peripheral edema, demonstrate a third heart sound on auscultation, have increased urine output, or accumulate ascites or pulmonary edema. Excessive crystalloid or colloid administration may result in a dilutional coagulopathy, which can be worsened by hypothermia if fluids are not properly warmed. Lack of fluid responsiveness (as defined previously) may indicate poor cardiac reserve or adequate resuscitation. EDM may show profiles of blood flow velocities consistent with euvolemia, whereas euvolemic mechanically ventilated patients have minimal PPV, SVV, and SPV on arterial waveform analysis. Changes in central venous pressure are neither sensitive nor specific for the identification of fluid responsiveness.[78] Inferior vena cava (IVC) diameter may be increased with minimal respiratory variation on bedside transthoracic echocardiogram (on standardized M-mode–based IVC variability measures). Multifrequency bioelectrical impedance analysis is currently used by some nephrologists to evaluate both extracellular and intracellular water volumes with proven accuracy.[79] Pharmacologic treatment of volume overload includes administration of diuretics such as furosemide (Lasix) or metolazone (Zaroxolyn) in patients with intact renal function.[80] Nonpharmacologic fluid removal (eg, hemodialysis) may be indicated in patients unresponsive to medications or intolerant to medication side effects who have signs of symptomatic renal failure.

SUMMARY

Optimal management of volume status before, during, and after abdominal surgery involves a combination of the recommendations discussed under ERAS protocols, iGDT in patients at moderate to high risk for perioperative complications, and a zero-balance goal in patients with significant physiologic reserve at low risk for complications (**Fig. 1**). Therapy may be titrated to fluid responsiveness or may be continued as long as weight gain is less than 2.5 kg (when dynamic measures are not being used). Measures such as mixed venous oxygen saturation, arterial lactate concentrations, or base deficit could be used as markers for globally adequate oxygen delivery. Ideally, patients are normotensive, with a cardiac index greater than 2.5 L/min/m^2 and a normal heart rate.

Future pathways for optimal fluid management may include the development of potentially noninvasive hemodynamic monitoring systems coupled with closed-loop fluid administration algorithms that would assess patients in the preoperative, intraoperative, and postoperative settings. At present, no single monitor can replace a vigilant anesthesiologist and surgeon working together to interpret hemodynamic data within the context of the patient's history and surgical procedure. Key decisions rely on experience with resource availability at the given perioperative setting and interventions with judicious intravenous fluid support.

REFERENCES

1. Lazarus-Barlow WS. On the initial rate of osmosis of blood-serum with reference to the composition of "physiological saline solution" in mammals. J Physiol 1896; 20(2-3):145–57.
2. Guidet B, Soni N, Della Rocca G, et al. A balanced view of balanced solutions. Crit Care 2010;14(5):325.
3. Kim SY, Huh KH, Lee JR, et al. Comparison of the effects of normal saline versus Plasmalyte on acid-base balance during living donor kidney transplantation using the Stewart and base excess methods. Transplant Proc 2013;45(6):2191–6.
4. Ho AM, Karmakar MK, Contardi LH, et al. Excessive use of normal saline in managing traumatized patients in shock: a preventable contributor to acidosis. J Trauma 2001;51(1):173–7.
5. Lobo DN, Bostock KA, Neal KR, et al. Effect of salt and water balance on recovery of gastrointestinal function after elective colonic resection: a randomized controlled trial. Lancet 2002;359(9320):1812–8.
6. Mecray PM, Barden RP, Ravdin IS. Nutritional edema: its effect on the gastric emptying time before and after gastric operations. Surgery 1937;1(1):53–64.
7. Tournadre JP, Allaouiche B, Malbert CH, et al. Metabolic acidosis and respiratory acidosis impair gastric-pyloric motility in anesthetized pigs. Anesth Analg 2000; 90(1):74–9.
8. Hansen PB, Jensen BL, Skott O. Chloride regulates afferent arteriolar contraction in response to depolarization. Hypertension 1998;32(6):1066–70.
9. Stone HH, Fulenwider JT. Renal decapsulation in the prevention of post-ischemic oliguria. Ann Surg 1977;186(3):343–55.
10. McCluskey SA, Karkouti K, Wijeysundera D, et al. Hyperchloremia after noncardiac surgery is independently associated with increased morbidity and mortality: a propensity-matched cohort study. Anesth Analg 2013;117(2):412–21.
11. Chowdhury AH, Cox EF, Francis ST, et al. A randomized, controlled, double-blind crossover study on the effects of 2-L infusions of 0.9% saline and Plasma-lyte® 148 on renal blood flow velocity and renal cortical tissue perfusion in healthy volunteers. Ann Surg 2012;256(1):18–24.

12. Powell-Tuck J, Gosling P, Lobo DN, et al. British consensus guidelines on intravenous fluid therapy for adult surgical patients (GIFTASUP). London: NHS National Library of Health; 2009.

13. Lobo DN, Awad S. Should chloride-rich crystalloids remain the mainstay of fluid resuscitation to prevent 'pre-renal' acute kidney injury?: con. Kidney Int 2014; 86(6):1096–105.

14. Hadimioglu N, Saadawy I, Saglam T, et al. The effect of different crystalloid solutions on acid-base balance and early kidney function after kidney transplantation. Anesth Analg 2008;107(1):264–9.

15. Shaw AD, Bagshaw SM, Goldstein SL, et al. Major complications, mortality, and resource utilization after open abdominal surgery: 0.9% saline compared to Plasma-Lyte. Ann Surg 2012;255(5):821–9.

16. Raghunathan K, Shaw AD, Bagshaw SM. Fluids are drugs: type, dose and toxicity. Curr Opin Crit Care 2013;19(4):290–8.

17. Finfer S, Bellomo R, Boyce N, et al. A comparison of albumin and saline for fluid resuscitation in the intensive care unit. N Engl J Med 2004;350(22): 2247–56.

18. Brunkhorst FM, Engel C, Bloos F, et al. Intensive insulin therapy and pentastarch resuscitation in severe sepsis. N Engl J Med 2008;358(2):125–39.

19. Annane D, Siami S, Jaber S, et al. Effects of fluid resuscitation with colloids vs crystalloids on mortality in critically ill patients presenting with hypovolemic shock: the CRISTAL randomized trial. JAMA 2013;310(17):1809–17.

20. Jacob M, Chappell D, Hofmann-Kiefer K, et al. The intravascular volume effect of Ringer's lactate is below 20%: a prospective study in humans. Crit Care 2012; 16(3):R86.

21. Hartog CS, Bauer M, Reinhart K. The efficacy and safety of colloid resuscitation in the critically ill. Anesth Analg 2011;112(1):156–64.

22. Wilkes MM, Navickis RJ, Sibbald WJ. Albumin versus hydroxyethyl starch in cardiopulmonary bypass surgery; a meta-analysis of postoperative bleeding. Ann Thorac Surg 2001;72(2):527–33.

23. Jonville-Bera AP, Autret-Leca E, Gruel Y. Acquired type I von Willebrand's disease associated with highly substituted hydroxyethyl starch. N Engl J Med 2001;345(8):622–3.

24. Schortgen R, Lacherade JC, Bruneel F, et al. Effects of hydroxyethyl starch and gelatin on renal function in severe sepsis: a multicentre randomised study. Lancet 2001;357(9260):911–6.

25. Cittanova ML, Leblanc I, Legendre C, et al. Effect of hydroxyethyl starch in brain-dead kidney donors on renal function in kidney-transplant recipients. Lancet 1996;348(9042):1620–2.

26. Rioux JP, Lessard M, De Bortoli B, et al. Pentastarch 10% (250 kDa/0.45) is an independent risk factor of acute injury following cardiac surgery. Crit Care Med 2009;37(4):1293–8.

27. Perel P, Roberts I, Ker K. Colloids versus crystalloids for fluid resuscitation in critically ill patients. Cochrane Database Syst Rev 2013;(2):CD000567.

28. Varadhan KK, Lobo DN. A meta-analysis of randomized controlled trials of intravenous fluid therapy in major elective open abdominal surgery: getting the balance right. Proc Nutr Soc 2010;69(4):488–98.

29. Brandstrup B, Tonnesen H, Beier-Holgersen R, et al. Effects of intravenous fluid restriction on postoperative complications: comparison of two perioperative fluid regimens: a randomized assessor-blinded multicenter trial. Ann Surg 2003; 238(5):641–8.

30. Cecconi M, Corredor C, Arulkumaran N, et al. Clinical review: goal-directed therapy - what is the evidence in surgical patients? The effect on different risk groups. Crit Care 2013;17(2):209.
31. Hamilton MA, Cecconi M, Rhodes A. A systematic review and meta-analysis on the use of preemptive hemodynamic intervention to improve postoperative outcomes in moderate and high-risk surgical patients. Anesth Analg 2011;112(6): 1392–402.
32. Pearse RM, Harrison DA, MacDonald N, et al. Effect of a perioperative, cardiac output-guided hemodynamic therapy algorithm on outcomes following major gastrointestinal surgery: a randomized clinical trial and systematic review. JAMA 2014;311(21):2181–90.
33. Gan TJ, Soppitt A, Maroof M, et al. Goal-directed intraoperative fluid administration reduces length of hospital stay after major surgery. Anesthesiology 2002;97(4): 820–6.
34. Pearse R, Dawson D, Fawcett J, et al. Early goal-directed therapy after major surgery reduces complications and duration of hospital stay. A randomized, controlled trial. Crit Care 2005;9(6):R687–93.
35. Cecconi M, Parsons AK, Rhodes A. What is a fluid challenge? Curr Opin Crit Care 2011;17(3):290–5.
36. Bennett-Guerrero E. Hemodynamic goal-directed therapy in high-risk surgical patients. JAMA 2014;311(21):2177–8.
37. Srinivasa S, Taylor MH, Sammour T, et al. Oesophageal Doppler-guided fluid administration in colorectal surgery: critical appraisal of published clinical trials. Acta Anaesthesiol Scand 2011;55(1):4–13.
38. Lassen K, Soop M, Nygren J, et al. Consensus review of optimal perioperative care in colorectal surgery: Enhanced Recovery After Surgery (ERAS) Group recommendations. Arch Surg 2009;144(10):961–9.
39. Brandstrup B, Svendsen PE, Rasmussen M, et al. Which goal for fluid therapy during colorectal surgery is followed by the best outcome: near-maximal stroke volume or zero fluid balance? Br J Anaesth 2012;109(2):191–9.
40. Srinivasa S, Taylor MH, Singh PP, et al. Randomized clinical trial of goal-directed fluid therapy within an enhanced recovery protocol for elective colectomy. Br J Surg 2013;100(1):66–74.
41. Yates DR, Davies SJ, Milner HE, et al. Crystalloid or colloid for goal-directed fluid therapy in colorectal surgery. Br J Anaesth 2014;112(2):281–9.
42. Lobo DN, Macafee DA, Allison SP. How perioperative fluid balance influences postoperative outcomes. Best Pract Res Clin Anaesthesiol 2006; 20(3):439–55.
43. Hannemann P, Lassen K, Hausel J, et al. Patterns in current anaesthesiological peri-operative practice for colonic resections: a survey in five northern European countries. Acta Anaesthesiol Scand 2006;50(9):1152–60.
44. Jacob M, Chappell D, Rehm M. The 'third space' – fact or fiction? Best Pract Res Clin Anaesthesiol 2009;23(2):145–57.
45. Shires T, Williams J, Brown F. Acute change in extracellular fluids associated with major surgical procedures. Ann Surg 1961;154:803–10.
46. Gustafsson UO, Scott MJ, Schwenk W, et al. Guidelines for perioperative care in elective colonic surgery: Enhanced Recovery After Surgery (ERAS®) Society recommendations. Clin Nutr 2012;31(6):783–800.
47. Nygren J, Thacker J, Carli F, et al. Guidelines for perioperative care in elective rectal/pelvic surgery: Enhanced Recovery After Surgery (ERAS®) Society recommendations. Clin Nutr 2012;31(6):801–16.

48. Lassen K, Coolsen MM, Slim K, et al. Guidelines for perioperative care for pancreaticoduodenectomy: Enhanced Recovery After Surgery (ERAS®) Society recommendations. Clin Nutr 2012;31(6):817–30.
49. Kingsnorth A, Bowley D. Fundamentals of surgical practice: a preparation guide for the intercollegiate MRCS examination. 3rd edition. New York: Cambridge University Press; 2011. p. 181–9.
50. Brady M, Kinn S, Stuart P. Preoperative fasting for adults to prevent perioperative complications. Cochrane Database Syst Rev 2003;(4):CD004423.
51. Awad S, Varadhan KK, Ljungqvist O, et al. A meta-analysis of randomised controlled trials on preoperative oral carbohydrate treatment in elective surgery. Clin Nutr 2013;32(1):34–44.
52. Holte K, Nielsen KG, Madsen JL, et al. Physiologic effects of bowel preparation. Dis Colon Rectum 2004;47(8):1397–402.
53. Bucher P, Mermillod B, Gervaz P, et al. Mechanical bowel preparation for elective colorectal surgery: a meta-analysis. Arch Surg 2004;139(12):1359–65.
54. Shoemaker WC, Appel PL, Kram HB. Hemodynamic and oxygen transport responses in survivors and nonsurvivors of high-risk surgery. Crit Care Med 1993;21(7):977–90.
55. Levy BF, Fawcett WJ, Scott MJ, et al. Intra-operative oxygen delivery in infusion volume-optimized patients undergoing laparoscopic colorectal surgery within an enhanced recovery programme: the effect of different analgesic modalities. Colorectal Dis 2012;14(7):887–92.
56. Hofer CK, Cannesson M. Monitoring fluid responsiveness. Acta Anaesthesiol Taiwan 2011;49(2):59–65.
57. Vincent JL, Weil MH. Fluid challenge revisited. Crit Care Med 2006;34(5):1333–7.
58. Hofer CK, Muller SM, Furrer L, et al. Stroke volume and pulse pressure variation for prediction of fluid responsiveness in patients undergoing off-pump coronary artery bypass grafting. Chest 2005;128(2):848–54.
59. Berkenstadt H, Margalit N, Hadani M, et al. Stroke volume variation as a predictor of fluid responsiveness in patients undergoing brain surgery. Anesth Analg 2001; 92(4):984–9.
60. Preisman S, Kogan S, Berkenstadt H, et al. Predicting fluid responsiveness in patients undergoing cardiac surgery: functional haemodynamic parameters including the respiratory systolic variation test and static preload indicators. Br J Anaesth 2005;95(6):746–55.
61. Reuter DA, Kirchner A, Felbinger TW, et al. Usefulness of left ventricular stroke volume variation to assess fluid responsiveness in patients with reduced cardiac function. Crit Care Med 2003;31(5):1399–404.
62. Biais M, Nouette-Gaulain K, Cottenceau V, et al. Uncalibrated pulse contour-derived stroke volume variation predicts fluid responsiveness in mechanically ventilated patients undergoing liver transplantation. Br J Anaesth 2008;101(6):761–8.
63. Cannesson M, Musard H, Desebbe O, et al. The ability of stroke volume variations obtained with Vigileo/FloTrac system to monitor fluid responsiveness in mechanically ventilated patients. Anesth Analg 2009;108(2):513–7.
64. Hofer CK, Senn A, Weibel L, et al. Assessment of stroke volume variation for prediction of fluid responsiveness using the modified FloTrac and PiCCOplus system. Crit Care 2008;12(3):R82.
65. Belloni L, Pisano A, Natale A, et al. Assessment of fluid-responsiveness parameters for off-pump coronary artery bypass surgery: a comparison among LiDCO, transesophageal echocardiography, and pulmonary artery catheter. J Cardiothorac Vasc Anesth 2008;22(2):243–8.

66. de Wilde RB, Geerts BF, van den Berg PC, et al. A comparison of stroke volume variation measured by the LiDCOplus and FloTrac-Vigileo system. Anaesthesia 2009;64(9):1004–9.

67. Marik PE, Cavallazzi R, Vasu T, et al. Dynamic changes in arterial waveform derived variables and fluid responsiveness in mechanically ventilated patients: a systematic review of the literature. Crit Care Med 2009;37(9):2642–7.

68. Harvey S, Young D, Brampton W, et al. Pulmonary artery catheters for adult patients in intensive care. Cochrane Database Syst Rev 2006;(3):CD003408.

69. Takala J. The pulmonary artery catheter: the tool versus treatments based on the tool. Crit Care 2006;10(4):162.

70. Noblett SE, Snowden CP, Shenton BK, et al. Randomized clinical trial assessing the effect of Doppler-optimized fluid management on outcome after elective colorectal resection. Br J Surg 2006;93(9):1069–76.

71. Abbas SM, Hill AG. Systematic review of the literature for the use of oesophageal Doppler monitor for fluid replacement in major abdominal surgery. Anaesthesia 2008;63(1):44–51.

72. Waldron NH, Miller TE, Thacker JK, et al. A prospective comparison of a noninvasive cardiac output monitor versus esophageal Doppler monitor for goal-directed fluid therapy in colorectal surgery patients. Anesth Analg 2014;118(5): 966–75.

73. Critchley LA, Critchley JA. A meta-analysis of studies using bias and precision statistics to compare cardiac output measurement techniques. J Clin Monit Comput 1999;15(2):85–91.

74. Peyton PJ, Chong SW. Minimally invasive measurement of cardiac output during surgery and critical care: a meta-analysis of accuracy and precision. Anesthesiology 2010;113(5):1220–35.

75. Kim SH, Lilot M, Sidhu KS, et al. Accuracy and precision of continuous noninvasive arterial pressure monitoring compared with invasive arterial pressure: a systematic review and meta-analysis. Anesthesiology 2014;120(5):1080–97.

76. Shamir M, Eidelman LA, Floman Y, et al. Pulse oximetry plethysmographic waveform during changes in blood volume. Br J Anaesth 1999;82(2):178–81.

77. Sandroni C, Cavallaro F, Marano C, et al. Accuracy of plethysmographic indices as predictors of fluid responsiveness in mechanically ventilated adults: a systematic review and meta-analysis. Intensive Care Med 2012;38(9):1429–37.

78. Marik PE, Cavallazzi R. Does the central venous pressure predict fluid responsiveness? An updated meta-analysis and a plea for some common sense. Crit Care Med 2013;41(7):1774–81.

79. Davenport A. Dialysis: bioimpedance spectroscopy for assessment of fluid overload. Nat Rev Nephrol 2013;9(5):252–4.

80. Goldstein S, Bagshaw S, Cecconi M, et al. Pharmacological management of fluid overload. Br J Anaesth 2014;113(5):756–63.

Optimal Analgesia During Major Open and Laparoscopic Abdominal Surgery

CrossMark

William J. Fawcett, MB BS, FRCA, FFPMRCA[a,b,*],
Gabriele Baldini, MD, MSc[c]

KEYWORDS

- Analgesia • Opioids • Local anesthetic • Acetaminophen
- Antiinflammatory agents • Alpha-2 agonists • Anticonvulsants
- N-Methyl-D-aspartate (NMDA) receptor antagonist

KEY POINTS

- Analgesia is a key element of enhanced recovery after surgery (ERAS) programs, particularly following abdominal surgery.
- Multimodal opioid-sparing analgesia is a cornerstone of all analgesic regimens, especially with the use of regular acetaminophen and antiinflammatories.
- Thoracic epidural analgesia is the principal technique for open surgery, but not for laparoscopic surgery, in which intrathecal or more peripherally placed local anesthetic (trunk blocks or wound blocks) is used.
- Several other adjuvants are described but evidence is less strong.
- Interest is growing in the potential for analgesic regimens affecting not only short-term benefits but also longer-term benefits, including rates of cancer recurrence.

INTRODUCTION

Analgesia plays a pivotal role in the management of patients undergoing open or laparoscopic abdominal surgery. Although the relief of pain is one of the most fundamental humanitarian roles for all health care professionals treating patients undergoing surgery, there is now a greater understanding of how this interacts with patient recovery. It has long been recognized that a good analgesic regimen permits not only patient comfort but also facilitates other benefits such as early mobilization and enteral feeding. In the last 20 years, fast-track surgery has evolved into the enhanced recovery after

[a] Department of Anaesthesia, Royal Surrey County Hospital, Egerton Road, Guildford GU2 7XX, UK; [b] Faculty of Health and Medical Sciences, Duke of Kent Building, University of Surrey, Guildford GU2 7TE, UK; [c] Department of Anesthesia, McGill University Health Centre, Montreal General Hospital, 1650 Avenue Cedar, Montreal, Quebec H3G 1A4, Canada
* Corresponding author. Department of Anaesthesia, Royal Surrey County Hospital, Egerton Road, Guildford GU2 7XX, UK.
E-mail address: wfawcett@nhs.net

Anesthesiology Clin 33 (2015) 65–78
http://dx.doi.org/10.1016/j.anclin.2014.11.005
anesthesiology.theclinics.com
1932-2275/15/$ – see front matter © 2015 Elsevier Inc. All rights reserved.

surgery (ERAS) program. Pivotal in the philosophy of ERAS is a reduction in the physiologic stress response to surgery and the associated catabolic response. In addition, there is growing evidence to suggest that patients on ERAS have reduced complications following surgery, which affects not only immediate survival but also long-term survival.[1] Although there are many elements to ERAS,[2] analgesic technique plays a large part. In addition, there is interest currently in how anesthetic technique in general, and analgesic technique in particular, may directly affect cancer outcome[3] by modulating immune function. This effect has been shown for breast and prostate surgery[4] but not so far for colorectal surgery.[5] This possibility is particularly relevant for this group of patients, many of whom are undergoing surgery for cancer.

Thus pain medicine has come a long way: correctly administered, it may not only give great relief to patients but may permit rapid return to normal activities and perhaps improve patients' long-term survival through reduction in early postoperative complications.[1,6]

More than 20 years ago, Kehlet and Dahl[7] described multimodal opioid-sparing analgesia, which is the cornerstone of the management of patients undergoing abdominal surgery. Using analgesic techniques acting via different mechanisms, side effects may be minimized and opioid consumption may be reduced. Although some opioid usage may be unavoidable, excess usage leads to a host of undesirable adverse effects: respiratory and cough suppression, postoperative nausea and vomiting (PONV), urinary retention, and delayed return of gastrointestinal (GI) function (**Box 1**). Following major abdominal surgery, the combination of these effects impairs the achievement of important ERAS milestones (**Fig. 1**) and can even be catastrophic; for example, hypoventilation, obtunded respiratory reflexes, and gastric stasis can predispose to passive regurgitation and pulmonary aspiration.

The most significant advance for patients undergoing GI surgery in the last 10 years has been the shift from open to laparoscopic surgery. There is a good evidence base for analgesia for the former, but the optimum analgesic modality for the latter is still debated.[8]

In addition, providing the best and safest analgesia requires more than a prescription. It is essential that regular postoperative input occurs from staff (usually specialist pain nurses) who assess the patients, monitor pain scores, and take appropriate action to relieve pain and treat any ensuing complications (such as hypotension).

OPIOID ANALGESIA

The use of morphine is not viewed as the gold standard for analgesia but has still become the gold standard for comparisons of effectiveness for practically all other

---

Box 1
Side effects of morphine

- Reduced gastrointestinal motility, leading to ileus
- Nausea and vomiting
- Cough suppression
- Respiratory depression with reduced sensitivity to $Paco_2$
- Urinary retention
- Euphoria, dysphoria, hallucination
- Histamine release (may cause itching, hypotension, and bronchospasm)
- Bradycardia
- Tolerance (over time)

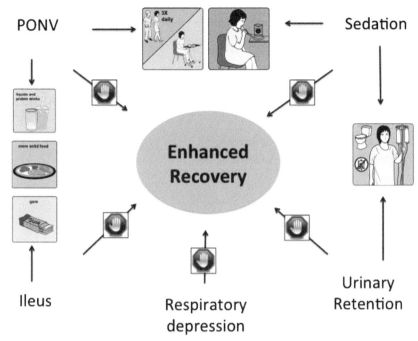

PONV

Sedation

Enhanced Recovery

Ileus

Respiratory depression

Urinary Retention

Fig. 1. Avoidance of complications to achieve ERAS.

methods of analgesia. However, for abdominal surgery, the mere mention of parenteral opioids such as morphine can produce an irrational fear. Whilst minimizing their use is desirable, that does not mean that their use has to be avoided. Leaving patients in unrelieved pain is not acceptable and opioids should be available as rescue analgesia if other methods fail. Moreover, early and limited use of morphine has little effect on outcome.[9] The use of short-acting opioids such as fentanyl in neuraxial block is discussed later. In addition because of its constipating effects, many providers avoid the use of oral moderate opioids, such as codeine, although drugs such as tramadol acting via opioid and other mechanisms (such as inhibition of reuptake of serotonin and norepinephrine) are used. In addition, in the last 5 years there has been an increasing debate about the relevance of opioid-induced hyperalgesia (OIH), in which there is a paradoxic effect from high-potency opioids (eg, perioperative remifentanil), and further opioid administration increases rather than reduces pain perception. OIH is a complex area and seems to be multifactorial, including both central and peripheral changes in nociceptive processing, the former involving N-methyl-D-aspartate (NMDA) receptors (discussed later), as well as genetic influences. The magnitude of the problem, including the patient's susceptibility, and potential treatments await further studies.[10,11]

If morphine is used it is often because other methods have failed. It is probably best administered intravenously as patient-controlled analgesia (PCA), permitting good control of pain in the early postoperative period, but with good knowledge of its side effects.

LOCAL ANESTHETIC TECHNIQUES
Epidural Analgesia

The mainstay of analgesia for GI surgery has been the thoracic epidural. There are several well-documented advantages (**Box 2**) but more recently its problems have

---

Box 2
Advantages of epidurals

- Attenuation of some aspects of the stress response
  - Neuroendocrine (sympathetic and pituitary activation)
  - Metabolic (eg, hyperglycemia, protein breakdown)
  - But no effect on inflammatory changes mediated by cytokines
- Improvement in pulmonary function
  - Reduced incidence of postoperative hypoxia
  - Reduced incidence of atelectasis and infection
- GI
  - Reduced ileus
  - Earlier return to diet
- Reduction in pulmonary thromboembolism
- Reduction in blood loss
- Some studies have shown reduction in myocardial infarction, renal failure, and mortality

---

been highlighted (**Box 3**). It is still considered the gold standard for open surgery, but for laparoscopic surgery there is less evidence to support its use and many clinicians have moved on to less invasive methods.

For open surgery, the placement of an epidural catheter for postoperative infusion is a straightforward theoretic concept and, when functioning optimally, provides superlative segmental analgesia for the first 48 to 72 hours. However, there are several areas that need to be addressed in this process:

Box 3
Disadvantages of epidurals

- Epidural failure
  - Wrong site (eg, lumbar and not thoracic)
  - Catheter not in epidural space (or migrated)
  - Inadequate drug dosages
- Hypotension
- Poor mobility
  - Motor block (especially with lumbar epidurals)
  - Sensory block
  - Hypotension
- Neurologic damage (temporary or permanent)
  - Space-occupying lesion of vertebral canal
  - Wrong drug injected
  - Direct trauma at insertion
- Dural puncture

1. Epidural positioning: the epidural needs to be placed appropriately for the type of surgery. Lumbar epidurals much less desirable because of their higher incidence of leg weakness.
2. The insertion technique used is important: the paramedian has been described as having advantages compared with the midline in terms of ease of identification of the epidural space and placement of the catheter with less paresthesia, but personal preference plays a large part in the technique used.
3. The drugs used. Local anesthetic alone was classically used, but in order to reduce excessive sympathetic and motor blockade and improve the quality of analgesia various other drugs have been added to the local anesthetic. These drugs include opioids (most commonly[12]) but also other adjuvants such as epinephrine or alpha-2 agonists (discussed later).
4. The postoperative management is fundamental in terms of titrating the epidural infusion and dealing with side effects, in particular hypotension and leg weakness (discussed later).
5. Contraindications to the insertion of an epidural catheter most commonly involve abnormalities of coagulation; historically thrombocytopenia and an increased International Normalized Ratio (INR) resulting from warfarin. Although there are no absolute agreed figures, many clinicians are reluctant to site an epidural with a platelet count of less than $75 \times 10^9/L$ or an INR of greater than 1.4. However, many coagulation-modifying drugs are used, including heparin (both unfractionated heparin and low-molecular-weight heparin), antiplatelet drugs (aspirin, thienopyridines, and glycoprotein IIb/IIIa receptor inhibitors), and the new oral anticoagulants (such as rivaroxaban and dabigatran) and thrombolytic drugs. Many of these drugs have no accepted laboratory test to confirm return of normal coagulation, have no antidote, and require knowledge of when the last dose was administered and in some cases (eg, rivaroxaban and dabigatran) renal function as well. However, there is no absolute evidence based on large studies confirming when it is safe to insert epidurals (vertebral canal hematomas are rare). Based on international guidelines and recommendations,[13,14] a suggested protocol is given in **Table 1**.

Poorly managed epidurals have potential to cause great harm and the management of their side effects and complications is paramount.

1. Poorly working or nonworking epidurals are common (up to 50% in some studies) and have recently been reviewed.[15] Patients are often denied other forms of analgesia (eg, systemic opioids) because of concern of causing respiratory depression and compounding the situation. Early identification of a nonworking epidural (primary failure) is essential to avoid returning patients to the ward with an ineffective analgesic modality. Effectiveness of epidural analgesia must be verified soon after the epidural catheter is placed, and ideally before the beginning of surgery or in the postanesthesia care unit. The problem then needs to be swiftly addressed by increasing the epidural rate, adding an adjuvant drug (eg, an epidural opioid), reinserting the epidural, or removing it and instituting an alternative analgesic regime, such as PCA morphine (**Fig. 2**).
2. Hypotension may commonly occur, caused by vasodilatation from sympathectomy, fluid depletion, or a combination of the two. Although the treatment of the fluid depletion is carefully titrated fluid management, the sympathectomy is more difficult to treat. There may be an early response to intravenous fluids but the effect may be transient and can result in excessive fluid administration, predisposing to edema, which is highly undesirable in both the lungs and any bowel anastomosis,

Table 1
Insertion of epidurals in patients receiving coagulation-modifying therapy

Drug Class	Safe to Insert Once Stopped	Comments
Heparin (unfractionated) prophylaxis dose	>4 h	Can confirm with normal APTT too
Heparin (fractionated) prophylaxis dose	>12 h	—
Heparin (fractionated) treatment dose	>24 h	—
Aspirin/dipyridamole	No precautions required	Irreversible platelet inhibition
Thienopyridines* (eg, clopidogrel)	1 wk	Irreversible platelet inhibition
Glycoprotein IIb/IIIa* inhibitors (eg, abciximab)	48 h	—
Warfarin	4–5 d	Check INR <1.4
Factor Xa inhibitors* (eg, rivaroxaban)	At least 24–48 h	Longer in elderly and/or reduced renal function
Thrombolytic drugs (eg, streptokinase)	10 d	—

Abbreviation: APTT, activated partial thromboplastin time.
   * The times quoted are for the specific drugs mentioned. Other drugs in that drug class may have different durations of action.

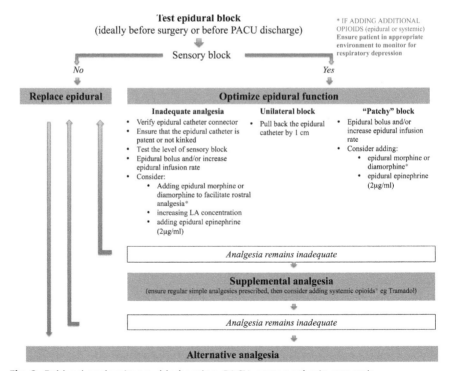

Fig. 2. Epidural analgesia: troubleshooting. PACU, postanesthesia care unit.

particularly if the epidural (and sympathectomy) is then stopped and there is further relative fluid overload as vascular tone begins to increase while the intravascular volume remains unchanged. A more logical approach is the use of vasoactive drugs to maintain perfusion pressure to the anastomosis,[16] but this requires the patient to be nursed in a more intensive environment (eg, critical care or high-dependency unit).

3. A catastrophic complication is vertebral canal and spinal cord compression from hematoma or abscess and its early recognition and management is of paramount importance. This condition usually presents with leg weakness and back pain. The epidural needs to be stopped immediately and, if there is no resolution of leg weakness, urgent imaging of the spine is required, with urgent spinal decompression required to prevent neurologic injury. It is paramount that good training and monitoring for this complication is in place.[17]

4. Accidental dural puncture should be a rare occurrence (0.5%) with appropriate training and skill. It can cause a severe postdural puncture headache and, rarely, more serious complications, including subdural hematoma. Severe postdural puncture headache is usually treated by autologous blood patching; commonly required in obstetric patients but much rarer in older patients undergoing major abdominal surgery.

Epidural analgesia has a considerable evidence base to support its use for open surgery. There is little to support its use on laparoscopic surgery,[8] for which it is regarded as unnecessary and even prolonging length of hospital stay (LOS),[9] although we consider the use of a thoracic epidural for patients having laparoscopic surgery who are at high risk for pulmonary complications, because epidurals may have a place in reducing these complications.[18] Another difficult issue from a practical standpoint is the unexpected prolonged laparoscopic cases or conversion to open surgery, for which an epidural may need to be sited postoperatively, with perhaps extra risks and/or issues with consent.

Intrathecal Analgesia

Intrathecal or spinal analgesia has functional similarities to epidural analgesia, but because it invariably involves a single-shot injection into the cerebrospinal fluid (rather than catheter placement) its duration of action is limited and its use is thus generally unsuitable for major open abdominal surgery. It is more logical for laparoscopic surgery, for which wound pain relief requirements are more modest, with many anesthesiologists having gained experience in intrathecal analgesia from other types of surgery (eg, cesarean sections). It also has a rapid onset of action, particularly the sympathetic blockade, which can be profound in the elderly, in the presence of hypovolemia, or with positioning the patient head down.

As with epidurals, a combination of local anesthetic (either hypobaric plain bupivacaine or hyperbaric bupivacaine) with an opioid (such as fentanyl, diamorphine, or morphine) is traditionally used. Some clinicians have tried shorter-acting local anesthetics (such as prilocaine) or adjuvants such as clonidine to enhance the quality of block and minimize side effects. In addition, similar contraindications for intrathecal analgesia and epidural analgesia exist, although given that spinals are more than 2.5 times as safe as epidurals for serious sequelae[17] (perhaps related to the smaller size of a spinal needle and the absence of passing a catheter) there is a more relaxed view of intrathecal analgesia compared with epidural analgesia in the presence of a coagulopathy.

The major side effect is hypotension, which can be rapid in onset and at times profound, and many clinicians choose to use intraoperative arterial access with invasive blood pressure transducing perioperatively. Vasopressors and/or sympathomimetics should always be at hand.

Outcomes

Evidence for spinal anesthesia in laparoscopic surgery over the last 5 years has increased. There are several studies confirming its safety efficacy both for 23-hour-stay surgery[19] and also its superiority compared with epidural analgesia, with a marked opioid-sparing effect and rapid return to GI function and reduced LOS.[9] Other clinicians have found less consistent results, albeit with better analgesia and reduced LOS, with either no effect on return to gut function and PONV[20] or with excessive respiratory depression with spinal morphine in the elderly.[21] There is little to support its use following prolonged laparoscopic or open surgery because the analgesia may have started to subside before the end of surgery. However, although it is regarded as a safer technique than epidural analgesia, it has risks and many clinicians think that even spinal analgesia may not be warranted in the future for laparoscopic surgery.

LOCAL ANESTHETIC DRUGS ADMINISTERED PERIPHERALLY

Although the use of local anesthetics administered centrally (eg, epidural or intrathecal) is effective, hypotension and reduced mobility are common and the potential for harm is great. Administering local anesthetics more peripherally on the pain pathway, such as with transversus abdominis plane (TAP) blocks, rectus sheath blocks, intraperitoneal instillation, and wound catheters, is considered safer in this regard. However, some of the techniques use large amounts of local anesthetic and the risk of high plasma levels of local anesthetic and the concomitant cardiac toxicity and neurotoxicity should not be underestimated. The location of lipid emulsion in clinical areas and knowledge of its administration to treat local anesthetic toxicity should be readily to hand.

TAP blocks were popularized nearly 10 years ago and have a growing evidence base to support their use. Local anesthetic is instilled between internal oblique and transversus abdominis muscles, preferably using ultrasonography. A blind technique was originally used, using a double-pop technique as a blunted needle passes through the external and internal oblique muscles. The needle is inserted in the lumbar triangle of Petit, the borders of which are the external oblique muscle anteriorly, the latissimus dorsi muscle posteriorly, and the iliac crest inferiorly. A large volume (20 mL) of local anesthetic provides block of the T10 to L1 dermatomes, and covers incision for specimen and some port sites. TAP blocks have been used in open and laparoscopic surgery, for which reductions in pain scores and morphine use (in the first 24 hours), time to tolerating diet, PONV, and LOS have been described.[22-24] Results from recent meta-analysis showed that preoperative TAP blocks provide greater analgesia than postoperative TAP blocks.[25] It is generally safe, although liver trauma has been described with inexpert clinicians.[26] Laparoscopy-guided TAP block has also been successfully used recently.[25,27,28] Subcostal TAP blocks are performed to provide analgesia in the upper quadrants of the abdominal wall.[29,30] The analgesic efficacy of TAP blocks can be prolonged by intermittent boluses or continuous infusion of local anesthetic through multihole catheters placed between the internal oblique and transversus abdominis muscle.[31-33]

Rectus sheath blocks have also used but the evidence base is mainly for gynecologic and urologic surgery and pediatric hernias. Like TAP blocks, they can be inserted by a loss of resistance or ultrasonography, although the surgeon can also insert them under direct vision. A catheter is commonly left in situ and local anesthetic can be administered either by bolus dosing or via infusion.

Wound catheters or surgical site analgesia have also been described for open surgery. These devices are multihole catheters placed in the preperitoneal space during layered closure, following which local anesthetic is administered via bolus or preferably by infusion for 48 hours or so.

The analgesic efficacy of these techniques has been compared with patients receiving systemic opioids, and recently with patients receiving thoracic epidural analgesia.[34,35] Results are varied, with Bertoglio and colleagues[34] reporting similar pain scores but less PONV and accelerated return of bowel function and reduced LOS compared with the epidural group, although these findings were not repeated in a later study by Jouve and colleagues.[35] Concerns of an increased wound infection rate seem to be unsubstantiated.

Intraperitoneal Local Anesthetic

Administering local anesthetic directly into the peritoneum was first described for open procedures more than 60 years ago but interest in this technique has been rekindled more recently for laparoscopic procedures such as gastric surgery, cholecystectomy, colonic resection, and gynecologic procedures. It is a promising technique, using 20 mL of 0.5% bupivacaine, and reductions in pain, morphine consumption, shoulder pain, and stress response activation have been described.[36,37]

SYSTEMIC ANALGESICS

In the quest to reduce systemic morphine consumption, several drugs with little or no opioid action have been successfully used.

Acetaminophen (Paracetamol)

Acetaminophen has been used for more than 125 years and is used worldwide with an excellent safety record, although hepatotoxicity, resulting from altered metabolism or prescription errors, has been recorded. Issues relating to variable bioavailability (particularly when administered rectally) have been solved with widespread use of an intravenous preparation, particularly valuable for GI patients who are unable to take medication orally. It is commonly used regularly for both open and laparoscopic surgery for 48 hours and has a good opioid-sparing effect. The maximum dose is 1 g 4 times per day for patients weighing more than 50 kg. There is some evidence to support a 2-g loading dose, with better pain relief and no increase in toxicity.

Antiinflammatory Drugs

The cyclooxygenase (COX) inhibitors are usually subdivided according to whether they are nonselective (ie, inhibit both the constitutive COX-1 isoform and the inducible COX-2 isoforms) or whether they inhibit principally the COX-2 isoform. Both drugs are commonly used, although care is required in the use of these drugs in patients with cardiac and cerebrovascular disease because of increased risk of thrombotic events. A more specific concern for GI patients is the increased risk of anastomotic leakage reported with both nonselective COX inhibitors (eg, diclofenac)[38] and COX-2 inhibitors after colonic surgery,[39] with a recent study suggesting that nonselective COX inhibitors were more likely to be implicated.[40] However, these drugs are still widely used, but their potential detrimental effects on healing, both in GI surgery and in other surgery (orthopedics), has led to reluctance by some clinicians to use these agents.

Intravenous Lidocaine

Intravenous lidocaine as an analgesic was described more than 50 years ago and has recently been reintroduced. A dose of 1.5 to 2 mg/kg is typically given before the surgical incision and then 1.5 to 2 mg/kg for up to 24 hours postoperatively, usually in a critical care or high-dependency environment. It has several beneficial effects apart from reducing opioid requirements (by up to two-thirds): there is a reduced duration of PONV, ileus, and hospital stay.[41,42] In addition, there are other systemic effects, such as reduced stress response as measured by total leukocyte count, C-reactive protein, and interleukin-6 (IL-6),[43] and possibly an anticancer effect too.[44] Many of these effects seem to be more marked for open surgery. There is good evidence to support its use, particularly as a second-line drug, and it is perhaps surprising that it is not more commonly used, although caution is urged concerning its safety given that some studies have observed toxic levels and others did not look for signs of toxicity.[41] Furthermore, its use in the postoperative period is limited because continuous cardiovascular monitoring is required.

Gabapentinoids (Gabapentin and Pregabalin)

These agents, which are familiar to chronic pain physicians, are now increasingly used for postoperative pain, with patients benefiting from reduced pain, opioid sparing, and a reduction in PONV. There is more evidence to support gabapentin because it is an older drug, but pregabalin has a better pharmacokinetic profile. There are many areas of debate, such as the dose and duration perioperatively, and perhaps most importantly how they affect the incidence of the progression to chronic pain syndromes. Common side effects include sedation and dizziness, and visual disturbances in the case of pregabalin, and these will probably limit their widespread clinical usefulness. A single dose of pregabalin 150 to 300 mg preoperatively is commonly used, but side effects are more common at the higher dose.[45,46]

N-Methyl-d-Aspartate Receptor Antagonists (Ketamine and Magnesium)

NMDA glutamate receptor activation is involved in several aspects of acute pain, including acute tolerance and hyperalgesia with central sensitization. Several drugs are antagonists at these excitatory receptors, including ketamine and magnesium, and both have been used to provide analgesia. Many anesthesiologists are more familiar with ketamine and its analgesic actions. NMDA glutamate receptor activation has been used to provide postoperative pain in several ways: mixed with morphine PCA (which has a more beneficial action for chest rather than abdominal surgery),[47] and also given intraoperatively, both as a bolus and infusion. As with the anticonvulsants agents, the optimal timing, dose, and duration is undecided, but when given at low doses (2 µg/kg/min after a 0.5-mg/kg bolus) morphine consumption was halved and the expected side effects, such as sedation, delusions, nightmares, and psychiatric disorders, were not an issue at these doses.[48] It also reduced the inflammatory response, as measured by IL-6.[49] Magnesium also has a documented place as an analgesic, but its other effects, such as potentiation of neuromuscular blockade and effects on cardiac conduction, will probably limits its use.[50]

Alpha-2 Agonists (Clonidine, Dexmedetomidine)

These agents reduce sympathetic outflow and norepinephrine release within the central and peripheral nervous systems, which has a multitude of effects including inhibiting pain pathways (and release of substance P). There are predictable side effects from their action and the Perioperative Ischemic Evaluation-2 trial highlighted these,[51] showing that clonidine was associated with significant excess in clinically significant hypotension, bradycardia, and (nonfatal) cardiac arrest. These side effects, as well as a lack of good-quality data on these agents, are sure to limit its usefulness, with optimum dose, timing, and routes of administration remaining largely unknown.

Peripheral Opioid Antagonists

Drugs such as alvimopan (a peripherally acting μ-opioid receptor antagonist) antagonize the peripheral adverse effects of opioids (eg, constipation), with the central analgesic effects unaffected. A few trials have shown benefit in open surgery, with reductions in time taken for return of GI function and LOS, but further work is needed to determine the usefulness of this approach, including its impact in laparoscopic surgery and cost-benefit analyses.[52]

Glucocorticoids

These agents, which are often used as perioperative antiemetics, have other actions too, including mild opioid-sparing effects,[53] reductions in length of stay, and modifications of the stress response, apparently without increasing complications (such as anastomotic leak). Further studies are underway to define their place within ERAS for abdominal surgery.[54]

SUMMARY

There are a multitude of analgesic techniques described and the combinations are therefore many. For open surgery, a thoracic epidural for 48 to 72 hours, with regular acetaminophen and antiinflammatories, is probably the treatment of choice provided there are no contraindications. For laparoscopic surgery, either intrathecal or local anesthesia in the wound combined with regular acetaminophen and antiinflammatory drugs is effective. If epidurals fail or are not used for open surgery, the best evidence is for intravenous lidocaine. For many of the other techniques described there is a weaker body of supporting evidence, but they are often used where local expertise has developed. Readers are directed to the PROSPECT (Procedure-specific Postoperative Pain Management) Web site at http://www.postoppain.org/ for the most recent evidence-based recommendations. Analgesia has come a long way from the immediate relief of postoperative pain: clinicians are now starting to determine how it may not only affect short-term outcome but may have a variety of effects on long-term outcome, including survival after major cancer surgery.[6]

REFERENCES

1. Khuri SF, Henderson WG, DePalma RG, et al. Determinants of long-term survival after major surgery and the adverse effect of postoperative complications. Ann Surg 2005;242(3):326–41 [discussion: 341–3].
2. Fearon KC, Ljungqvist O, Von Meyenfeldt M, et al. Enhanced recovery after surgery: a consensus review of clinical care for patients undergoing colonic resection. Clin Nutr 2005;24(3):466–77.
3. Snyder GL, Greenberg S. Effect of anaesthetic technique and other perioperative factors on cancer recurrence. Br J Anaesth 2010;105(2):106–15.
4. Myles PS, Peyton P, Silbert B, et al. Perioperative epidural analgesia for major abdominal surgery for cancer and recurrence-free survival: randomised trial. BMJ 2011;342:d1491.

5. Day A, Smith R, Jourdan I, et al. Retrospective analysis of the effect of postoperative analgesia on survival in patients after laparoscopic resection of colorectal cancer. Br J Anaesth 2012;109(2):185–90.
6. Fawcett WJ, Mythen MG, Scott MJ. Enhanced recovery: more than just reducing length of stay? Br J Anaesth 2012;109(5):671–4.
7. Kehlet H, Dahl JB. The value of "multimodal" or "balanced analgesia" in postoperative pain treatment. Anesth Analg 1993;77(5):1048–56.
8. Levy BF, Tilney HS, Dowson HM, et al. A systematic review of postoperative analgesia following laparoscopic colorectal surgery. Colorectal Dis 2010;12(1):5–15.
9. Levy BF, Scott MJ, Fawcett W, et al. Randomized clinical trial of epidural, spinal or patient-controlled analgesia for patients undergoing laparoscopic colorectal surgery. Br J Surg 2011;98(8):1068–78.
10. Colvin LA, Fallon MT. Opioid-induced hyperalgesia: a clinical challenge. Br J Anaesth 2010;104(2):125–7.
11. Zhao M, Joo DT. Enhancement of spinal N-methyl-D-aspartate receptor function by remifentanil action at delta-opioid receptors as a mechanism for acute opioid-induced hyperalgesia or tolerance. Anesthesiology 2008;109(2):308–17.
12. Finucane BT, Ganapathy S, Carli F, et al. Prolonged epidural infusions of ropivacaine (2 mg/mL) after colonic surgery: the impact of adding fentanyl. Anesth Analg 2001;92(5):1276–85.
13. Gogarten W, Vandermeulen E, Van Aken H, et al. Regional anaesthesia and antithrombotic agents: recommendations of the European Society of Anaesthesiology. Eur J Anaesthesiol 2010;27(12):999–1015.
14. Horlocker TT, Wedel DJ, Rowlingson JC, et al. Regional anesthesia in the patient receiving antithrombotic or thrombolytic therapy: American Society of Regional Anesthesia and Pain Medicine Evidence-Based Guidelines (third edition). Reg Anesth Pain Med 2010;35(1):64–101.
15. Hermanides J, Hollmann MW, Stevens MF, et al. Failed epidural: causes and management. Br J Anaesth 2012;109(2):144–54.
16. Gould TH, Grace K, Thorne G, et al. Effect of thoracic epidural anaesthesia on colonic blood flow. Br J Anaesth 2002;89(3):446–51.
17. Third National Audit Project of the Royal College of Anaesthetists (NAP3): major complications of central neuraxial block. Available at: http://www.rcoa.ac.uk/system/files/CSQ-NAP3-Full_1.pdf. Accessed December 8, 2014.
18. Popping DM, Elia N, Marret E, et al. Protective effects of epidural analgesia on pulmonary complications after abdominal and thoracic surgery: a meta-analysis. Arch Surg 2008;143(10):990–9 [discussion: 1000].
19. Levy BF, Scott MJ, Fawcett WJ, et al. 23-hour-stay laparoscopic colectomy. Dis Colon Rectum 2009;52(7):1239–43.
20. Virlos I, Clements D, Beynon J, et al. Short-term outcomes with intrathecal versus epidural analgesia in laparoscopic colorectal surgery. Br J Surg 2010;97(9):1401–6.
21. Wongyingsinn M, Baldini G, Stein B, et al. Spinal analgesia for laparoscopic colonic resection using an enhanced recovery after surgery programme: better analgesia, but no benefits on postoperative recovery: a randomized controlled trial. Br J Anaesth 2012;108(5):850–6.
22. Zafar N, Davies R, Greenslade GL, et al. The evolution of analgesia in an 'accelerated' recovery programme for resectional laparoscopic colorectal surgery with anastomosis. Colorectal Dis 2010;12(2):119–24.
23. Johns N, O'Neill S, Ventham NT, et al. Clinical effectiveness of transversus abdominis plane (TAP) block in abdominal surgery: a systematic review and meta-analysis. Colorectal Dis 2012;14(10):e635–42.

24. De Oliveira GS Jr, Castro-Alves LJ, Nader A, et al. Transversus abdominis plane block to ameliorate postoperative pain outcomes after laparoscopic surgery: a meta-analysis of randomized controlled trials. Anesth Analg 2014;118(2):454–63.

25. Favuzza J, Delaney CP. Outcomes of discharge after elective laparoscopic colorectal surgery with transversus abdominis plane blocks and enhanced recovery pathway. J Am Coll Surg 2013;217(3):503–6.

26. Lancaster P, Chadwick M. Liver trauma secondary to ultrasound-guided transversus abdominis plane block. Br J Anaesth 2010;104(4):509–10.

27. Favuzza J, Brady K, Delaney CP. Transversus abdominis plane blocks and enhanced recovery pathways: making the 23-h hospital stay a realistic goal after laparoscopic colorectal surgery. Surg Endosc 2013;27(7):2481–6.

28. Keller DS, Stulberg JJ, Lawrence JK, et al. Process control to measure process improvement in colorectal surgery: modifications to an established enhanced recovery pathway. Dis Colon Rectum 2014;57(2):194–200.

29. Niraj G, Kelkar A, Jeyapalan I, et al. Comparison of analgesic efficacy of subcostal transversus abdominis plane blocks with epidural analgesia following upper abdominal surgery. Anaesthesia 2011;66(6):465–71.

30. Wu Y, Liu F, Tang H, et al. The analgesic efficacy of subcostal transversus abdominis plane block compared with thoracic epidural analgesia and intravenous opioid analgesia after radical gastrectomy. Anesth Analg 2013;117(2):507–13.

31. Allcock E, Spencer E, Frazer R, et al. Continuous transversus abdominis plane (TAP) block catheters in a combat surgical environment. Pain Med 2010;11(9): 1426–9.

32. Kadam VR, Moran JL. Epidural infusions versus transversus abdominis plane (TAP) block infusions: retrospective study. J Anesth 2011;25(5):786–7.

33. Niraj G, Kelkar A, Hart E, et al. Comparison of analgesic efficacy of four-quadrant transversus abdominis plane (TAP) block and continuous posterior TAP analgesia with epidural analgesia in patients undergoing laparoscopic colorectal surgery: an open-label, randomised, non-inferiority trial. Anaesthesia 2014;69(4): 348–55.

34. Bertoglio S, Fabiani F, Negri PD, et al. The postoperative analgesic efficacy of preperitoneal continuous wound infusion compared to epidural continuous infusion with local anesthetics after colorectal cancer surgery: a randomized controlled multicenter study. Anesth Analg 2012;115(6):1442–50.

35. Jouve P, Bazin JE, Petit A, et al. Epidural versus continuous preperitoneal analgesia during fast-track open colorectal surgery: a randomized controlled trial. Anesthesiology 2013;118(3):622–30.

36. Kahokehr A, Sammour T, Shoshtari KZ, et al. Intraperitoneal local anesthetic improves recovery after colon resection: a double-blinded randomized controlled trial. Ann Surg 2011;254(1):28–38.

37. Kahokehr A, Sammour T, Soop M, et al. Intraperitoneal local anaesthetic in abdominal surgery - a systematic review. ANZ J Surg 2011;81(4):237–45.

38. Klein M, Andersen LP, Harvald T, et al. Increased risk of anastomotic leakage with diclofenac treatment after laparoscopic colorectal surgery. Dig Surg 2009;26(1): 27–30.

39. Holte K, Andersen J, Jakobsen DH, et al. Cyclo-oxygenase 2 inhibitors and the risk of anastomotic leakage after fast-track colonic surgery. Br J Surg 2009; 96(6):650–4.

40. Gorissen KJ, Benning D, Berghmans T, et al. Risk of anastomotic leakage with non-steroidal anti-inflammatory drugs in colorectal surgery. Br J Surg 2012; 99(5):721–7.

41. Vigneault L, Turgeon AF, Cote D, et al. Perioperative intravenous lidocaine infusion for postoperative pain control: a meta-analysis of randomized controlled trials. Can J Anaesth 2011;58(1):22–37.
42. Sun Y, Li T, Wang N, et al. Perioperative systemic lidocaine for postoperative analgesia and recovery after abdominal surgery: a meta-analysis of randomized controlled trials. Dis Colon Rectum 2012;55(11):1183–94.
43. Sridhar P, Sistla SC, Ali SM, et al. Effect of intravenous lignocaine on perioperative stress response and post-surgical ileus in elective open abdominal surgeries: a double-blind randomized controlled trial. ANZ J Surg 2014. [Epub ahead of print].
44. Lirk P, Berger R, Hollmann MW, et al. Lidocaine time- and dose-dependently demethylates deoxyribonucleic acid in breast cancer cell lines in vitro. Br J Anaesth 2012;109(2):200–7.
45. Ramaswamy S, Wilson JA, Colvin L. Non-opioid-based adjuvant analgesia in perioperative care. Cont Educ Anaesth Crit Care Pain 2013;13:152–7.
46. Zhang J, Ho KY, Wang Y. Efficacy of pregabalin in acute postoperative pain: a meta-analysis. Br J Anaesth 2011;106(4):454–62.
47. Carstensen M, Moller AM. Adding ketamine to morphine for intravenous patient-controlled analgesia for acute postoperative pain: a qualitative review of randomized trials. Br J Anaesth 2010;104(4):401–6.
48. Zakine J, Samarcq D, Lorne E, et al. Postoperative ketamine administration decreases morphine consumption in major abdominal surgery: a prospective, randomized, double-blind, controlled study. Anesth Analg 2008;106(6):1856–61.
49. Dale O, Somogyi AA, Li Y, et al. Does intraoperative ketamine attenuate inflammatory reactivity following surgery? A systematic review and meta-analysis. Anesth Analg 2012;115(4):934–43.
50. Fawcett WJ, Haxby EJ, Male DA. Magnesium: physiology and pharmacology. Br J Anaesth 1999;83(2):302–20.
51. Devereaux PJ, Sessler DI, Leslie K, et al. Clonidine in patients undergoing noncardiac surgery. N Engl J Med 2014;370(16):1504–13.
52. Vaughan-Shaw PG, Fecher IC, Harris S, et al. A meta-analysis of the effectiveness of the opioid receptor antagonist alvimopan in reducing hospital length of stay and time to GI recovery in patients enrolled in a standardized accelerated recovery program after abdominal surgery. Dis Colon Rectum 2012;55(5):611–20.
53. Waldron NH, Jones CA, Gan TJ, et al. Impact of perioperative dexamethasone on postoperative analgesia and side-effects: systematic review and meta-analysis. Br J Anaesth 2013;110(2):191–200.
54. Srinivasa S, Kahokehr AA, Yu TC, et al. Preoperative glucocorticoid use in major abdominal surgery: systematic review and meta-analysis of randomized trials. Ann Surg 2011;254(2):183–91.

Pathophysiology of Major Surgery and the Role of Enhanced Recovery Pathways and the Anesthesiologist to Improve Outcomes

Michael J. Scott, MB ChB, MRCP, FRCA, FFICM[a,b,]*,
Timothy E. Miller, MB ChB, FRCA[c]

KEYWORDS

- Enhanced recovery pathway • Fast-track surgery • Anesthesia • Perioperative care
- Pathophysiology of surgery • Stress response to surgery
- Metabolic response to surgery • Minimally invasive surgery

KEY POINTS

- Enhanced recovery pathways aim to reduce the stress response and improve the metabolic response to surgery restoring the patient to preoperative function more quickly.
- It is increasingly recognized that rapid, uncomplicated, recovery reduces not only the cost and length of stay of the patient episode but medical and possibly surgical related complications. Provided defined discharge criteria are met readmission rates are not increased.
- Minimally invasive surgery is a key component of enhanced recovery to reduce the primary injury of tissue damage and blood loss, which both drive the stress response and metabolic response to surgery.
- All elements of an enhanced recovery pathway are important because they interact positively with each other, a term likened to the sum of small gains.
- The anesthesiologist plays a key role in optimizing surgical outcomes by controlling a patient's physiology throughout the perioperative pathway.

[a] Department of Anesthesia and Perioperative Medicine, Royal Surrey County Hospital NHS Foundation Trust, Egerton Road, Surrey, Guildford GU1 7XX, United Kingdom; [b] Surrey Perioperative Anesthesia Critical Care Research Group (SPACeR), University of Surrey, Surrey, Guildford GU2 7XH, United Kingdom; [c] Department of Anesthesiology, Duke University Medical Center, BOX 3094, HAFS 5677, Durham, NC 27710, USA
* Corresponding author. Department of Anesthesia and Perioperative Medicine, Royal Surrey County Hospital NHS Foundation Trust, Egerton Road, Surrey, Guildford GU1 7XX.
E-mail address: mjpscott@btinternet.com

Anesthesiology Clin 33 (2015) 79–91
http://dx.doi.org/10.1016/j.anclin.2014.11.006   anesthesiology.theclinics.com
1932-2275/15/$ – see front matter © 2015 Elsevier Inc. All rights reserved.

INTRODUCTION

This article provides an overview of the pathophysiologic process of major surgery and how the perioperative management of patients within an enhanced recovery pathway (ERP) can improve recovery after surgery with the aim of reducing stress and complications and improve postoperative function and outcomes.[1–4] A detailed presentation of the biochemical, neuroendocrine, and immunologic changes is beyond the scope of this article.

ERPs, or fast-track surgery, were originally implemented by Henrik Kehlet in colorectal surgery in Denmark in the late 1990s.[5] He asked the fundamental question: why is the patient still in hospital after surgery? He noted that although the causes were multifactorial the common end points were that patients did not have return of gut function and had poor postoperative mobility and function. He devised a protocolized pathway aimed at addressing these issues by reducing any small element that had a negative impact on recovery and promoting early enteral feeding and mobility. The main elements to reduce the stress response and alter the metabolic response to surgery were formalized in a Consensus Guideline by the Enhanced Recovery After Surgery (ERAS) Society in 2005 by Fearon and colleagues for colorectal surgery. Since then the colorectal guidelines have been revised twice by the ERAS Society with the view of keeping the evidence up to date. For instance, in the 2012 guidelines there was an important change in direction recognizing that in laparoscopic colorectal surgery the benefits of thoracic epidural anesthesia (TEA) seen in open colorectal surgery were not directly transferable to laparoscopic surgery.[6]

There are now multinational guideline groups developing guidelines across all surgical specialties and so far evidence-based guidelines have been published or are being developed in pancreatectomy,[7] gastric resection,[8] cystectomy,[9] pelvic and rectal surgery,[10] gynecology, and esophagectomy. The spread and adoption of ERPs has been rapid and some centers in the United Kingdom now have ERPs in all elective surgical specialties, and emergency orthopedic and abdominal surgery.

The ERAS elements are shown in **Fig. 1**, grouped into preoperative, intraoperative, and postoperative factors. The elements themselves and evidence base behind them are not listed here because they are covered elsewhere in this issue and in the article by Gustafsson and coworkers.[6] The ERAS elements can be further categorized into the following groups with some appearing in more than one group:

1. **Preadmission:** counseling, assessment, and optimization
2. **Standards of care:** antibiotic prophylaxis, thromboprophylaxis, prevention of postoperative nausea and vomiting, maintenance of normothermia
3. **Elements to reduce the pathophysiologic insult:** avoidance of bowel preparation, avoidance of nasogastric tubes, minimally invasive surgery, short-acting anesthetic agents, TEA in open surgery, no drains, early removal of catheters
4. **Elements to avoid postoperative gut dysfunction and ileus:** avoidance of salt and water overload, minimally invasive surgery, stimulation of gut motility, nonopioid oral analgesia and nonsteroidal anti-inflammatory drugs, regional anesthesia
5. **Elements to improve the metabolic response to surgery:** avoidance of prolonged starvation, carbohydrate loading, early enteral feeding
6. **Audit:** compliance and outcome

A key issue to ensure the success of an ERP is compliance with all the elements.[11] Gustafsson's group using a large database showed that with increasing compliance with the number of ERAS elements there was a proportional reduction in length of

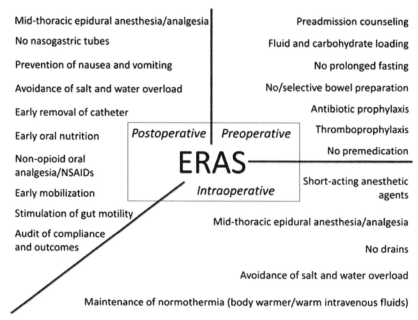

Fig. 1. Enhanced recovery after surgery elements. NSAID, nonsteroidal anti-inflammatory drugs.

stay and complications.[12] It is therefore important to have regular audit and compliance even in centers with established ERPs.

OVERVIEW OF CELLULAR INJURY AND THE STRESS AND METABOLIC RESPONSE TO SURGERY

Primary cellular injury during the perioperative process can be caused by direct surgical injury (from trauma, heating, vaporization, traction, and so forth) or indirect injury from changes in global or local perfusion impairing oxygen and nutrient delivery.

Secondary injury is caused by the effect of locally released inflammatory mediators or the systemic effect of cytokines, inflammatory mediators, or hormones, often termed the stress response to surgery. The consequential injury that results if left untreated is a patient who is catabolic, immobile, feeling weak, and with gut dysfunction. This compounds the injury, delays healing, may lead to complications. The stress response is an evolutionary response to limit further injury, conserve fluid, and mobilize substrates. The benefit the stress response confers to the patient within modern surgery with the availability of modern medical treatments (eg, intravenous fluid, which can maintain or restore altered physiologic parameters to normal) is questionable and in some instances may even impede recovery (**Tables 1** and **2**).

PRIMARY INJURY
Direct Cellular Injury

Surgical access, tissue dissection, mobilization, and extraction
The stress response to surgery is proportional to the type of injury and duration of insult. This results in localized tissue trauma, and cytokine and inflammatory mediator release, which drive a complex bundle of metabolic, hormonal, and immunologic processes in the body, the so-called stress response. Minimizing this process can

Table 1
Primary and secondary injury following surgery

Primary injury	Direct	Surgical access (wound/organ mobilization)
		Organ removal (dissection/tissue injury)
	Indirect	Blood loss, perfusion, anesthetic technique
Secondary injury	Directly mediated	Cytokine, hormonal, neural
	Consequential	Fasting immobilization

have a profound effect on how the body responds to surgery. However, some surgical procedures have more impact than others, even through similar surgical access sites, because the organ being removed or operated on can trigger a large systemic inflammatory response or impair gut function, which can impair the restoration of normal homeostasis (eg, open two-stage esophagectomy). The development of laparoscopic and robotic-assisted surgery has led to a reduction in the total abdominal wall wound area for patients and reduced intra-abdominal tissue damage by using surgical planes with modern instruments for dissection, which in turn reduces blood loss (**Figs. 2** and **3**). In addition to reducing direct injury, the pain requirements after

Table 2
Key pathophysiologic differences between laparoscopic and open surgery

	Laparoscopic Surgery	Open Surgery
Cardiovascular risk	Equal to open surgery	Equal to laparoscopic surgery
Oxygen delivery	Can be reduced compared with open surgery because of increased aortic afterload and head down or head up position	Can be increased because of epidural block causing vasodilatation
Oxygen consumption driven by cellular injury	Minimized compared with open surgery depending on tissue damage	Depends on primary and secondary cellular injury
Pain after surgery	Severe pain settles after 12–24 h so can be addressed with oral analgesia	Severe pain up to 72 h
Fluid shifts	Minimized after 6 h unless bleeding or gut ileus	Depends on surgery, up to 24 h postoperatively
Postoperative fluid requirements	Intravenous fluid rarely needed beyond 24 h	Intravenous fluids often carried on for duration of epidural
Systemic inflammatory response syndrome	Reduced compared with open surgery	Substantial because of surgical cuts and bowel handling
Gut ileus	Reduced, less surgical bowel handling; lower total intravenous fluid volumes	Can be prolonged
Renal function	Renal perfusion reduced during surgery	Renal perfusion reduced
Mobility after surgery	Good	Often impaired by pain and pumps
Lung function after surgery	Improved compared with open surgery	Can have reduced functional residual capacity, especially if inadequate analgesia or abdominal distention

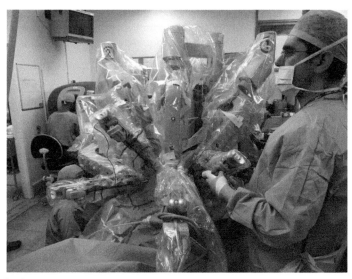

Fig. 2. Robotic surgery.

minimally invasive surgery are such that at 24 hours most visceral pain has diminished so that analgesic requirements can be met with oral analgesics rather than the more complex forms of analgesia used in open surgery, such as TEA or rectus sheath and wound catheters. The reduction of pain also reduces the total surgical stress response through reduction in the neural pathways (see later). Although minimally invasive surgery is increasing there are still many operations where open surgery remains the standard. Advances in surgical technique and the use of modern instruments in open surgery, such as harmonic scalpel, have also led to less tissue injury and blood loss. The fluid shifts as a result are reduced, which in modern ERPs where early enteral

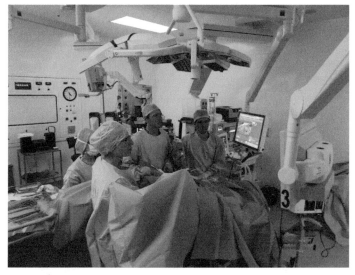

Fig. 3. Laparoscopic surgery.

feeding is promoted has led to simplification of fluid therapy and the reduction in the use of postoperative intravenous fluids. Importantly, reducing the amount of tissue injury also reduces the increased metabolic requirement for oxygen postoperatively (**Box 1**).

Indirect Cellular Injury

Indirect cellular injury during surgery is caused by changes in blood supply or oxygen and nutrient delivery.

Blood loss

Blood loss reduces global oxygen delivery, which can lead to reduction in localized tissue oxygen delivery. Total oxygen delivery is determined by the combination of cardiac output, hemoglobin concentration, and oxygen saturation. Local oxygen delivery can be further complicated by changes in local perfusion, the causes of which are discussed next. Blood loss also triggers a systemic inflammatory response syndrome (SIRS), particularly if intravascular volume is compromised to cause organ dysfunction.[13,14] It is likely this effect is proportional to the total volume of blood loss. Thus, blood loss of up to 5 mL/kg is well tolerated, but increasing losses after this have a greater physiological impact.

Local perfusion and microvascular changes

Local perfusion to organs can be affected by a multitude of factors. Retraction of tissue, clamping or coagulation of blood vessels, and mobilization of the gut can alter local perfusion and delivery of oxygen and nutrients to the cells causing cellular dysfunction. Local perfusion may also be affected during pneumoperitoneum because of direct pressure effects and changes in oxygen delivery[15] and effects on vital organs.[16] Even after surgery there is evidence that microcirculatory blood flow around surgical sites, such as anastomosis, can be impaired for a significant period postoperatively even in the face of normal global oxygen delivery.[17]

Box 1
Key points to reduce the stress and metabolic effects of surgery

Surgical factors

- Reduce primary surgical injury.
- Reduce blood loss.

Anesthetic factors

- Individualized control of patient's physiology during surgery to optimize outcomes.
- Optimal analgesia using regional and local anesthetics, multimodal analgesia, and avoidance of drains to reduce neural activation of stress response. Aim is to reduce total opioid use to avoid risk of gut ileus.
- Individualized fluid therapy to maintain cellular perfusion, reduce extracellular fluid flux, and avoid salt and water overload, which can lead to gut ileus.

Postoperative goals

- Early gut function and enteral feeding to get benefit of hormonal effects of duodenal feeding, maintain gut perfusion, reduced surgical insult, avoid nasogastric tubes, regular small quantities of nutrition.
- Early mobilization to reduce complications, such as chest infection and deep vein thrombosis; stimulate muscle function to maintain strength and reduce insulin resistance.

Anesthetic technique

Anesthetic agents and techniques can have direct and indirect effects on cellular function. The physiologic effects of intermittent positive pressure ventilation have a multitude of effects. Hepatosplanchnic blood flow and renal blood flow are reduced and there is a change in intrathoracic pressure affecting preload and afterload, all of which can lead to alterations in cardiac output and blood pressure with subsequent changes at a microvascular and cellular level. In the presence of Thoracic Epidural Anesthesia (TEA) the gut is pressure dependent such that even if the cardiac output is good a mean arterial pressure less than 60 mm Hg may lead to hypoperfusion.[18]

Most anesthetic drugs reduce vasomotor tone and interfere with autoregulatory mechanisms to maintain local pressure and flow. Remifentanil, which is popular as a continuous opioid infusion for rapid awakening, can reduce venous tone and pulse pressure. TEA and spinal anesthesia effect arteriolar and venous tone because of a sympathetic block, which leads to vasodilatation and hypotension unless corrected by the anesthetist. Vasopressors can restore these physiologic effects but if used inappropriately they can also cause problems particularly if vasoconstriction is maintained in the face of hypovolemia. Boluses can lead to erratic changes in blood pressure and venous tone because there is variation in arteriolar and venous effect of vasopressors depending on the patient and their intravascular volume status.

Fluid therapy is an important component of Enhanced Recovery under the control of the anesthesiologist. Fluid therapy has a direct effect on intravascular volume and cardiac output with a resultant effect on oxygen and nutrient delivery to the tissues. There are also complex effects downstream on the microcirculation and vascular beds. There are 2 dedicated chapters on fluid therapy and the use of advanced hemodynamic monitoring in this series so the reader is referred to these and this subject is not covered further in this chapter.

The position of the patient during surgery (head up, head down, legs up, legs down) effects intravascular volume and perfusion pressure gradients across tissues. Factors influencing local tissue perfusion by effects on vasomotor tone, vascular volume, or localized blood supply include the following:

Surgical and operative factors
1. Surgical retraction, dissection, mobilization, and extraction
2. Blood loss
3. Pneumoperitoneum

Anesthetic factors
1. Induction of anesthesia
2. Intermittent positive pressure ventilation
3. Ventilatory strategy and positive end-expiratory pressure
4. Patient position: head up, head down, legs up
5. Anesthetic agents
6. Opioids, particularly remifentanil infusions
7. Epidural or spinal anesthesia
8. Vasopressor use: type and dose and whether delivered by infusion or bolus
9. Fluid therapy: can effect central compartment and microvascular flow

SECONDARY INJURY

Secondary injury from surgery is classically described as the stress response. This process releases local cytokine and inflammatory mediators driving a complex process of metabolic, hormonal, and immunologic processes in the whole body. The peak cytokine response and duration is proportional to primary surgical injury and blood loss. These can be minimized by surgical technique. The hormonal and metabolic effects in response to surgery are one of the key factors that an ERP attempts to modify, principally by achieving early gut function (to reverse the catabolic response to surgery) and restoring the patient to independent mobility. Neural effects can also be minimized by appropriate analgesic techniques to reduce the central effects of pain and improve mobility, function, and sleep postoperatively.

Directly Mediated Effects

Cytokine
Cellular injury causes the release of cytokines and inflammatory mediators, such as interleukin IL-6, IL-1, IL-8, tumor necrosis factor-α, and C-reactive protein. This causes local inflammation and stimulation of afferent neurons, which carry impulses through the spinal cord up to the brain. There is release of corticotrophin from the hypothalamus and activation of the locus-coeruleus-noradrenergic systems. Both systems have a positive feedback on each other. The coeruleus-noradrenergic system stimulates the sympathetic nervous system and catecholamine release from the adrenal medulla. Circulating catecholamines have a varied effect on organs and tissue throughout the body. The effect on β cells of the pancreas is to inhibit the secretion of insulin, which is an anabolic hormone.

Hormonal
Hormonal effects after surgery are complex and variable. The key issue for surgical outcome is that the body develops a state of insulin resistance. Insulin is needed for the passage of glucose and amino acids into cells, so this has a direct effect on cellular function and crucially, healing of damaged tissue. Several studies have shown that the degree of insulin resistance is proportional to the magnitude of surgery. Insulin resistance can usually be overcome with administration of more endogenous insulin.[19] Glycemic control has been shown to be an important predictor of complications.[20] Glycemic control within the range of 8 to 10 mmol/L with the use of exogenous insulin is normal practice on intensive care units with the Leuven study showing improved outcomes[21]; however, overaggressive management of blood sugar levels was shown to increase mortality.[22] Early feeding (hormonal effects) and mobility (muscle effect) help to reverse the state of insulin resistance.

Neural
The neural mechanism of the stress response is mediated by receptors activated by tissue injury and subsequent inflammation. Surgical access causes damage to skin and muscle injury, and injury to intra-abdominal organs and the peritoneum cause visceral fiber activation. The ascending pathways cause release of corticotrophin from the hypothalamus and activation of the locus-coeruleus-noradrenergic systems as outlined previously. The key issue for the anesthesiologist is that the use of local, truncal, and regional anesthetic techniques can alter this part of the stress response.[23,24]

Consequential Effects

The result of the stress response, pain and gut dysfunction after surgery, leads to a state of fasting and immobility that can further exacerbate an altered metabolic state of insulin resistance, which reduces the availability of glucose and amino acids for cellular function and repair. Unfortunately, this process is often exacerbated by medical intervention. For instance, the normal treatment of ileus can be insertion of a nasogastric tube and intravenous fluids (often with high sodium), which can lead to further bowel edema and prolong the period of ileus. The abdominal distention leads to pressure on the diaphragm and pulmonary basal hypoventilation, which leads to hypoxia and increased risk of pulmonary infection and a SIRS response. Therefore, a multimodal strategy to prevent ileus is extremely important. The key factors to reduce ileus are reducing surgical manipulation and handling of the gut; maintaining gut perfusion during the perioperative period; avoiding fluid excess, particularly above 30 mL/kg total fluid gain; avoiding salt overload; and reducing opioids to a minimum.

Fasting

Inappropriate postoperative fasting leads to metabolic changes in the body at the time when the body has a high energy requirement to heal injury and maintain immune function. European Society for Clinical Nutrition and Metabolism (ESPEN) guidelines for surgical patients are to reduce periods of fasting to a minimum.

Immobility

The cause of postoperative immobility is usually multifactorial. Patients may be in pain and not able to mobilize, or feel weak and not be able to mobilize without help. Interventions, such as surgical drains, continuous pumps delivering intravenous fluids, and analgesic methods (eg, TEA), make it difficult for patients to move independently. The pathophysiologic result is that the lack of muscle use and the catabolic response of surgery lead to further weakness and muscle loss. Immobility is also a risk factor for developing deep vein thrombosis, which can lead to pulmonary embolus. Respiratory function is also compromised, particularly after abdominal surgery where there is often basal atelectasis and loss of functional residual capacity. The problem is compounded if the patient has poor analgesia or has abdominal distention caused by ileus. This can lead to the development of postoperative chest infection, which in turn can lead to a SIRS response and sepsis (**Fig. 4**).

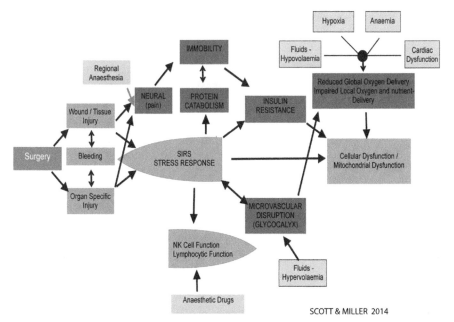

Fig. 4. Diagram showing overview and interrelationship of surgical injury, the stress response, immune response, and cellular dysfunction. Other factors that compound cellular dysfunction are included and key intervention points delivered by the anesthetist. NK, natural killer; SIRS, systemic inflammatory response syndrome.

THE ENHANCED RECOVERY PATHWAY AND ROLE OF THE ANESTHESIOLOGIST

The anesthesiologist is in a position to have significant input into the entire ERP. The ERP starts preoperatively with counseling of the patient. There is increasing recognition of the importance of preoperative assessment, informed decision-making, and risk assessment to ensure the patient is placed on the correct perioperative care pathway. This decision-making process may also be not to operate and for the patient to follow a different clinical treatment modality, such as radiotherapy or chemotherapy. Prehabilitation aims to improve outcomes after surgery by improving the patient's physiologic reserve (discussed elsewhere in this issue).[25]

The anesthesiologist must deliver a suitable anesthetic from which the patient can awaken rapidly with minimal pain, avoiding postoperative nausea and vomiting, and in a fluid-optimized state. Reducing secondary injury is done by modulating the stress response by effective analgesia and early oral intake of food, which stops the catabolic response and promotes anabolism and healing. To achieve this optimal analgesia and fluid therapy are the key components delivered by the anesthetist. By ensuring effective analgesia the stress response is minimized and the patient can mobilize, which in turn leads to reduced pulmonary and thromboembolic complications. Individualized fluid therapy ensures cells have adequate oxygen and nutrient delivery, which in turn avoids cellular dysfunction and complications. The gut perfusion is maintained and enables early feeding, and avoiding fluid overload reduces the risk of ileus. Early feeding and anabolism ensures optimal healing and leads to reduced complications and earlier return to preoperative function. This has led to the description of the trimodal approach delivery of enhanced recovery for anesthesiologists whereby the anesthesiologist delivers individualized fluid therapy and optimal analgesia and most of the other nonsurgical enhanced recovery elements are protocolized in the perioperative care pathway (**Fig. 5**).[26]

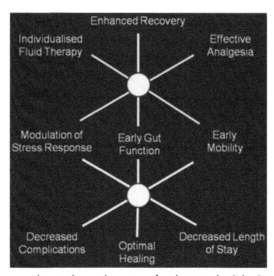

Fig. 5. Trimodal approach to enhanced recovery for the anesthesiologist. (*From* Mythen M, Scott M. Anaesthetic contributions in enhanced recovery. Chapter 4. In: Francis N, Kennedy RH, Ljungqvist O, et al, editors. Manual of fast track recovery for colorectal surgery. London: Springer Science & Business Media; 2012; with permission.)

EVIDENCE BASE FOR ENHANCED RECOVERY PATHWAYS

The adoption of ERPs has now spread across the globe. The evidence base has been growing in open and minimally invasive surgery. The key benefits of ERPs are reducing patient stay (without increase in readmission), improving consistency of length of stay, and improving patient outcomes by reducing complications and restoring patients to preoperative function more quickly.

In the United Kingdom data from the Hospital Episodes Statistics (www.hscic. gov.uk) has shown that since the introduction of ERPs in colorectal, gynecologic, musculoskeletal, and urologic surgery there has been a year on year reduction in length of stay in hospital (LOSH) with no increase in readmission rates. The number of hospitals with unusually high LOSH has been reduced. It is estimated the program has released 118,000 bed-days in the United Kingdom per annum.

A meta-analysis by Varadhan's group in 2010 showed ERPs reduce length of stay in colorectal surgery without increasing admissions.[27] There have been 10 meta-analyses since including newer and similar studies with different conclusions. A critical appraisal of these meta analysis by Chambers and colleagues[28] for ERPs in colorectal surgery concludes that using ERPs there is a reduction in LOSH of 2.5 days. Ultrashort lengths of stay showing the benefit of combining minimally invasive surgery and ERPs have been published with no increase in complications and with good patient satisfaction.[29] There is increasing evidence that good compliance with ERPs can lead to a reduction in complications.[30,31]

Measuring the stress response, immune function, and insulin resistance after surgery and interpreting the results can be difficult. The LAFA study looked at four groups of surgical patients undergoing colorectal surgery: (1) open surgery within an ERP, (2) open surgery without an ERP, (3) laparoscopic surgery within an ERP, and (4) laparoscopic surgery without an ERP.[32] IL-6 and C-reactive protein levels were highest in the open surgery group, as expected. The biggest impact on improving postoperative immune function (measured by effect on HLA-DR) was having laparoscopic surgery and the addition of an ERP improved this further. The open surgical group also demonstrated an improved response within an ERP.

Insulin resistance is difficult to measure in the perioperative setting. In 2012 Ren's group published data from almost 600 patients undergoing surgery either within an ERP or not. They measured insulin resistance using homeostatic model assessment for insulin resistance (HOMA-IR) and showed reduced insulin resistance within the ERP group. Cortisol and cytokines, such as IL-6, IL-1, and tumor necrosis factor-α, were also reduced in the ERP group.[33]

SUMMARY

The pathophysiologic changes during the perioperative surgical pathway are varied and complex. The process is driven by primary surgical injury. ERPs aim to reduce the resulting secondary injury by using a group of evidence-based elements. All the elements in an ERP aim to return the patient to independent mobility with early enteral feeding and restoration of preoperative function as quickly as possible. It is difficult to identify the benefits of each ERP element individually and it is the sum of all the small gains that make the pathway successful. ERPs reduce length of stay, and improve the consistency and quality of the surgical care pathway. There is increasing evidence that there is a reduction in complications and improvement in long-term outcomes. The anesthesiologist plays a key role in delivering care in an ERP by controlling the patient's physiology during surgery and the perioperative period. The anesthesiologist is responsible for two key elements that affect outcome: fluid therapy and optimal analgesia. The surgeon is responsible for reducing primary injury (see **Box 1**).

Clinicians are entering a new era of surgery and perioperative care where it is now recognized that the whole perioperative pathway has an impact on short- and long-term outcome after major abdominal surgery.

REFERENCES

1. Fawcett WJ, Mythen MG, Scott MJ. Enhanced recovery: more than just reducing length of stay? Br J Anaesth 2012;109:671–4.
2. Khuri SF, Henderson WG, DePalma RG. Determinants of long-term survival after major surgery and the adverse effect of postoperative complications. Ann Surg 2005;242:326–41.
3. Moonesinghe SR, Harris S, Mythen MG, et al. Survival after postoperative morbidity: a longitudinal observational cohort study†. Br J Anaesth 2014. [Epub ahead of print].
4. Day AR, Middleton G, Smith RV, et al. Time to adjuvant chemotherapy following colorectal cancer resection is associated with an improved survival. Colorectal Dis 2014;16:368–72.
5. Kehlet H, Wilmore DW. Evidence-based surgical care and the evolution of fast-track surgery. Ann Surg 2008;248:189–98.
6. Gustafsson UO, Scott MJ, Schwenk W, et al. Guidelines for perioperative care in elective colonic surgery: Enhanced Recovery After Surgery (ERAS®) Society Recommendations. World J Surg 2012;37:259–84.
7. Lassen K, Coolsen MM, Slim K, et al. Guidelines for perioperative care for pancreaticoduodenectomy: Enhanced Recovery After Surgery (ERAS®) Society recommendations. Clin Nutr 2012;31:817–30.
8. Mortensen K, Nilsson M, Slim K, et al. Consensus guidelines for enhanced recovery after gastrectomy: Enhanced Recovery After Surgery (ERAS®) Society recommendations. Br J Surg 2014;101:1209–29.
9. Cerantola Y, Valerio M, Persson B, et al. Guidelines for perioperative care after radical cystectomy for bladder cancer: Enhanced Recovery After Surgery (ERAS(®)) society recommendations. Clin Nutr 2013;32:879–87.
10. Nygren J, Thacker J, Carli F, et al. Guidelines for perioperative care in elective rectal/pelvic surgery: Enhanced Recovery After Surgery (ERAS(®)) Society recommendations. World J Surg 2013;37:285–305.
11. Maessen J, Dejong CH, Hausel J, et al. A protocol is not enough to implement an enhanced recovery programme for colorectal resection. Br J Surg 2007;94:224–31.
12. Gustafsson UO, Hausel J, Thorell A, et al. Adherence to the enhanced recovery after surgery protocol and outcomes after colorectal cancer surgery. Arch Surg 2011;146:571–7.
13. Stephan RN, Kupper TS, Geha AS, et al. Hemorrhage without tissue trauma produces immunosuppression and enhances susceptibility to sepsis. Arch Surg 1987;122:62–8.
14. Ayala A, Perrin MM, Meldrum DR, et al. Hemorrhage induces an increase in serum TNF which is not associated with elevated levels of endotoxin. Cytokine 1990;2:170–4.
15. Levy BF, Fawcett WJ, Scott MJ, et al. Intra-operative oxygen delivery in infusion volume-optimized patients undergoing laparoscopic colorectal surgery within an enhanced recovery programme: the effect of different analgesic modalities. Colorectal Dis 2012;14:887–92.

16. Demyttenaere S, Feldman LS, Fried GM. Effect of pneumoperitoneum on renal perfusion and function: a systematic review. Surg Endosc 2007;21:152–60.
17. Schröder W, Stippel D, Gutschow C, et al. Postoperative recovery of microcirculation after gastric tube formation. Arch Surg 2004;389:267–71.
18. Gould TH, Grace K, Thorne G, et al. Effect of thoracic epidural anaesthesia on colonic blood flow. Br J Anaesth 2002;89:446–51.
19. Brandi LS, Frediani M, Oleggini M, et al. Insulin resistance after surgery: normalization by insulin treatment. Clin Sci 1990;79:443–50.
20. Frioud A, Comte-Perret S, Nguyen S, et al. Blood glucose level on postoperative day 1 is predictive of adverse outcomes after cardiovascular surgery. Diabetes Metab 2010;36:36–42.
21. Egi M, Finfer S, Bellomo R. Glycemic control in the ICU. Chest 2011;140:212–20.
22. NICE-SUGAR Study Investigators, Finfer S, Chittock DR, et al. Intensive versus conventional glucose control in critically ill patients. N Engl J Med 2009;360: 1283–97.
23. Sheeran P, Hall GM. Cytokines in anaesthesia. Br J Anaesth 1997;78:201–19.
24. Carli F, Halliday D. Continuous epidural blockade arrests the postoperative decrease in muscle protein fractional synthetic rate in surgical patients. Anesthesiology 1997;86:1033–40.
25. Mayo NE, Feldman L, Scott S, et al. Impact of preoperative change in physical function on postoperative recovery: argument supporting prehabilitation for colorectal surgery. Surgery 2011;150:505–14.
26. Francis N, Kennedy RH, Ljungqvist O, et al. Manual of fast track recovery for colorectal surgery. In: Francis N, Kennedy RH, Ljungqvist O, et al, editors. London: Springer Science & Business Media; 2012.
27. Varadhan KK, Neal KR, Dejong CH, et al. The enhanced recovery after surgery (ERAS) pathway for patients undergoing major elective open colorectal surgery: a meta-analysis of randomized controlled trials. Clin Nutr 2010;29:434–40.
28. Chambers D, Paton F, Wilson P, et al. An overview and methodological assessment of systematic reviews and meta-analyses of enhanced recovery programmes in colorectal surgery. BMJ Open 2014;4:e005014.
29. Scott MJP, Levy BF, Rockall TA, et al. 23-hour-stay laparoscopic colectomy. Dis Colon Rectum 2009;52:1239–43.
30. Jones C, Kelliher L, Dickinson M, et al. Randomized clinical trial on enhanced recovery versus standard care following open liver resection. Br J Surg 2013;100: 1015–24.
31. Markar SR, Karthikesalingam A, Low DE. Enhanced recovery pathways lead to an improvement in postoperative outcomes following esophagectomy: systematic review and pooled analysis. Dis Esophagus 2014. [Epub ahead of print].
32. Veenhof AA, Vlug MS, van der Pas MH, et al. Surgical stress response and postoperative immune function after laparoscopy or open surgery with fast track or standard perioperative care: a randomized trial. Ann Surg 2012;255:216–21.
33. Ren L, Zhu D, Wei Y, et al. Enhanced Recovery After Surgery (ERAS) program attenuates stress and accelerates recovery in patients after radical resection for colorectal cancer: a prospective randomized controlled trial. World J Surg 2012;36:407–14.

Anesthesia for Colorectal Surgery

Gabriele Baldini, MD, MSc[a],*, William J. Fawcett, MB BS, FRCA, FFPMRCA[b]

KEYWORDS

- Colon surgery • Rectum surgery • Optimization • Analgesia • Anesthesia
- Fluid therapy • Goal-directed therapy

KEY POINTS

- Anesthesiologists play a pivotal role in facilitating recovery of patients undergoing colorectal surgery, as many Enhanced Recovery After Surgery (ERAS) elements are under their direct control.
- Successful implementation of ERAS programs requires that anesthesiologists become more involved in perioperative care and more aware about the impact of anesthetic techniques on surgical outcomes and recovery.
- A key area for achieving a successful outcome is the strict adherence to the principle of aggregation of marginal gains.
- Anesthesia considerations for patients with colorectal cancer and those undergoing emergency colorectal surgery are discussed.

INTRODUCTION

Anesthesiologists play a pivotal role in facilitating recovery of patients undergoing colorectal surgery, as many Enhanced Recovery After Surgery (ERAS) elements are under their direct control. Successful implementation of ERAS programs requires firstly that anesthesiologists become more involved in perioperative care and more aware about the impact of anesthetic techniques on surgical outcomes and recovery. Second, there are many evidenced-based steps within ERAS protocols. Although some of these steps may have greater impact than others, a key area for achieving a successful outcome for these patients is the strict adherence to these individual steps: the principle of aggregation of marginal gains.[1] This article reviews anesthetic and analgesic care of patients undergoing elective colorectal surgery in the context of an ERAS program. Anesthesia considerations for patients with colorectal cancer and emergency colorectal surgery are also discussed.

The authors have no conflict of interest.

[a] Department of Anesthesia, Montreal General Hospital, McGill University Health Centre, 1650 Avenue Cedar, Montreal, Quebec H3G 1A4, Canada; [b] Royal Surrey County Hospital, Postgraduate School, University of Surrey, Guildford GU2 7XX, UK
* Corresponding author.
E-mail address: gabriele.baldini@mcgill.ca

Anesthesiology Clin 33 (2015) 93–123
http://dx.doi.org/10.1016/j.anclin.2014.11.007   **anesthesiology.theclinics.com**

PREOPERATIVE PATIENT EDUCATION

Preoperative patient education is an essential component of any ERAS program. Preoperative patient education and preparation has positive effects on outcomes such as pain, psychological distress, and indices of recovery, including hospital stay, even if the intervention is relatively brief and not individualized. Patient expectation may also play a role in postoperative outcome.[2,3] As the enhanced recovery approach may differ from patients' and their caregivers' expectations, it is important to specify the active role the patient is expected to play. Specifications include explicit written information, at an appropriate literacy level, specifying daily goals for nutritional intake and ambulation in the perioperative period, discharge criteria, and expected hospital stay.

PREOPERATIVE EVALUATION, RISK STRATIFICATION, AND OPTIMIZATION

Preoperative evaluation and risk stratification are valuable only if they allow subsequent patient optimization, leading to reduced postoperative mortality and morbidity. Thirty-day mortality after colorectal surgery varies among countries and institutions,[4] and ranges between 2% and 6%.[5,6] Data from 182 hospitals participating in the American College of Surgeons National Surgery Quality Improvement Program (NSQIP) showed that in 28,863 patients undergoing colorectal surgery, overall 30-day mortality was 3.9%.[7] After emergency surgery, 30-day mortality is 3 to 4 times higher than after elective surgery.[5,8] Overall morbidity ranges between 21% and 30%,[7] and is higher after rectal surgery than after colon surgery.[9] Of interest, patients developing complications within 30 days from surgery have a 69% lower chance of surviving at 8 years.[10]

General[7,11] and organ-specific[12–16] preoperative scoring systems and assessment of functional capacity[17,18] can help to predict and stratify preoperative risk. The preoperative evaluation is also an opportunity to improve long-term health besides surgery, such as counseling patients who may benefit from long-term β-blockers, stopping smoking, or tightening glycemic control. Although a substantive discussion about cardiopulmonary risk assessment and reduction is beyond the scope of this article, current guidelines and algorithms are available for assessment and reduction of perioperative risk related to cardiac disease,[19] anemia,[20] pulmonary complications,[21] obesity,[22] obstructive sleep apnea,[23] and diabetes.[24] Preoperative evaluation and risk stratification of elderly patients is complex, and should also measure cognitive function, estimate the risk of postoperative delirium and postoperative falls, and estimate functional capacity and the patient's frailty.[25] Secondary adrenal suppression should be suspected in patients with inflammatory bowel diseases on long-term systemic steroids. Steroids should be continued at the same dose throughout the perioperative period (including the morning of surgery), with higher doses (stress dose) administered only to hypotensive patients in whom arterial hypotension is unrelated to other causes (eg hypovolemia, sepsis).[26]

Preoperative smoking cessation has been shown to improve outcomes,[27] but the optimal duration of preoperative abstinence still remains unclear. It is acknowledged that the implementation of such an approach in clinical practice is not always feasible because of limited hospital resources, lack of organization, and waiting time before the operation. Nevertheless, perioperative caregivers should take the opportunity to emphasize the importance of smoking cessation and be more proactive in helping patients to quit smoking. Preoperative alcohol cessation can improve organ dysfunction, but the effect on postoperative outcomes remains unclear.[28]

Patients undergoing colorectal surgery are commonly malnourished, as undernutrition ranges from approximately 10% to 40% depending on the nutrition risk tool used.

Poor nutritional status is associated with higher morbidity after surgery.[29] Patients with moderate and severe undernutrition benefit from preoperative nutrition, preferably using the enteral route, for 7 to 10 days before major surgery.[30] In patients with less severe malnutrition, including those with diminished oral intake resulting from their underlying disease, oral nutritional supplements are added to their normal diet. Preoperative parenteral nutrition is indicated in severely malnourished patients[31] in whom enteral nutrition is not feasible or not tolerated.[30] Combination with enteral nutrition might be beneficial in patients who need supplemental nutritional support and in whom energy needs cannot be met (<60% of caloric requirements) by the enteral route. Preoperative immune-enhancing nutrition has been shown to reduce postoperative complications after gastrointestinal surgeries, especially for infections,[32] but these results need to be confirmed in a context of a multimodal ERAS program. Moreover, adverse effects have been reported in critically ill patients.[32]

The perioperative period may be associated with rapid physical deconditioning, requiring a period of recovery during which patients are fatigued and quality-of-life and activities are curtailed. Patients with poor baseline exercise tolerance and physical conditioning are at increased risk for serious perioperative complications and prolonged disability,[17] and improving functional capacity by increasing physical activity before surgery may be protective.[33] Physical fitness can be improved in the time that patients are waiting for scheduled surgery, as modest improvements in aerobic capacity can be seen in older adults after training only 1 hour per day, 4 times a week, for 4 weeks. The strategy of augmenting physical capacity with preoperative exercise in combination with nutritional counseling and protein supplementation in anticipation of an upcoming stressor is termed prehabilitation, as opposed to rehabilitation, which begins only after the injury or surgery has occurred.[34] Several small trials have suggested that prehabilitation is effective for improving physical fitness and is safe, although evidence for improved clinical outcomes related to preoperative exercise is limited.[35] Detailed preoperative evaluation and optimization take time and are not always feasible, especially in patients undergoing emergency surgery or colorectal cancer surgery. More studies evaluating the role of optimizing preoperative conditions to a point to delay surgery in patients undergoing oncologic colorectal surgery are warranted (**Table 1**).

PREOPERATIVE FASTING AND PREOPERATIVE ORAL CARBOHYDRATE DRINKS

There is no scientific evidence to support a policy of routine NPO (nothing by mouth) after midnight.[36] Fasting from midnight increases insulin resistance,[37] depletes glycogen reserves,[38] increases patient discomfort,[39] and decreases intravascular volume, mainly in patients receiving mechanical bowel preparation (MBP).[40] In fact, functional intravascular deficit after fasting time, as indicated by guidelines[41] or after 8 hours' fasting,[42] is minimally affected in patients undergoing elective surgeries without MBP.[41,42] Current preoperative fasting guidelines for adult patients undergoing elective surgery recommend a 2-hour fast for liquids and a 6-hour fast for solids.[43] Radiologic studies have further supported the safety of allowing clear fluids up to 2 hours before the induction of anesthesia, showing complete gastric emptying within 90 minutes.[44] These recommendations do not apply to patients with delayed gastric emptying (eg, gastroparesis, gastrointestinal obstruction, upper gastrointestinal tract malignancy). Patients should receive detailed information on what they are allowed to drink and until what time. In addition, written materials should be supplied with information on minimizing fasting times to facilitate the implementation of fasting guidelines.

Table 1
Preoperative risk stratification, evaluation, and optimization

Preoperative Risk Stratification

Scoring systems that predict overall morbidity and mortality
  POSSUM-CR[11]
  ACS NSQIP colorectal risk calculator[7]
  Walking tests[a,17]
  CPET[18]
Examples of organ-specific scoring systems
  Revised Cardiac Risk[12]
  Cardiac Risk Calculator[15]
  Modified Clinical Pulmonary Infection Score[14]
  Postoperative pneumonia risk index[13]
  General Surgery Acute Kidney Injury Risk Index[16]

Preoperative Risk Evaluation and Optimization

Preoperative Risk Evaluation	Preoperative Optimization

Cardiovascular function
  Revised Cardiac Risk[12]
  Cardiac Risk Calculator[15]
  METs[16,19]
	ACC/AHA guidelines[19]

Renal function
  General Surgery Acute Kidney Injury Risk
    Index
	—

Respiratory function
  Modified Clinical Pulmonary Infection
    Score[14]
  Postoperative pneumonia risk index[13]
	American College of Physicians guidelines[21]

Diabetic patients
  Hb_{A1c} >6.0%[24] (even in nondiabetic
    patients[115])
	American Association of Clinical
	  Endocrinologists and American Diabetes
	  Association guideline[24]
	  Exercise
	  Weight loss
	  Glycemic control

Anemia
  Determine the cause of the anemia[20]
	American Anesthesiology Society
	  recommendations[20]
	  Optimize preoperative Hb levels
	  Perioperative blood management strategies

Nutritional status[30]
Evaluation of
  Energy intake
  Recent weight loss or gain
  Body fat, muscle mass, presence or
    absence of fluid accumulation
  Grip strength'
Biochemical nutritional indices
  Serum albumin
  Serum prealbumin
Tools to assess nutritional risk
  Nutritional Risk Screening (NRS-2002)
  Subjective Global Assessment (SGA)
  Malnutrition Universal Screening Tool
    (MUST)
  Nutritional Risk Index (NRI)
Severe nutritional risk[31]
  Weight loss 10%–15% within 6 mo or
  BMI <18.5 kg/m^2
  Subjective Global Assessment Grade C or
  Serum albumin 30 g/L (with no evidence
    of hepatic or renal dysfunction)
	Nutritional support
	Mild nutritional risk
	  Nutritional supplements added to normal diet
	Moderate to severe nutritional risk[31]
	  Enteral nutrition for 7–10 d (even if surgery
	    has to be delayed)
	  Consider combination with parenteral
	    route if >60% of calorie requirement
	    cannot be met
	  Parenteral route if enteral nutrition is not
	    feasible for 5–7 d
	Immune-enhancing nutrition[31,32]
	Prehabilitation[34]

(continued on next page)

Table 1
(continued)

Preoperative Risk Evaluation and Optimization	
Preoperative Risk Evaluation	**Preoperative Optimization**

Frailty (frailty phenotype)[25]
  Weight loss
  Weakness
  Exhaustion
  Slowness
  Low physical activity
	Prehabilitation[34]

Smoking and alcohol abuse	Smoking cessation
	  Multidisciplinary approach
	  Preoperative counseling + NRT
	  The beneficial effect of smoking cessation is correlated with the length of the period of abstinence. Reduction of postoperative complications is seen after at least 3 wk of abstinence before surgery

Functional capacity
  METs[19]
  Walking test[a,17]
  CPET[18]
	Preoperative exercise[34,35]
	Prehabilitation[34]

Secondary adrenal suppression	Continue administration of steroids throughout the perioperative period, including the morning of surgery, at the same dose A higher dose of steroid (stress dose) is required in hypotensive patients, in whom hypotension is unrelated to other causes (eg, hypovolemia, sepsis)[26]

Abbreviations: ACC/AHA, American College of Cardiology/American Heart Association; BMI, body mass index; CPET, cardiopulmonary exercise tests; Hb, hemoglobin; METs, metabolic equivalents; NRT, nicotine replacement therapy.

[a] Six-minute or 2-minute walking test and shuttle-walking test.

Administration of oral carbohydrate (CHO) drinks with a relatively high concentration (12.5%) of complex CHO (maltodextrin), 100 g (800 mL) the evening before elective surgery, and a further 50 g (400 mL) 2 to 3 hours before induction of anesthesia, has been shown to attenuate the catabolic stress response to surgery. This effect seems particularly related to the CHO dose administered 2 to 3 hours before the induction of anesthesia.[45] As a consequence, insulin resistance is decreased, protein breakdown reduced, and muscle strength improved.[46,47] This might turn in a faster surgical recovery as indicated by the results of a recent Cochrane meta-analysis showing a 1 day reduction in hospital stay after abdominal surgery.[48] Preoperative oral CHO drinks are safe and do not increase the risk of aspiration, even in patients with uncomplicated type 2 diabetes[49] and obese patients.[50]

ANESTHETIC MANAGEMENT
Antibiotic Prophylaxis

Antibiotic prophylaxis for patients undergoing colorectal surgery should cover the aerobic and anaerobic flora of the bowel. It should begin within 30 to 60 minutes before surgical incision, be completed before surgical incision, and last no more than 24 hours. Intraoperative dosing is required for surgical procedures lasting more than 2 antibiotic half-lives or with extensive blood loss. First-choice recommended agents are cefazolin plus metronidazole, or a second-generation cephalosporin with aerobic and anaerobic activities (cefoxitin or cefotetan) for patients undergoing elective colorectal surgery. In patients with type 1 allergic reactions to β-lactamine, cefazolin and metronidazole should be replaced with gentamicin (5 mg/kg) and clindamycin (900 mg).[51] In patients with a high risk of methicillin-resistant *Staphylococcus aureus* (MRSA) colonization or known MRSA colonization, vancomycin should be used in combination with cefazolin, as cefazolin is more effective than vancomycin in preventing surgical-site infections (SSIs) caused by methicillin-susceptible *S aureus*.[51] MBP combined with oral neomycin sulfate plus oral erythromycin base, or with oral neomycin sulfate plus oral metronidazole, and in combination with intravenous antibiotic prophylaxis has been shown to further reduce SSIs. However, the increased risk of gastrointestinal symptoms associated with this regimen can offset the former benefit.[51] Furthermore, the use of MBP causes undesirable side effects, and is no longer routinely indicated in patients undergoing colonic surgery within an ERAS program.[52] Although in many institutions surgeons and infection disease determine the choice of antibiotic based on local microbiological data and international guidelines, anesthesiologists still remain responsible for administering antibiotics before skin incision and ensuring adequate redosing when indicated.

Premedication

Patients should not routinely receive anxiolytic agents. The choice, timing, and dose of anxiolytics have to be tailored according to the patient's age, comorbidities, and medications. The type and duration of surgery need also to be considered. Long-acting anxiolytic medications can prolong immediate surgical recovery, interfering with patient mobilization and early postoperative nutrition. The use of short-acting medications to reduce anxiety associated with surgery and provide comfort during painful intervention before the induction of anesthesia, such as insertion of epidural or arterial cannulation, is recommended.[53] Benzodiazepines can cause undesirable side effects such as postoperative delirium and postoperative cognitive dysfunction that can prolong convalescence, especially in the elderly.[53] Morphine and meperidine are no longer used as premedicants, owing to their prolonged duration of action and side effects. Premedicatiing with α_2-agonists such as clonidine and dexmedetomidine has been shown to attenuate surgical stress, but side effects such as arterial hypotension and sedation that might impair early recovery must be considered.[53] Their role as premedication agents in the context of an ERAS program remains unknown.

Intraoperative Anesthetic Management

Intraoperative anesthetic management of patients undergoing colorectal surgery within an ERAS program aims to provide adequate anesthesia and analgesia, attenuate surgical stress, maintain organ perfusion and oxygenation, and facilitate early feeding and postoperative mobilization.

Anesthetic agents and cerebral monitoring

Few studies have evaluated the impact of different anesthesia techniques (intravenous anesthesia versus inhalational anesthesia) on postoperative outcomes in colorectal surgery. Contrasting results are available, and recommendations cannot be made. However, it seems intuitive to use short-acting inhalation agents such as desflurane and sevoflurane to facilitate rapid emergence from anesthesia. In patients at high risk of postoperative nausea and vomiting (PONV), total intravenous anesthesia with propofol is advised. The use of nitrous oxide (50%–70%) should be avoided, especially during laparoscopic surgery, as prolonged use of nitrous oxide can cause bowel distension and significantly increase the risk of PONV despite the administration of prophylactic antiemetic agents.[54,55] Cerebral monitoring can reduce awareness in high-risk surgical patients, and improve postanesthetic recovery.[56] Monitoring the depth of anesthesia can be particularly useful in elderly patients (>65 years old), as titrating anesthetic agents to maintain bispectral index values between 40 and 60 reduces the incidence of postoperative delirium and postoperative cognitive dysfunction.[57]

Attenuation of surgical and inflammatory stress

The attenuation of the physiologic stress response to surgery and the associated sequelae (such as insulin resistance and protein catabolism) is widely regarded as a key area within ERAS programs.[58] Many of the elements of ERAS pathways have already been very successful in this area, such as laparoscopic surgery and preoperative oral CHO loading. Intraoperative strategies attenuating surgical stress and the inflammatory response to surgery have been also shown to facilitate surgical recovery.[58] It is well established that perioperative epidural analgesia with local anesthetic attenuates the catabolic response to surgery, but poorly influences the inflammatory response.[59] Similar results have been reported after spinal anesthesia. The anti-inflammatory effect seems more related to the systemic effect of local anesthetics than to the neuraxial blockade per se, as demonstrated by the anti-inflammatory properties of intravenous lidocaine. Continuous infusion of intraoperative intravenous lidocaine has been shown to reduce postoperative pain, opioid consumption, and opioid side effects.[60] Glucocorticoids were also found to be beneficial in colorectal patients.[61–63] β-Blockers can be particularly useful to blunt the acute sympathetic response induced by pneumoperitoneum in patients undergoing laparoscopic colorectal surgery. Furthermore, they possess anticatabolic properties, as shown in burn patients in whom they attenuate catabolism.[64] Core temperature needs to be monitored and normothermia maintained throughout the perioperative period, as prevention of hypothermia attenuates circulating levels of catecholamines and reduces postoperative complications.[65,66]

Intraoperative analgesia

Several factors must be considered when choosing the type of analgesia for patients undergoing colorectal surgery. The choice depends on the surgical approach (laparotomy or laparoscopy), the site of the incision (midline, transverse, semicurve, or Pfannenstiel-like incision), the type of surgery (colon or rectum), and patient comorbidities. Perioperative analgesia should aim to provide optimal intraoperative and postoperative pain control, with minimal side effects, with the ultimate goal of facilitating early oral feeding and postoperative mobilization.

Thoracic epidural analgesia (TEA) has been shown to reduce the requirement of anesthetic, systemic opioids, and neuromuscular blockade agents, and attenuate the catabolic stress response to surgery.[59] The impact of TEA on surgical outcomes remains debatable. Although the results of the MASTER trial did not show any benefit of combining epidural analgesia with general anesthesia, a recent meta-analysis of 125 randomized controlled trials (RCTs) (N = 9044) found that epidural analgesia in combination with general anesthesia reduces 30-day mortality and morbidity by 40%, independently of the type of surgery.[67] The use of short-acting opioids such as fentanyl and remifentanil is suggested. However, opioid-inducing hyperalgesia (OIH) has been reported, especially after remifentanil infusion. The use of N-methyl-D-aspartate (NMDA) glutamate receptor antagonists, such as ketamine or magnesium, to prevent OIH remains controversial.[68] Intravenous lidocaine has shown to provide adequate analgesia, reduce anesthetic requirement, opioids needs and hasten recovery in open[60] and laparoscopic surgery.[69] Intrathecal morphine with local anesthetics in combination with general anesthesia has also been successfully used, especially in patients undergoing laparoscopic surgery.[70,71] Other analgesic adjuvants such as ketamine, β-blockers, and α_2-agonists are useful alternatives to spare anesthetic and opioid requirements.[53] However, their role as part of multimodal analgesic interventions to improve postoperative outcomes has not been extensively evaluated, especially in colorectal patients and in the setting of an ERAS program. Based on the PROSPECT (Procedure Specific Postoperative Pain Management) recommendations,[72] a guide to the choice of analgesia in colorectal surgery is proposed in **Fig. 1**.

Intraoperative ventilation

Intraoperative lung-protective ventilation has been shown to be beneficial even in patients undergoing abdominal surgery with normal lungs (**Table 2**).[73] Early studies failed to demonstrate reduction of systemic and local inflammatory markers in the early postoperative period (1–5 hours) in patients receiving intraoperative lung-protective ventilation with low tidal volumes (V_T = 6–8 mL/kg) and adequate positive endexpiratory pressure (PEEP) (10–12 cm H_2O), in comparison with patients receiving standard ventilation with V_T of 10 to 15 mL/kg and without PEEP (see **Table 2**). However, results from 2 recent RCTs have shown a reduction in postoperative respiratory complications and shorter hospital stay in patients receiving lung-protective ventilation with low tidal volumes (V_T = 6–8 mL/kg), adequate PEEP (6–10 cm H_2O), and lung recruitment maneuvers (see **Table 2**). Most of the studies included only patients undergoing open abdominal surgery. Similar benefits could be hypothesized, especially in patients undergoing laparoscopic colorectal surgery, in whom the effects of the pneumoperitoneum in combination with steep Trendelenburg position can significantly increase the risk of atelectasis and ventilator-induced lung injury. Further studies are warranted to confirm the role of intraoperative protective ventilation in this specific population. Oxygen therapy (fraction of inspired oxygen [Fio_2]) should be titrated to the most favorable concentration that ensures optimal tissue oxygenation based on the evaluation of oxygen saturation, arterial partial oxygen pressure (Pao_2/Fio_2 ratio), and serum lactates. The use of intraoperative high Fio_2 (Fio_2 = 0.8) to prevent SSI has shown conflicting results. However, patients undergoing colorectal surgery might particularly benefit from this intervention.[74] It must be borne in mind that hyperoxia can cause damage attributable to the production of oxygen free radicals.

Myorelaxation

Short-acting or intermediate-acting muscle relaxants are recommended in patients undergoing colorectal surgery. Cisatracurium should be used in patients with impaired liver or kidney function. Deep neuromuscular blockade (posttetanic count 1–2) facilitates surgical exposure, especially during laparoscopic procedures,[75] and could be particularly useful during laparoscopic rectal surgery. Neuromuscular function should be monitored (train-of-four [TOF], double-burst, or tetanic stimulation patterns) to avoid residual paralysis (TOF <0.9) and postoperative hypoxia.[76,77] Clinical assessment of neuromuscular function underestimates residual paralysis and increases the risk of postoperative respiratory complications, even when sugammadex is used.[78] Qualitative (visual or tactile) assessment is less sensitive than quantitative assessment (acceleromyography) in identifying patients with residual paralysis. Anticholinesterases should be administered 15 to 20 minutes before tracheal extubation and with a TOF count of 4.[77] Sugammadex has been shown to provide faster and more reliable

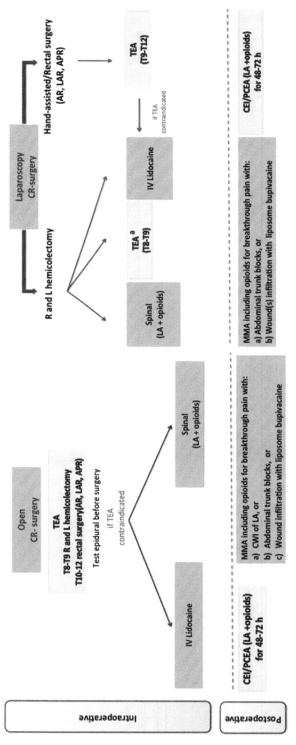

Fig. 1. A guide to the choice of analgesia in colorectal surgery. APR, abdominal perineal resection; AR, anterior resection of the rectum; CEA, continuous epidural analgesia; CR, colorectal surgery; CWI, continuous wound infusion; IV, intravenous; L, left; LA, local anesthetic; LAR, low anterior resection of the rectum; MMA, multimodal analgesia; PCEA, patient-controlled epidural analgesia; R, right; TEA, thoracic epidural analgesia. [a] In patients at high risk of pulmonary complications[122] and in those with high probability of conversion to laparotomy.

Table 2
Intraoperative ventilation and postoperative outcomes

	Protective Lung Ventilation (PV) Versus Standard Ventilation (SV)							
	Wrigge et al, 2000	Wrigge et al, 2004	Choi et al, 2006	Determann et al, 2008	Weingarten et al, 2010	Treschan et al, 2012	Severgnini et al, 2013	Futier et al, 2013
Study design (N)	RCT (39)	RCT (64)	RCT (40)	RCT	RCT	RCT (n = 101)	RCT (56)	RCT (400)
Population	Open, abdominal	Open, abdominal (30) and thoracic (34)	Open >5 h	Open, general surgery	Open, major abdominal	ASA >2, age >50 y Open >3 h	Open abdominal >2 h	High-risk[a] Open (79%)/ laparoscopic (21%) >2 h
Colorectal patients, n (%)	NR	NR	0	1	NR	2	NR	87 (21)
Analgesia (%)	IV opioids	IV opioids	Epidural	Epidural	IV opioids	Epidural (83) IV opioids (17)	Epidural (67) IV/SC opioids (33)	Epidural (40%) IV opioids (60%)
Fluid managements	1.5 L of crystalloid				Not standardized	500 mL bolus of RL 2–4 mL/kg/h Crystalloid (3:1) or colloids (2:1) to replace EBL	12–15 mL/kg/ h	Not standardized
Protective lung ventilation, PV (n)								
V_T (mL/kg)-IBW	6	6	6	6	6	6	7	8
PEEP (cmH_2O)	10	10	10	10	12	5	10	6–8

RM (Y/N)	No	No	No	No	Yes	No	Yes	Yes, every 30 min
Fio₂ (%)	0.3	0.3 and 1ᵃ (OLV)	0.4	0.4	0.5	0.5	0.4	0.46
Standard ventilation, SV (n)								
V$_T$ (mL/kg) -IBW	15	12–15	12	12	10	12	9	10–12
PEEP (cmH$_2$O)	0	0	0	0	0	5	0	0
RM	No	No	No	No	No	No	No	No
Fio₂ (%)	0.3	0.3 and 1ᵃ (OLV)	0.4	0.4	0.5	0.5	0.4	0.47
Primary outcome	Intraoperative cytokine plasma level	Intraoperative cytokine plasma and tracheal aspirates levels	Intraoperative BAL: coagulation (TAT), MPO, IL and cytokines levels	Intraoperative CC16	Intraoperative Pao₂/Fio₂	(TWA) FVC (TWA) FEV₁ over 5 d	mCPIS	Major pulmonary and extrapulmonary complications over 7 d
Results	No difference	No difference	TAT and MPO ↓ PV group; No differences in other cytokines	No difference	↑ PV group	No difference	↓ PV group at POD 1 and POD 3	↓ PV group (RR = 0.4, 95% CI 0.24–0.68)

Abbreviations: ASA, American Society of Anesthesiologists score; BAL, bronchoalveolar lavage; CC16, Clara cell protein; CI, confidence interval; EBL, estimated blood loss; IBW, ideal body weight; IV, intravenous; mCPIS, Modified Clinical Pulmonary Infection Score[14]; MPO, myeloperoxidase; NR, not reported; OLV, one-lung ventilation; POD, postoperative day; RCT, randomized controlled trial; RL, Ringer lactate; RM, recruitment maneuvers; RR, relative risk; SC, subcutaneous; TAT, thrombin-antithrombin; (TWA) FEV₁, time-weighted average forced expiratory volume in 1 second; (TWA) FVC, time-weighted average forced vital capacity.

ᵃ Postoperative pneumonia risk index greater than 2.[13]

Adapted from Coppola S, Froio S, Chiumello D. Protective lung ventilation during general anesthesia: is there any evidence? Crit Care 2014;18(2):210.

reversal than anticholinesterase agents and without muscarinic side effects, thus facilitating earlier tracheal extubation and potentially reducing postoperative respiratory complications as a result of residual muscle paralysis.[79]

Prevention of hypothermia

Intraoperative hypothermia increases the risk of postoperative complications and prolongs emergence from anesthesia. In colorectal patients, unintentional perioperative hypothermia (core temperature <35°C) has been recently associated with an increased mortality and morbidity.[65] Laparoscopic surgery does not reduce the risk of perioperative hypothermia, as hypothermia is mainly caused by anesthesia.[80] Maintenance of intraoperative normothermia with the use of active and passive warming devices together with aggressive postoperative management of shivering and residual hypothermia decreases the incidence of wound infections, blood loss, myocardial ischemia, and protein breakdown. Although not always feasible, preoperative warming strategies 20 to 30 minutes before induction of anesthesia has been shown to attenuate redistribution hypothermia, and could be indicated for patients at high risk of hypothermia, such as elderly and malnourished patients. Core temperature should be monitored and maintained higher than 36°C in the intraoperative and immediate postoperative period.[66]

Intraoperative hemodynamic management

Maintenance of optimal organ perfusion is essential in colorectal patients to prevent organ dysfunction and protect bowel anastomosis. Colonic blood flow is poorly autoregulated, and the perfusion of the colon mainly depends on mean arterial pressure, more so than cardiac output. Several considerations must be taken into account when administering intravenous fluids in the context of an ERAS program.[81] The minimization of preoperative fasting, select use of MBP, a more rational and evidence-based intravenous fluid administration, and early resumption of oral intake have significantly reduced the amount of perioperative intravenous fluids (**Table 3**).

Intraoperative fluid management of patients undergoing colorectal surgery remains controversial. However, it is well established that intravenous fluid overload or splanchnic hypoperfusion increases postoperative complications and delays the recovery of gastrointestinal function.[82] Static hemodynamic measures such as central venous pressure or pulmonary arterial wedge are inaccurate in measuring preload[83,84] and predicting fluid responsiveness.[85] Early studies showed that intravenous fluid administration and inotropic agents based on optimization of cardiac output and targeting predetermined hemodynamic goals (goal-directed therapy [GDT]) reduced postoperative complications, accelerated the recovery of bowel function, and shortened the length of hospital stay in patients undergoing colorectal surgery.[86–89] However, the last 2 RCTs found that GDT was not beneficial, as low-risk patients treated with a more restrictive fluid regimen and within an ERAS program had morbidity and surgical recovery similar to those of patients treated with GDT.[90,91] These data were also confirmed by a recent meta-analysis.[92] The value of GDT might be more evident in high-risk patients undergoing colorectal procedures with extensive blood loss (estimated blood loss >7 mL/kg).[93–97] Inotropes can be considered in patients with reduced cardiac contractility (cardiac index <2.5 L/m^2) to ensure optimal oxygen delivery. Esophageal Doppler has been mainly used to guide fluid therapy in colorectal patients. However, GDT based on pulse contour analysis and aiming to minimize stroke volume variations during the respiratory cycle of mechanically ventilated patients has also been shown to decrease morbidity and accelerate recovery, especially in high-risk patients.[93,96,98,99] Intraoperative and postoperative central venous oxygen

Table 3
Intraoperative intravenous fluid management

Intraoperative Fluid Replacement	Intravenous Fluid Administration: a Physiologic and Evidence-Based Approach (70 kg, Elective, No MBP, 2 h Fasting, 2 h Laparoscopic SR surgery, EBL = 500 mL)
Preoperative fasting	Intravascular volume is minimally reduced after overnight fasting[41,42] 30% of patients do not have an intravascular preoperative deficit[41]
MBP	Avoided in colonic surgery 1000–2000 mL if MBP is used
Preloading in patients receiving epidural or spinal analgesia	Intravenous fluids do not prevent hypotension induced by neuraxial blockade Vasopressors are the first choice to treat hypotension induced by neuraxial blockade
Intravascular volume expansion (anesthesia-related)	In normovolemic patients, intravenous fluids are not necessary and vasopressors are the first choice to treat hypotension induced by anesthesia
Maintenance	Replacement of insensible losses (iso-oncotic crystalloids, avoid 0.9% normal saline) Insensible loss during maximal bowel exposure are not higher than 1 mL/kg/h[82] Open surgery: 3–5 mL/kg/h Laparoscopic surgery: <3 mL/kg/h GDT: in high-risk patients or in patients undergoing surgery with extensive blood loss (>7 mL/kg)
Third space	Nil A primarily fluid-consuming third space has never been identified[82]
Urine/GI loss	1:1 iso-oncotic crystalloids according to clinical estimation
Blood/type 2 shifting[a]	1:1 colloid, or 3:1 iso-oncotic crystalloids (in patients with AKI) Intravascular deficit should be measured (GDT high-risk patients) GDT: in high-risk patients or in patients undergoing surgery with extensive blood loss (>7 mL/kg)
Total (mL)	1000–3200

Abbreviations: AKI, acute kidney injury; GDT, goal-directed therapy; GI, gastrointestinal; MBP, mechanical bowel preparation.

[a] Type 2 shifting refers to extravascular shift of fluids that occurs during the surgical trauma owing to an increased endothelial permeability secondary to (1) the release of inflammatory mediators and (2) the release of atrial natriuretic peptide during iatrogenic acute hypervolemia.[82]

saturation–guided fluid administration has not been shown to affect postoperative complications.[100] Intraoperative cardiac output monitoring is also useful to guide fluid therapy during hemodynamic changes induced by pneumoperitoneum and patient positioning, and avoids unnecessary fluid administration. Arterial hypotension induced by general anesthesia or epidural analgesia should be treated with vasopressors when administration of intravenous fluid fails to increase stroke volume by more than 10%,[52,94,101] as low-dose vasopressors do not impair colonic oxygenation.[102]

Crystalloid solutions should be used to replace extracellular losses, such as urine loss, insensible blood loss, and gastrointestinal loss, while in presence of objective measures of hypovolemia iso-oncotic colloid solution should be used to replace intravascular volume.[82] Crystalloid isotonic balanced solutions should be preferred and 0.9% saline solutions avoided.[103] Hyperchloremia caused by the use of 0.9% saline solutions has been associated with kidney dysfunction,[104–106] prolonged hospital stay, and increased 30-day mortality (odds ratio 1.58, 95% confidence interval 1.25–1.98).[104] Recent data have suggested that the use of hydroxyethyl starch (HES) solutions can increase the risk of death and acute kidney injury in critically ill patients,[107,108] but these results have not been confirmed in the perioperative setting.[109] Moreover, the use of large volumes of HES 130/0.4 (2605 ± 512 mL) during major urologic procedures has been shown to impair hemostasis and increase blood loss in comparison with crystalloid solutions.[110] Nevertheless, intraoperative crystalloids-based fluid regimens increase the risk of fluid overload.[110]

Acute intraoperative anemia results in increased mortality.[111] Blood loss reported during open and rectal surgery is higher than during laparoscopic and colonic surgery, respectively. Anemia thresholds triggering red blood cell transfusions cannot be currently recommended, as hemoglobin levels resulting in tissue hypoxia are patient-specific.[111] The decision to transfuse should be made on an individual basis, depending on the clinical context, serum lactate levels, central oxygen venous saturation, and patient comorbidities. Administration of red blood cell transfusion and bone marrow–stimulating agents to treat anemia failed to improve outcomes. Furthermore, it must be also considered that blood transfusions are associated with an increased risk of morbidity and mortality.[111] Optimization of preoperative hemoglobin levels and implementation of blood management programs might reduce red blood cell transfusion, minimize blood loss, and improve postoperative outcomes,[111] especially in patients at high risk of intraoperative transfusion.[112]

Prevention of postoperative nausea and vomiting

PONV prophylaxis is a key component of an ERAS program for patients undergoing colorectal surgery, as avoidance of PONV facilitates early feeding and accelerates recovery. The risk of PONV can be predicted by the Apfel score, based on the presence of the following risk factors: female, nonsmoking status, history of PONV, and opioid use.[113] Several PONV prophylaxis strategies are available, which include minimal preoperative fasting, CHO loading, adequate hydration, prophylactic administration of antiemetic agents, multimodal analgesic strategies to spare opioids and opioid side effects, use of regional analgesia techniques, total intravenous anesthesia, and avoidance of nitrous oxide. The use of high oxygen concentration has a weak effect in reducing PONV.[74] In patients with more than 2 risk factors a multimodal approach, including pharmacologic and nonpharmacologic antiemetic techniques, is required.[114] Detailed information about PONV prophylaxis can be found in the recently updated consensus guidelines for the management of PONV.[114]

Glycemic control

Perioperative hyperglycemia is associated with an increased risk of morbidity and mortality. Preoperative hemoglobin A_{1c} levels (>6.0%) can identify patients at risk of perioperative hyperglycemia and can predict postoperative complications even in nondiabetic patients.[115] Reduced preoperative fasting times, preoperative oral CHO, use of epidural anesthesia, and adequate analgesia facilitate glucose control by reducing insulin resistance. Although the optimal glucose level remains to be determined, it is recommended to maintain random blood sugar lower than 10 mmol/L.[52,94]

POSTOPERATIVE ANALGESIA

Postoperative pain after colorectal surgery is complex in nature (**Fig. 2**). A multimodal analgesic approach including opioid and nonopioid analgesics, in combination with regional analgesia techniques when indicated, is advised to provide optimal analgesia and reduce opioid side effects, aiming at facilitating early feeding and postoperative

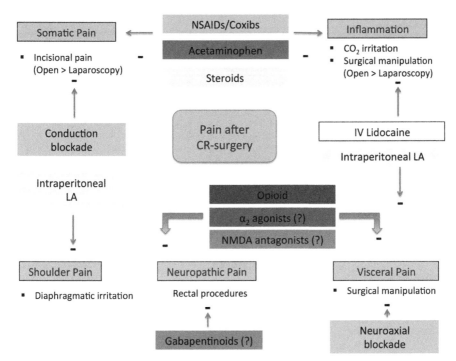

Fig. 2. Complexity of pain in colorectal surgery. The analgesic efficacy of some analgesic medications (?) remains to be proven in colorectal patients. -, inhibitory effect; CR, colorectal surgery; IV, intravenous; LA, local anesthetic; NMDA, N-Methyl-D-aspartate receptor; NSAIDs, nonsteroidal anti-inflammatory drugs.

mobilization. The role of preemptive analgesic strategies, such as preoperative administration of acetaminophen, cyclooxygenase-2 (COX-2) inhibitors, NMDA antagonists, and/or gabapentinoids, remains unclear, especially in the context of an ERAS program for colorectal surgery.[116] Epidural analgesia remains the only preemptive analgesic technique that consistently reduces postoperative pain, analgesic consumption, and time to rescue analgesia.[116] Perioperative opioids are still necessary, but should be used as rescue analgesia if other methods fail. An opioid-free multimodal analgesic strategy would be appealing, but more studies are warranted to establish its feasibility, efficacy, and safety. Establishing the impact of analgesia techniques on surgical outcomes remains challenging, as surgical recovery depends on many perioperative factors including patient comorbidities, type of surgery, type of perioperative care (ERAS versus traditional care), and the occurrence of postoperative complications. Common analgesic techniques used in colorectal surgery and their application in the ERAS setting are summarized in **Table 4**. Indications and contraindications are discussed in this issue in one of the article "Optimal analgesia during major open and laparoscopic abdominal surgery" by Fawcett and Baldini.

Analgesia for Open Colorectal Surgery

TEA with local anesthetic and small doses of lipophilic opioids remains the gold standard for postoperative pain after open colorectal surgery. Adding epinephrine (1.5–2.0 µg/mL) to an epidural mixture of local anesthetic improves postoperative analgesia, especially during mobilization and coughing, and reduces pruritus.[117]

Table 4
Common analgesic techniques used in colorectal surgery

Analgesia	Technique and Dose	Comments and Potential Complications
Thoracic epidural analgesia (TEA)	T8–T9 for R and L hemicolectomy T10–T12 for sigmoid-rectal surgery[a] Intraoperative: 5 mL bupivacaine 0.25%–0.5% intermittent boluses or 5 mL/h continuous infusion Postoperative (CEI or PCEA): bupivacaine 0.05%–0.125% or ropivacaine 0.2%, with fentanyl 2–3 µg/mL or hydromorphone 5–7.5 µg/mL	Arterial hypotension Bladder dysfunction Lower limb weakness Consider adding epidural epinephrine (2 µg/mL) if epidural block is patchy or weak
Spinal analgesia	10 mg 0.5% isobaric bupivacaine or 15 mg 0.5% hyperbaric bupivacaine Intrathecal morphine: <70 y 200–250 µg >70 y 150 µg	Arterial hypotension Pruritus Bladder dysfunction Respiratory depression
Intravenous lidocaine	Intraoperative and in PACU 1.5 mg/kg bolus or within 30 min before induction of anesthesia followed by 2 mg/kg/h until the end of surgery. Infusion can be extended in PACU	Local anesthetic toxicity Intravenous lidocaine infusion requires continuous cardiovascular monitoring
Continuous wound infusion of local anesthetic	In most of the studies a multihole catheter is positioned along the surgical incision between the peritoneum and the fascia (preperitoneal) Ropivacaine 0.2% 8–10 mL in the wound followed by Ropivacaine 0.2% 5–8 mL/h for 48 h	Local anesthetic toxicity The ideal anatomic location where multihole catheters are to be placed has not yet been clearly determined
TAP block US-guided or surgically performed Subcostal approach (upper abdominal surgery) Lateral approach (lower abdominal) Posterior approach (lower abdomen)	Unilateral or bilateral Single shot 15–20 mL of 0.25%–0.375% bupivacaine or levobupivacaine Intermittent boluses through multihole catheters 15–20 mL of local anesthetic every 6 h per site Continuous infusion through multihole catheters 6–8 mL/h of 0.25% bupivacaine or 0.2% ropivacaine	Few complications have been reported, especially when the TAP block is performed under direct US guidance; these include intrahepatic and intraperitoneal injections. Local anesthetic toxicity should be also considered, especially when multiples or continuous TAP blocks are performed Pain: reduced static pain score and opioid consumption *(continued on next page)*

Table 4
(*continued*)

Analgesia	Technique and Dose	Comments and Potential Complications
		Reduction of opioid side effects: inconclusive evidence
		Duration of the analgesic effect is limited (≤24 h)
		The analgesic effect is volume and dose dependent
		Dermatomal spread is limited (1.5 dermatomes)
		Preoperative TAP block provides better analgesia than postoperative TAP block
		Single-shot posterior TAP block or continuous TAP block has been used to prolong analgesia (>24 h)
Rectus sheath block US-guided	Bilateral Single shot 15–20 mL of 0.25%–0.375% bupivacaine or levobupivacaine Intermittent boluses through a multihole catheter 15–20 mL of 0.25% bupivacaine or levobupivacaine per site	Provide analgesia for the whole midline of the abdomen Shorter analgesic effect then TAP block
Liposomal bupivacaine	266 mg in 40 mL 0.9% normal saline	Use in the context of MMA phase IV studies. Limited evidence

Abbreviations: CEI, continuous epidural analgesia; MMA, multimodal analgesia; PACU, postanesthesia care unit; PCEA, patient-controlled epidural analgesia; TAP, transversus abdominis plane block; TEA, thoracic epidural analgesia; US, ultrasound.

[a] Supplementary analgesia is needed in patients undergoing abdominal perianal resection, in whom perianal pain (S1–S3 dermatomes) is not covered by TEA.

Supplementary analgesia is required in patients undergoing abdominal perianal resection, in whom perianal pain (S1–S3 dermatomes) is not controlled by TEA. Evidence supporting the use of epidural clonidine is inconclusive, and the risk of arterial hypotension and sedation is increased.[118] It remains unclear as to whether TEA improves postoperative surgical outcomes, especially in the context of an ERAS program. Compared with parenteral opioids, epidural infusion of low-dose local anesthetic and short-acting opioids has been shown to provide better postoperative static and dynamic analgesia for the first 72 hours,[119] accelerate the recovery of gastrointestinal function,[120] reduce insulin resistance,[121] and impact positively on cardiovascular and respiratory complications.[67,122] However, arterial hypotension, urinary retention, pruritus, and lower limb weakness are common side effects.[123] Arterial hypotension induced by TEA reduces splanchnic circulation,[124] and it does not respond to intravenous fluid administration.[101] Nevertheless, improvement of mean arterial pressure with small doses of vasopressors restores splanchnic perfusion[101] and does not impair colonic oxygen delivery.[102] Orthostatic hypotension associated with postoperative epidural analgesia does not impair the ability to ambulate.[125] When TEA analgesia is contraindicated, intraoperative and postoperative intravenous lidocaine infusion or spinal analgesia with intrathecal morphine can be used. Although systemic local anesthetic toxicity is rare, postoperative intravenous lidocaine infusion requires continuous cardiovascular monitoring. Abdominal trunk blocks, such as transversus abdominis plane (TAP) block[126,127] and rectus sheath block, or continuous wound infusion of local anesthetic,[128,129] can be performed at the end of surgery with the purpose of improving postoperative pain, reducing opioid side effects, and hastening recovery (see **Fig. 1**, **Table 4**).

Analgesia for Laparoscopic Colorectal Surgery

The use of TEA for patients undergoing laparoscopic colorectal surgery remains controversial. If the only purpose of using TEA is to control postoperative pain, its use seems unnecessary or sometimes disadvantageous,[130] especially in a context of an ERAS program.[131,132] Although pain scores can be statistically lower in the first 24 hours after surgery, patients not receiving TEA still report adequate analgesia (nutritional risk score <4).[133] The use of TEA remains valuable in patients at high risk of postoperative respiratory complications,[122] in those with high probability of conversion to laparotomy, and in patients with an 8- to 10-cm Pfannenstiel-like incision after laparoscopic rectal surgery, especially in the first 24 hours.[134] TEA seems to facilitate the recovery of bowel function, even after laparoscopic procedures,[135] when compared with patients receiving systemic opioids and without an ERAS program. However, faster recovery of bowel function does not necessarily translate into faster surgical recovery, as colorectal patients treated with TEA in the context of an ERAS program have a longer hospital stay[71] and medical recovery[132] than those receiving spinal analgesia or systemic opioids. Alternative and safer analgesic techniques have been shown to provide similar analgesia without delaying discharge. These approaches include intrathecal morphine with local anesthetic,[71] intravenous lidocaine,[60] the use of ultrasound-guided abdominal trunk blocks,[136] and intraperitoneal local anesthetic.[133,137] TAP block under direct laparoscopic vision has also been successfully used.[138–140] Continuous would infusion of local anesthetic has been successfully used in one feasibility study (see **Fig. 1**, **Table 4**).[141]

Coanalgesia

Nonsteroidal anti-inflammatory drugs (NSAIDs), including COX-2 inhibitors and acetaminophen (orally, per rectum, and intravenously) are commonly used as part of multimodal analgesic regimens as opioid-sparing strategies. Intravenous preparations are particularly valuable in the perioperative period, as oral and rectal bioavailability is unpredictable after gastrointestinal surgery. Furthermore, suppositories are not usually administered in patients with rectal anastomosis. Recent concerns have been raised about the risk of anastomotic leakage and the use of NSAIDs or COX-2 inhibitors after colorectal surgeries based on experimental, retrospective, observational, and case-series studies.[142] This effects seems to be class specific (the risk of anastomotic leakage is higher with NSAIDs than COX-2 inhibitors),[143] molecule specific (diclofenac is associated with the highest risk)[142] and time dependent.[143] Large RCTs are needed to confirm these results. Although not statistically significant, a trend toward higher risk of developing anastomotic leakage after bowel surgery was reported in a recent meta-analysis of 6 RCTs (480 patients) of patients receiving at least 1 dose of NSAIDs or COX-2 inhibitors within 48 hours of surgery (Peto odds ratio

2.16; 95% confidence interval 0.85–5.53).[144] Caution should be used in patients at high risk of anastomotic leakage. α_2-Agonists, glucocorticoids, gabapentinoids, and ketamine have been poorly studied in colorectal patients, and their use in other types of surgery has shown conflicting results. Wound infiltration with long-acting multivesicular liposome formulation of bupivacaine as part of multimodal analgesic regimens has also shown promising results.[145,146]

SPECIAL CONSIDERATIONS FOR PATIENTS UNDERGOING ONCOLOGIC COLORECTAL SURGERY

Most patients undergo colorectal surgery because of precancer or cancer lesions. In the last years, many in vitro and in vivo experimental studies and retrospective human studies have attempted to establish the impact of many perioperative factors on oncologic outcomes. Associations have been reported but causation has never been proved. Nutritional status and factual capacity of colorectal patients are negatively affected by neoadjuvant chemotherapy and cancer cachexia. In this context, prehabilitation might positively affect surgical recovery.[34] Side effects and complications associated with specific chemotherapy agents must be considered. Opioids have been shown to have an immunosuppressive effect, mainly suppressing natural killer cell activity, but the effect on cancer recurrence and metastasis remains unknown. NSAIDs might have a direct and indirect anticancer effect.[147] Intravenous lidocaine has also shown an antitumor effect at plasma concentrations observed in clinical practice.[148] By contrast, in a small sample of patients, dexamethasone has been recently associated with cancer recurrence after elective colectomy.[149] Minimizing opioid consumption, and favoring regional anesthesia techniques and nonopioid analgesics might be even more valuable in patients with cancer. Allogeneic blood transfusions have also been associated with worse oncologic outcomes.[150] At present, there is insufficient evidence to justify changing anesthesia and analgesia practice or perioperative care in the prevention of cancer recurrence or metastasis in patients with colorectal cancer.

SPECIAL CONSIDERATIONS FOR PATIENTS UNDERGOING EMERGENCY COLORECTAL SURGERY

Indications for emergency colorectal surgery include colon perforation, bowel obstruction, bowel ischemia, bleeding, and anastomotic leakage. Early optimization of hemodynamics to ensure optimal oxygen delivery and early antibiotic therapy when indicated are key elements, especially before the induction of anesthesia. Dehydration, hypovolemia, and electrolyte derangements are commonly observed in patients with bowel obstruction. Septic patients with peritonitis secondary to bowel perforation, intra-abdominal abscess, or anastomotic leakage should be treated according to international guidelines.[151] In these patients, advanced hemodynamic monitoring to guide fluid therapy is recommended,[96] and administration of inotrope and vasopressors might be required. For these reasons, the insertion of arterial and central lines before the induction of anesthesia is advised. Aspiration through nasogastric tubes (when already inserted), preoxygenation, and rapid sequence induction of anesthesia with cricoid pressure is required because of the high risk of pulmonary aspiration. If not carefully titrated, administration of induction agents can catastrophically induce hypotension, especially in septic patients with an already reduced vascular tone and increased vascular permeability. Assessment of fluid responsiveness is critical, as unnecessary administration of crystalloids to treat hemodynamically unstable patients causes interstitial edema and increases morbidity. Colloids should be avoided in septic patients.[108] Markers of systemic organ hypoperfusion such as

Table 5
ERAS elements under direct control of the anesthesiologist: key points

ERAS Elements Under Direct Control of Anesthesiologist	Key Points
Patient education	Preoperative patient education is an essential component of any ERAS program
	It is important to specify the active role the patient is expected to play in the perioperative period
	Written or visual information at an appropriate literacy level, specifying daily goals for nutritional intake and postoperative ambulation, discharge criteria, and expected hospital stay should be provided
Preoperative evaluation, risk stratification, and optimization	Optimize preoperative conditions associated with poor outcomes include patient comorbidities, nutritional status, anemia, and functional capacity
	Intense smoking cessation interventions including NRT and individual counseling for at least 3–4 wk before surgery to reduce postoperative complications
	More studies evaluating the role of optimizing preoperative conditions to a point to delay surgery in patients undergoing oncologic colorectal surgery are warranted
Preoperative fasting and preoperative oral carbohydrate (CHO) drinks	There is no scientific evidence to support policy of routine NPO after midnight
	Fasting from midnight increases insulin resistance and depletes glycogen reserves. These effects are magnified by the stress response induced by surgery
	Current preoperative fasting guidelines for adult patients undergoing elective surgery recommend a 2-h fast for liquids and a 6-h fast for solids
	Preoperative oral CHO drinks are safe, reduce insulin resistance, and improve patients' well-being
Antibiotic prophylaxis	Antibiotic prophylaxis for patients undergoing colorectal surgery must cover aerobic and anaerobic flora, according to international guidelines
	Antibiotic prophylaxis should be completed within 1 h before surgical incision. Intraoperative dosing depends on the half-life of the antibiotic used and on the surgical blood loss. It should not last more than 24 h
Premedication	Patients should not routinely receive anxiolytic agents
	The use of short-acting anxiolytic agents is advised to facilitate invasive procedures uncomfortable for patients (epidural, arterial lines, etc)
	Benzodiazepine should be avoided in patients older than 65 y
Anesthetic agents and cerebral monitoring	The use of short-acting inhalation or intravenous agents is advised
	TIVA with propofol should be considered in patients at high risk of PONV
	Avoid N_2O
	Monitoring depth of anesthesia reduces anesthetic requirement, minimizes anesthetic hemodynamic effects, and can be particularly useful in elderly patients to facilitate recovery
Attenuation of surgical and inflammatory stress	Attenuation of surgical stress is a key element in enhancing recovery
	The use of regional anesthesia techniques, glucocorticoids, intravenous lidocaine, and prevention of hypothermia has been shown to attenuate the stress response associated with surgery

(continued on next page)

Table 5
(continued)

ERAS Elements Under Direct Control of Anesthesiologist	Key Points
Intraoperative analgesia	Regional anesthesia techniques, including TEA and spinal anesthesia, reduces anesthetic and systemic opioid requirements The analgesic and anti-inflammatory properties of intravenous lidocaine has been shown to reduce anesthetic and opioid consumption, reduce opioid side effects, and hasten recovery Ketamine, α_2-agonists, and other analgesic adjuvants have shown opioid-sparing properties, but their role in colorectal patients and in the context of an ERAS program has not been studied
Intraoperative ventilation	Intraoperative lung-protective ventilation with low tidal volumes (V_T = 6–8 mL/kg, IBW), adequate PEEP (6–10 cmH_2O), and lung recruitment maneuvers is beneficial (reduced inflammation and better outcomes) even in patients with uninjured lungs undergoing abdominal surgery Intraoperative oxygen therapy (Fio_2) should be titrated to the most favorable concentration that ensures optimal tissue oxygenation based on the evaluation of oxygen saturation, arterial partial oxygen pressure (Pao_2/Fio_2 ratio), and serum lactates The use of intraoperative high-inspired oxygen fraction (Fio_2 = 0.8) to prevent surgical-site infections has shown conflicting results. However, patients undergoing colorectal surgery might particularly benefit from this intervention
Myorelaxation	Short- or intermediate-acting muscle relaxants are recommended Adequate muscle relaxation is essential to guarantee optimal surgical conditions, especially during laparoscopic colorectal surgery Neuromuscular blockade must be monitored (TOF, double-burst, or tetanic stimulation pattern) throughout the intraoperative period. Quantitative assessment (acceleromyography) of neuromuscular function is more reliable than qualitative assessment (visual or tactile) in identifying patients with residual paralysis
Prevention of hypothermia	Core temperature must be monitored and hypothermia (core temperature <36°C) avoided
Intraoperative hemodynamic management	In colorectal patients treated within an ERAS program, minimization of preoperative fasting, avoidance of MBP, a more rational and evidence-based intravenous fluid administration, and early resumption of oral intake have significantly reduced the amount of perioperative intravenous fluids needed GDT seems beneficial in high-risk patients and in patients undergoing surgery with extensive blood loss (>7 mL/kg) Iso-oncotic crystalloid solutions should be used and 0.9% saline solutions avoided Colloid should be avoided in patents with preexisting renal diseases and in septic patients Anemia thresholds triggering blood transfusions cannot be currently recommended, as hemoglobin levels resulting in tissue hypoxia are patient-specific The decision to transfuse blood should be made on an individual basis, depending on the clinical context, serum lactate levels, central oxygen venous saturation, and patient comorbidities
PONV prophylaxis	PONV prophylaxis is an essential to facilitate early feeding Patients at high risk of PONV can be identified PONV prophylaxis guidelines must be followed

(continued on next page)

Table 5 *(continued)*	
ERAS Elements Under Direct Control of Anesthesiologist	**Key Points**
Glycemic control	Hyperglycemia is associated with worse outcomes Preoperative hemoglobin A_{1c} >6.0% can predict hyperglycemia and postoperative complications even in nondiabetic patients Maintain glycemia <10 mmol/L
Postoperative analgesia	The choice of the analgesia depends on the surgical approach (laparotomy or laparoscopy), the site of the surgical incision (midline, transverse, semicurve, or Pfannenstiel-like incision), the type of surgery (colon or rectum), and patient comorbidities TEA remains the goal standard for postoperative pain control for patients undergoing open colorectal surgery. However, TEA increases the risk of arterial hypotension Spinal analgesia with intrathecal morphine, abdominal trunk blocks, intravenous lidocaine, continuous wound infiltration of local anesthetic, and wound infiltration with liposome bupivacaine are valuable analgesic techniques, especially for laparoscopic colorectal surgery A multimodal analgesic approach is recommended with the aim of providing optimal analgesia and reducing opioid consumption and side effects, with the ultimate goal of facilitating early feeding and early postoperative mobilization

Abbreviations: GDT, goal-directed therapy; IBW, ideal body weight; MBP, mechanical bowel preparation; NPO, nothing by mouth; NRT, nicotine replacement therapy; PEEP, positive end-expiratory pressure; PONV, postoperative nausea and vomiting; TEA, thoracic epidural analgesia; TIVA, total intravenous anesthesia; TOF, train-of-four.

serum lactate, base excess, and low oxygen venous saturation might help to guide fluid therapy, but alternative explanations other than hypoperfusion should be also considered, especially in anemic patients, septic patients, and patients receiving catecholamines.[152] Titrating anesthetic depth based on cerebral monitoring helps to minimize the hemodynamic effects of the anesthetic agents. Regional anesthesia techniques are frequently contraindicated because of coagulopathy and infections. Postoperative monitoring in high-dependency units or intensive care units may be required. Early-warning scoring systems can help to identify patients who require advanced postoperative care.[153]

Key points summarizing each ERAS element for patients undergoing elective colorectal are listed in **Table 5**.

REFERENCES

1. Durrand JW, Batterham AM, Danjoux GR. Pre-habilitation. I: aggregation of marginal gains. Anaesthesia 2014;69(5):403–6.
2. Kiecolt-Glaser JK, Page GG, Marucha PT, et al. Psychological influences on surgical recovery. Perspectives from psychoneuroimmunology. Am Psychol 1998; 53(11):1209–18.
3. Mondloch MV, Cole DC, Frank JW. Does how you do depend on how you think you'll do? A systematic review of the evidence for a relation between patients' recovery expectations and health outcomes. CMAJ 2001;165(2):174–9.

4. Pearse RM, Moreno RP, Bauer P, et al. Mortality after surgery in Europe: a 7 day cohort study. Lancet 2012;380(9847):1059–65.
5. Pearse RM, Harrison DA, James P, et al. Identification and characterisation of the high-risk surgical population in the United Kingdom. Crit Care 2006;10(3):R81.
6. Morris CK, Ueshima K, Kawaguchi T, et al. The prognostic value of exercise capacity: a review of the literature. Am Heart J 1991;122(5):1423–31.
7. Cohen ME, Bilimoria KY, Ko CY, et al. Development of an American College of Surgeons National Surgery Quality Improvement Program: morbidity and mortality risk calculator for colorectal surgery. J Am Coll Surg 2009;208(6):1009–16.
8. Sjo OH, Larsen S, Lunde OC, et al. Short term outcome after emergency and elective surgery for colon cancer. Colorectal Dis 2009;11(7):733–9.
9. Lucas DJ, Pawlik TM. Quality improvement in gastrointestinal surgical oncology with American College of Surgeons National Surgical Quality Improvement Program. Surgery 2014;155(4):593–601.
10. Khuri SF, Henderson WG, DePalma RG, et al. Determinants of long-term survival after major surgery and the adverse effect of postoperative complications. Ann Surg 2005;242(3):326–41 [discussion: 341–3].
11. Tekkis PP, Poloniecki JD, Thompson MR, et al. Operative mortality in colorectal cancer: prospective national study. BMJ 2003;327(7425):1196–201.
12. Lee TH, Marcantonio ER, Mangione CM, et al. Derivation and prospective validation of a simple index for prediction of cardiac risk of major noncardiac surgery. Circulation 1999;100(10):1043–9.
13. Arozullah AM, Khuri SF, Henderson WG, et al. Development and validation of a multifactorial risk index for predicting postoperative pneumonia after major noncardiac surgery. Ann Intern Med 2001;135(10):847–57.
14. Pelosi P, Barassi A, Severgnini P, et al. Prognostic role of clinical and laboratory criteria to identify early ventilator-associated pneumonia in brain injury. Chest 2008;134(1):101–8.
15. Gupta PK, Gupta H, Sundaram A, et al. Development and validation of a risk calculator for prediction of cardiac risk after surgery. Circulation 2011;124(4):381–7.
16. Kheterpal S, Tremper KK, Heung M, et al. Development and validation of an acute kidney injury risk index for patients undergoing general surgery: results from a national data set. Anesthesiology 2009;110(3):505–15.
17. Lee L, Schwartzman K, Carli F, et al. The association of the distance walked in 6 min with pre-operative peak oxygen consumption and complications 1 month after colorectal resection. Anaesthesia 2013;68(8):811–6.
18. Smith TB, Stonell C, Purkayastha S, et al. Cardiopulmonary exercise testing as a risk assessment method in non cardio-pulmonary surgery: a systematic review. Anaesthesia 2009;64(8):883–93.
19. Fleisher LA, Beckman JA, Brown KA, et al. 2014 ACC/AHA Guideline on Perioperative Cardiovascular Evaluation and Management of Patients Undergoing Noncardiac Surgery. J Am Coll Cardiol 2014;64(22):e77–137.
20. Goodnough LT, Shander A. Patient blood management. Anesthesiology 2012;116(6):1367–76.
21. Qaseem A, Snow V, Fitterman N, et al. Risk assessment for and strategies to reduce perioperative pulmonary complications for patients undergoing noncardiothoracic surgery: a guideline from the American College of Physicians. Ann Intern Med 2006;144(8):575–80.
22. Ebert TJ, Shankar H, Haake RM. Perioperative considerations for patients with morbid obesity. Anesthesiol Clin 2006;24(3):621–36.

23. American Society of Anesthesiologists Task Force on Perioperative Management of patients with obstructive sleep apnea. Practice guidelines for the perioperative management of patients with obstructive sleep apnea: an updated report by the American Society of Anesthesiologists Task Force on Perioperative Management of patients with obstructive sleep apnea. Anesthesiology 2014;120(2):268–86.

24. Moghissi ES, Korytkowski MT, DiNardo M, et al. American Association of Clinical Endocrinologists and American Diabetes Association consensus statement on inpatient glycemic control. Diabetes Care 2009;32(6):1119–31.

25. Chow WB, Rosenthal RA, Merkow RP, et al. Optimal preoperative assessment of the geriatric surgical patient: a best practices guideline from the American College of Surgeons National Surgical Quality Improvement Program and the American Geriatrics Society. J Am Coll Surg 2012;215(4):453–66.

26. Kelly KN, Domajnko B. Perioperative stress-dose steroids. Clin Colon Rectal Surg 2013;26(3):163–7.

27. Mills E, Eyawo O, Lockhart I, et al. Smoking cessation reduces postoperative complications: a systematic review and meta-analysis. Am J Med 2011;124(2):144–54.e8.

28. Tonnesen H, Nielsen PR, Lauritzen JB, et al. Smoking and alcohol intervention before surgery: evidence for best practice. Br J Anaesth 2009;102(3):297–306.

29. Garth AK, Newsome CM, Simmance N, et al. Nutritional status, nutrition practices and post-operative complications in patients with gastrointestinal cancer. J Hum Nutr Diet 2010;23(4):393–401.

30. Miller KR, Wischmeyer PE, Taylor B, et al. An evidence-based approach to perioperative nutrition support in the elective surgery patient. JPEN J Parenter Enteral Nutr 2013;37(5 Suppl):39S–50S.

31. Weimann A, Braga M, Harsanyi L, et al. ESPEN Guidelines on Enteral Nutrition: surgery including organ transplantation. Clin Nutr 2006;25(2):224–44.

32. Burden S, Todd C, Hill J, et al. Pre-operative nutrition support in patients undergoing gastrointestinal surgery. Cochrane Database Syst Rev 2012;(11):CD008879.

33. Carli F, Zavorsky GS. Optimizing functional exercise capacity in the elderly surgical population. Curr Opin Clin Nutr Metab Care 2005;8(1):23–32.

34. Gillis C, Li C, Lee L, et al. Prehabilitation versus rehabilitation: a randomized control trial in patients undergoing colorectal resection for cancer. Anesthesiology 2014;121(5):937–47.

35. O'Doherty AF, West M, Jack S, et al. Preoperative aerobic exercise training in elective intra-cavity surgery: a systematic review. Br J Anaesth 2013;110(5):679–89.

36. Maltby JR. Fasting from midnight–the history behind the dogma. Best Pract Res Clin Anaesthesiol 2006;20(3):363–78.

37. Ljungqvist O. Jonathan E. Rhoads lecture 2011: Insulin resistance and enhanced recovery after surgery. JPEN J Parenter Enteral Nutr 2012;36(4):389–98.

38. Martindale RG, McClave SA, Taylor B, et al. Perioperative nutrition: what is the current landscape? JPEN J Parenter Enteral Nutr 2013;37(5 Suppl):5S–20S.

39. Hausel J, Nygren J, Lagerkranser M, et al. A carbohydrate-rich drink reduces preoperative discomfort in elective surgery patients. Anesth Analg 2001;93(5):1344–50.

40. Holte K, Nielsen KG, Madsen JL, et al. Physiologic effects of bowel preparation. Dis Colon Rectum 2004;47(8):1397–402.

41. Bundgaard-Nielsen M, Jorgensen CC, Secher NH, et al. Functional intravascular volume deficit in patients before surgery. Acta Anaesthesiol Scand 2010;54(4):464–9.

42. Muller L, Briere M, Bastide S, et al. Preoperative fasting does not affect haemodynamic status: a prospective, non-inferiority, echocardiography study. Br J Anaesth 2014;112(5):835–41.
43. American Society of Anesthesiologists Committee. Practice guidelines for preoperative fasting and the use of pharmacologic agents to reduce the risk of pulmonary aspiration: application to healthy patients undergoing elective procedures: an updated report by the American Society of Anesthesiologists Committee on Standards and Practice Parameters. Anesthesiology 2011;114(3):495–511.
44. Lobo DN, Hendry PO, Rodrigues G, et al. Gastric emptying of three liquid oral preoperative metabolic preconditioning regimens measured by magnetic resonance imaging in healthy adult volunteers: a randomised double-blind, crossover study. Clin Nutr 2009;28(6):636–41.
45. Gjessing PF, Hagve M, Fuskevag OM, et al. Single-dose carbohydrate treatment in the immediate preoperative phase diminishes development of postoperative peripheral insulin resistance. Clin Nutr 2014. [Epub ahead of print].
46. Ljungqvist O. Modulating postoperative insulin resistance by preoperative carbohydrate loading. Best Pract Res Clin Anaesthesiol 2009;23:401–9.
47. Awad S, Varadhan KK, Ljungqvist O, et al. A meta-analysis of randomised controlled trials on preoperative oral carbohydrate treatment in elective surgery. Clin Nutr 2013;32(1):34–44.
48. Smith MD, McCall J, Plank L, et al. Preoperative carbohydrate treatment for enhancing recovery after elective surgery. Cochrane Database Syst Rev 2014;8:CD009161.
49. Gustafsson UO, Nygren J, Thorell A, et al. Pre-operative carbohydrate loading may be used in type 2 diabetes patients. Acta Anaesthesiol Scand 2008; 52(7):946–51.
50. Maltby JR, Pytka S, Watson NC, et al. Drinking 300 mL of clear fluid two hours before surgery has no effect on gastric fluid volume and pH in fasting and nonfasting obese patients. Can J Anaesth 2004;51(2):111–5.
51. Bratzler DW, Dellinger EP, Olsen KM, et al. Clinical practice guidelines for antimicrobial prophylaxis in surgery. Am J Health Syst Pharm 2013;70(3):195–283.
52. Gustafsson UO, Scott MJ, Schwenk W, et al. Guidelines for perioperative care in elective colonic surgery: Enhanced Recovery After Surgery (ERAS((R))) Society recommendations. World J Surg 2013;37(2):259–84.
53. Baldini G, Carli F. Anesthetic and adjunctive drugs for fast-track surgery. Curr Drug Targets 2009;10(8):667–86.
54. Scheinin B, Lindgren L, Scheinin TM. Peroperative nitrous oxide delays bowel function after colonic surgery. Br J Anaesth 1990;64(2):154–8.
55. Myles PS, Leslie K, Chan MT, et al. The safety of addition of nitrous oxide to general anaesthesia in at-risk patients having major non-cardiac surgery (ENIGMA-II): a randomised, single-blind trial. Lancet 2014;384(9952):1446–54.
56. Punjasawadwong Y, Phongchiewboon A, Bunchungmongkol N. Bispectral index for improving anaesthetic delivery and postoperative recovery. Cochrane Database Syst Rev 2014;(6):CD003843.
57. Chan MT, Cheng BC, Lee TM, et al. BIS-guided anesthesia decreases postoperative delirium and cognitive decline. J Neurosurg Anesthesiol 2013;25(1):33–42.
58. Kehlet H, Wilmore DW. Evidence-based surgical care and the evolution of fast-track surgery. Ann Surg 2008;248(2):189–98.
59. Carli F, Kehlet H, Baldini G, et al. Evidence basis for regional anesthesia in multidisciplinary fast-track surgical care pathways. Reg Anesth Pain Med 2011; 36(1):63–72.

60. Marret E, Rolin M, Beaussier M, et al. Meta-analysis of intravenous lidocaine and postoperative recovery after abdominal surgery. Br J Surg 2008;95(11):1331–8.
61. Waldron NH, Jones CA, Gan TJ, et al. Impact of perioperative dexamethasone on postoperative analgesia and side-effects: systematic review and meta-analysis. Br J Anaesth 2013;110(2):191–200.
62. Vignali A, Di Palo S, Orsenigo E, et al. Effect of prednisolone on local and systemic response in laparoscopic vs. open colon surgery: a randomized, double-blind, placebo-controlled trial. Dis Colon Rectum 2009;52(6):1080–8.
63. Zargar-Shoshtari K, Sammour T, Kahokehr A, et al. Randomized clinical trial of the effect of glucocorticoids on peritoneal inflammation and postoperative recovery after colectomy. Br J Surg 2009;96(11):1253–61.
64. Herndon DN, Hart DW, Wolf SE, et al. Reversal of catabolism by beta-blockade after severe burns. N Engl J Med 2001;345(17):1223–9.
65. Billeter AT, Hohmann SF, Druen D, et al. Unintentional perioperative hypothermia is associated with severe complications and high mortality in elective operations. Surgery 2014;156(5):1245–52.
66. Forbes SS, Eskicioglu C, Nathens AB, et al. Evidence-based guidelines for prevention of perioperative hypothermia. J Am Coll Surg 2009;209(4):492–503.e1.
67. Popping DM, Elia N, Van Aken HK, et al. Impact of epidural analgesia on mortality and morbidity after surgery: systematic review and meta-analysis of randomized controlled trials. Ann Surg 2014;259(6):1056–67.
68. Liu Y, Zheng Y, Gu X, et al. The efficacy of NMDA receptor antagonists for preventing remifentanil-induced increase in postoperative pain and analgesic requirement: a meta-analysis. Minerva Anestesiol 2012;78(6):653–67.
69. Kaba A, Laurent SR, Detroz BJ, et al. Intravenous lidocaine infusion facilitates acute rehabilitation after laparoscopic colectomy. Anesthesiology 2007;106(1):11–8 [discussion: 15–6].
70. Wongyingsinn M, Baldini G, Stein B, et al. Spinal analgesia for laparoscopic colonic resection using an enhanced recovery after surgery programme: better analgesia, but no benefits on postoperative recovery: a randomized controlled trial. Br J Anaesth 2012;108(5):850–6.
71. Levy BF, Scott MJ, Fawcett W, et al. Randomized clinical trial of epidural, spinal or patient-controlled analgesia for patients undergoing laparoscopic colorectal surgery. Br J Surg 2011;98(8):1068–78.
72. PROcedure SPECific postoperative pain managemenT (PROSPECT). Available at: http://www.postoppain.org/. Accessed February 28, 2013.
73. Coppola S, Froio S, Chiumello D. Protective lung ventilation during general anesthesia: is there any evidence? Crit Care 2014;18(2):210.
74. Hovaguimian F, Lysakowski C, Elia N, et al. Effect of intraoperative high inspired oxygen fraction on surgical site infection, postoperative nausea and vomiting, and pulmonary function: systematic review and meta-analysis of randomized controlled trials. Anesthesiology 2013;119(2):303–16.
75. Martini CH, Boon M, Bevers RF, et al. Evaluation of surgical conditions during laparoscopic surgery in patients with moderate vs deep neuromuscular block. Br J Anaesth 2014;112(3):498–505.
76. Murphy GS, Brull SJ. Residual neuromuscular block: lessons unlearned. Part I: definitions, incidence, and adverse physiologic effects of residual neuromuscular block. Anesth Analg 2010;111(1):120–8.
77. Brull SJ, Murphy GS. Residual neuromuscular block: lessons unlearned. Part II: methods to reduce the risk of residual weakness. Anesth Analg 2010;111(1):129–40.

78. Kotake Y, Ochiai R, Suzuki T, et al. Reversal with sugammadex in the absence of monitoring did not preclude residual neuromuscular block. Anesth Analg 2013; 117(2):345–51.
79. Abrishami A, Ho J, Wong J, et al. Sugammadex, a selective reversal medication for preventing postoperative residual neuromuscular blockade. Cochrane Database Syst Rev 2009;(4):CD007362.
80. Danelli G, Berti M, Perotti V, et al. Temperature control and recovery of bowel function after laparoscopic or laparotomic colorectal surgery in patients receiving combined epidural/general anesthesia and postoperative epidural analgesia. Anesth Analg 2002;95(2):467–71.
81. Mythen MG, Swart M, Acheson N, et al. Perioperative fluid management: consensus statement from the enhanced recovery partnership. Perioper Med (Lond) 2012;1:2.
82. Chappell D, Jacob M, Hofmann-Kiefer K, et al. A rational approach to perioperative fluid management. Anesthesiology 2008;109(4):723–40.
83. Marik PE, Baram M, Vahid B. Does central venous pressure predict fluid responsiveness? A systematic review of the literature and the tale of seven mares. Chest 2008;134(1):172–8.
84. Kumar A, Anel R, Bunnell E, et al. Pulmonary artery occlusion pressure and central venous pressure fail to predict ventricular filling volume, cardiac performance, or the response to volume infusion in normal subjects. Crit Care Med 2004;32(3):691–9.
85. Osman D, Ridel C, Ray P, et al. Cardiac filling pressures are not appropriate to predict hemodynamic response to volume challenge. Crit Care Med 2007;35(1):64–8.
86. Noblett SE, Snowden CP, Shenton BK, et al. Randomized clinical trial assessing the effect of Doppler-optimized fluid management on outcome after elective colorectal resection. Br J Surg 2006;93(9):1069–76.
87. Wakeling HG, McFall MR, Jenkins CS, et al. Intraoperative oesophageal Doppler guided fluid management shortens postoperative hospital stay after major bowel surgery. Br J Anaesth 2005;95(5):634–42.
88. Gan TJ, Soppitt A, Maroof M, et al. Goal-directed intraoperative fluid administration reduces length of hospital stay after major surgery. Anesthesiology 2002; 97(4):820–6.
89. Conway DH, Mayall R, Abdul-Latif MS, et al. Randomised controlled trial investigating the influence of intravenous fluid titration using oesophageal Doppler monitoring during bowel surgery. Anaesthesia 2002;57(9):845–9.
90. Srinivasa S, Taylor MH, Singh PP, et al. Randomized clinical trial of goal-directed fluid therapy within an enhanced recovery protocol for elective colectomy. Br J Surg 2013;100(1):66–74.
91. Brandstrup B, Svendsen PE, Rasmussen M, et al. Which goal for fluid therapy during colorectal surgery is followed by the best outcome: near-maximal stroke volume or zero fluid balance? Br J Anaesth 2012;109(2):191–9.
92. Srinivasa S, Lemanu DP, Singh PP, et al. Systematic review and meta-analysis of oesophageal Doppler-guided fluid management in colorectal surgery. Br J Surg 2013;100(13):1701–8.
93. Pearse RM, Harrison DA, MacDonald N, et al. Effect of a perioperative, cardiac output-guided hemodynamic therapy algorithm on outcomes following major gastrointestinal surgery: a randomized clinical trial and systematic review. JAMA 2014;311(21):2181–90.
94. Nygren J, Thacker J, Carli F, et al. Guidelines for perioperative care in elective rectal/pelvic surgery: Enhanced Recovery After Surgery (ERAS(R)) Society recommendations. World J Surg 2013;37(2):285–305.

95. Grocott MP, Dushianthan A, Hamilton MA, et al. Perioperative increase in global blood flow to explicit defined goals and outcomes after surgery: a Cochrane systematic review. Br J Anaesth 2013;111(4):535–48.

96. Hamilton MA, Cecconi M, Rhodes A. A systematic review and meta-analysis on the use of preemptive hemodynamic intervention to improve postoperative outcomes in moderate and high-risk surgical patients. Anesth Analg 2011;112(6): 1392–402.

97. Miller TE, Roche AM, Mythen M. Fluid management and goal-directed therapy as an adjunct to Enhanced Recovery After Surgery (ERAS). Can J Anaesth 2014.

98. Benes J, Chytra I, Altmann P, et al. Intraoperative fluid optimization using stroke volume variation in high risk surgical patients: results of prospective randomized study. Crit Care 2010;14(3):R118.

99. Benes J, Giglio M, Brienza N, et al. The effects of goal-directed fluid therapy based on dynamic parameters on post-surgical outcome: a meta-analysis of randomized controlled trials. Crit Care 2014;18:584.

100. Jammer I, Ulvik A, Erichsen C, et al. Does central venous oxygen saturation-directed fluid therapy affect postoperative morbidity after colorectal surgery? A randomized assessor-blinded controlled trial. Anesthesiology 2010;113(5): 1072–80.

101. Gould TH, Grace K, Thorne G, et al. Effect of thoracic epidural anaesthesia on colonic blood flow. Br J Anaesth 2002;89(3):446–51.

102. Hiltebrand LB, Koepfli E, Kimberger O, et al. Hypotension during fluid-restricted abdominal surgery: effects of norepinephrine treatment on regional and micro-circulatory blood flow in the intestinal tract. Anesthesiology 2011;114(3): 557–64.

103. Powell-Tuck J, Gosling P, Lobo DN, et al. British Consensus Guidelines on Intravenous Fluid Therapy for Adult Surgical Patients (GIFTASUP). London: NHS National Library of Health; 2009.

104. McCluskey SA, Karkouti K, Wijeysundera D, et al. Hyperchloremia after noncardiac surgery is independently associated with increased morbidity and mortality: a propensity-matched cohort study. Anesth Analg 2013;117(2):412–21.

105. Yunos NM, Bellomo R, Hegarty C, et al. Association between a chloride-liberal vs chloride-restrictive intravenous fluid administration strategy and kidney injury in critically ill adults. JAMA 2012;308(15):1566–72.

106. Shaw AD, Bagshaw SM, Goldstein SL, et al. Major complications, mortality, and resource utilization after open abdominal surgery: 0.9% saline compared to Plasma-Lyte. Ann Surg 2012;255(5):821–9.

107. Myburgh JA, Finfer S, Bellomo R, et al. Hydroxyethyl starch or saline for fluid resuscitation in intensive care. N Engl J Med 2012;367(20):1901–11.

108. Perner A, Haase N, Guttormsen AB, et al. Hydroxyethyl starch 130/0.42 versus Ringer's acetate in severe sepsis. N Engl J Med 2012;367(2):124–34.

109. Gillies MA, Habicher M, Jhanji S, et al. Incidence of postoperative death and acute kidney injury associated with i.v. 6% hydroxyethyl starch use: systematic review and meta-analysis. Br J Anaesth 2014;112(1):25–34.

110. Rasmussen KC, Johansson PI, Hojskov M, et al. Hydroxyethyl starch reduces coagulation competence and increases blood loss during major surgery: results from a randomized controlled trial. Ann Surg 2014;259(2):249–54.

111. Hare GM, Freedman J, David Mazer C. Review article: risks of anemia and related management strategies: can perioperative blood management improve patient safety? Can J Anaesth 2013;60(2):168–75.

112. Bernard AC, Davenport DL, Chang PK, et al. Intraoperative transfusion of 1 U to 2 U packed red blood cells is associated with increased 30-day mortality, surgical-site infection, pneumonia, and sepsis in general surgery patients. J Am Coll Surg 2009;208(5):931–7, 937.e1–2; [discussion: 938–9].

113. Apfel CC, Laara E, Koivuranta M, et al. A simplified risk score for predicting postoperative nausea and vomiting: conclusions from cross-validations between two centers. Anesthesiology 1999;91(3):693–700.

114. Gan TJ, Diemunsch P, Habib AS, et al. Consensus guidelines for the management of postoperative nausea and vomiting. Anesth Analg 2014;118(1): 85–113.

115. Gustafsson UO, Thorell A, Soop M, et al. Haemoglobin A1c as a predictor of postoperative hyperglycaemia and complications after major colorectal surgery. Br J Surg 2009;96(11):1358–64.

116. Ong CK, Lirk P, Seymour RA, et al. The efficacy of preemptive analgesia for acute postoperative pain management: a meta-analysis. Anesth Analg 2005; 100(3):757–73.

117. Niemi G, Breivik H. The minimally effective concentration of adrenaline in a low-concentration thoracic epidural analgesic infusion of bupivacaine, fentanyl and adrenaline after major surgery. A randomized, double-blind, dose-finding study. Acta Anaesthesiol Scand 2003;47(4):439–50.

118. Chan AK, Cheung CW, Chong YK. Alpha-2 agonists in acute pain management. Expert Opin Pharmacother 2010;11(17):2849–68.

119. Werawatganon T, Charuluxanun S. Patient controlled intravenous opioid analgesia versus continuous epidural analgesia for pain after intra-abdominal surgery. Cochrane Database Syst Rev 2005;(1):CD004088.

120. Shi WZ, Miao YL, Yakoob MY, et al. Recovery of gastrointestinal function with thoracic epidural vs. systemic analgesia following gastrointestinal surgery. Acta Anaesthesiol Scand 2014;58(8):923–32.

121. Uchida I, Asoh T, Shirasaka C, et al. Effect of epidural analgesia on postoperative insulin resistance as evaluated by insulin clamp technique. Br J Surg 1988; 75(6):557–62.

122. Popping DM, Elia N, Marret E, et al. Protective effects of epidural analgesia on pulmonary complications after abdominal and thoracic surgery: a meta-analysis. Arch Surg 2008;143(10):990–9 [discussion: 1000].

123. Block BM, Liu SS, Rowlingson AJ, et al. Efficacy of postoperative epidural analgesia: a meta-analysis. JAMA 2003;290(18):2455–63.

124. Richards ER, Kabir SI, McNaught CE, et al. Effect of thoracic epidural anaesthesia on splanchnic blood flow. Br J Surg 2013;100(3):316–21.

125. Gramigni E, Bracco D, Carli F. Epidural analgesia and postoperative orthostatic haemodynamic changes. Eur J Anaesthesiol 2013;30(7):398–404.

126. Abdallah FW, Chan VW, Brull R. Transversus abdominis plane block: a systematic review. Reg Anesth Pain Med 2012;37(2):193–209.

127. Abdallah FW, Laffey JG, Halpern SH, et al. Duration of analgesic effectiveness after the posterior and lateral transversus abdominis plane block techniques for transverse lower abdominal incisions: a meta-analysis. Br J Anaesth 2013; 111(5):721–35.

128. Ventham NT, O'Neill S, Johns N, et al. Evaluation of novel local anesthetic wound infiltration techniques for postoperative pain following colorectal resection surgery: a meta-analysis. Dis Colon Rectum 2014;57(2):237–50.

129. Ventham NT, Hughes M, O'Neill S, et al. Systematic review and meta-analysis of continuous local anaesthetic wound infiltration versus epidural analgesia for

postoperative pain following abdominal surgery. Br J Surg 2013;100(10): 1280–9.

130. Halabi WJ, Kang CY, Nguyen VQ, et al. Epidural analgesia in laparoscopic colorectal surgery: a nationwide analysis of use and outcomes. JAMA Surg 2014; 149(2):130–6.

131. Rawal N. Epidural technique for postoperative pain: gold standard no more? Reg Anesth Pain Med 2012;37(3):310–7.

132. Hubner M, Blanc C, Roulin D, et al. Randomized clinical trial on epidural versus patient-controlled analgesia for laparoscopic colorectal surgery within an enhanced recovery pathway. J Am Coll Surg 2013;216(6):1124–34.

133. Joshi GP, Bonnet F, Kehlet H, et al. Evidence-based postoperative pain management after laparoscopic colorectal surgery. Colorectal Dis 2013;15(2):146–55.

134. Wongyingsinn M, Baldini G, Charlebois P, et al. Intravenous lidocaine versus thoracic epidural analgesia: a randomized controlled trial in patients undergoing laparoscopic colorectal surgery using an enhanced recovery program. Reg Anesth Pain Med 2011;36(3):241–8.

135. Khan SA, Khokhar HA, Nasr AR, et al. Effect of epidural analgesia on bowel function in laparoscopic colorectal surgery: a systematic review and meta-analysis. Surg Endosc 2013;27(7):2581–91.

136. De Oliveira GS Jr, Castro-Alves LJ, Nader A, et al. Transversus abdominis plane block to ameliorate postoperative pain outcomes after laparoscopic surgery: a meta-analysis of randomized controlled trials. Anesth Analg 2014;118(2): 454–63.

137. Kahokehr A, Sammour T, Shoshtari KZ, et al. Intraperitoneal local anesthetic improves recovery after colon resection: a double-blinded randomized controlled trial. Ann Surg 2011;254(1):28–38.

138. Favuzza J, Brady K, Delaney CP. Transversus abdominis plane blocks and enhanced recovery pathways: making the 23-h hospital stay a realistic goal after laparoscopic colorectal surgery. Surg Endosc 2013;27(7):2481–6.

139. Favuzza J, Delaney CP. Outcomes of discharge after elective laparoscopic colorectal surgery with transversus abdominis plane blocks and enhanced recovery pathway. J Am Coll Surg 2013;217(3):503–6.

140. Keller DS, Stulberg JJ, Lawrence JK, et al. Process control to measure process improvement in colorectal surgery: modifications to an established enhanced recovery pathway. Dis Colon Rectum 2014;57(2):194–200.

141. Boulind CE, Ewings P, Bulley SH, et al. Feasibility study of analgesia via epidural versus continuous wound infusion after laparoscopic colorectal resection. Br J Surg 2013;100(3):395–402.

142. Klein M. Postoperative non-steroidal anti-inflammatory drugs and colorectal anastomotic leakage. NSAIDs and anastomotic leakage. Dan Med J 2012; 59(3):B4420.

143. Gorissen KJ, Benning D, Berghmans T, et al. Risk of anastomotic leakage with non-steroidal anti-inflammatory drugs in colorectal surgery. Br J Surg 2012;99: 721–7.

144. Burton TP, Mittal A, Soop M. Nonsteroidal anti-inflammatory drugs and anastomotic dehiscence in bowel surgery: systematic review and meta-analysis of randomized, controlled trials. Dis Colon Rectum 2013;56(1):126–34.

145. Candiotti KA, Sands LR, Lee E, et al. Liposome bupivacaine for postsurgical analgesia in adult patients undergoing laparoscopic colectomy: results from prospective phase IV sequential cohort studies assessing health economic outcomes. Curr Ther Res Clin Exp 2014;76:1–6.

146. Cohen SM. Extended pain relief trial utilizing infiltration of Exparel(R), a long-acting multivesicular liposome formulation of bupivacaine: a Phase IV health economic trial in adult patients undergoing open colectomy. J Pain Res 2012; 5:567–72.
147. Ash SA, Buggy DJ. Does regional anaesthesia and analgesia or opioid analgesia influence recurrence after primary cancer surgery? An update of available evidence. Best Pract Res Clin Anaesthesiol 2013;27(4):441–56.
148. Lirk P, Berger R, Hollmann MW, et al. Lidocaine time- and dose-dependently demethylates deoxyribonucleic acid in breast cancer cell lines in vitro. Br J Anaesth 2012;109(2):200–7.
149. Singh PP, Lemanu DP, Taylor MH, et al. Association between preoperative glucocorticoids and long-term survival and cancer recurrence after colectomy: follow-up analysis of a previous randomized controlled trial. Br J Anaesth 2014;113(Suppl 1):i68–73.
150. Acheson AG, Brookes MJ, Spahn DR. Effects of allogeneic red blood cell transfusions on clinical outcomes in patients undergoing colorectal cancer surgery: a systematic review and meta-analysis. Ann Surg 2012;256(2):235–44.
151. Dellinger RP, Levy MM, Rhodes A, et al. Surviving Sepsis Campaign: international guidelines for management of severe sepsis and septic shock, 2012. Intensive Care Med 2013;39(2):165–228.
152. Veenstra G, Ince C, Boerma EC. Direct markers of organ perfusion to guide fluid therapy: when to start, when to stop. Best Pract Res Clin Anaesthesiol 2014; 28(3):217–26.
153. Ludikhuize J, Smorenburg SM, de Rooij SE, et al. Identification of deteriorating patients on general wards; measurement of vital parameters and potential effectiveness of the Modified Early Warning Score. J Crit Care 2012;27(4):424.e7–13.

Anesthesia for Hepatobiliary Surgery

Chris Snowden, MBBS, FRCA, MD[a,b,]*, James Prentis, MBBS, FRCA[a]

KEYWORDS

- Hepatobiliary • Anesthesia • Hepatectomy • Enhanced recovery • Intrathecal
- Opiate

KEY POINTS

- Reduced mortality after hepatobiliary surgery is related to improved patient selection, introduction of preoperative embolization techniques, improved intraoperative surgical techniques/equipment, and reduced operative blood loss.
- Alternative therapies (eg, radiofrequency ablation) are being introduced in patients who are unable to tolerate extensive hepatic resections.
- Lowering the central venous pressure during hepatic resection reduces blood loss but must be optimized to avoid hypovolemia and excessive use of vasoconstrictor medication.
- Intrathecal opiates may provide an alternative postoperative pain control regimen to epidural analgesia, especially where there is abnormal coagulation.

INTRODUCTION

Hepatobiliary (HPB) surgery, variably defined to include pancreatic surgery, and liver and pancreas transplantation, has become a major surgical specialty with explicit training opportunities, mainly as a response to poor surgical outcomes in the early 1970s. The subsequent improvement in HPB surgical outcomes (now usually <5% mortality) has been associated with:

1. The concentration of HPB surgery to large volume centers
2. Better preoperative treatment, including radiologic venous embolization and chemoradiotherapy regimes
3. Introduction of newer surgical techniques and equipment to minimize blood loss (eg, Cavitron ultrasonic aspirator [CUSA] or harmonic scalpel to dissect the liver parenchyma).

The authors have no disclosures.
[a] Department of Perioperative and Critical Care Medicine, Freeman Hospital, Freeman Road, Newcastle upon Tyne NE7 7DN, UK; [b] Institute of Cellular Medicine, The Medical School, University of Newcastle upon Tyne, Framlington Place, Newcastle upon Tyne NE1 4LP, UK
* Corresponding author. Department of Perioperative and Critical Care Medicine, Freeman Hospital, Freeman Road, Newcastle upon Tyne NE7 7DN, UK.
E-mail address: Chris.Snowden@nuth.nhs.uk

Anesthesiology Clin 33 (2015) 125–141
http://dx.doi.org/10.1016/j.anclin.2014.11.008
1932-2275/15/$ – see front matter © 2015 Elsevier Inc. All rights reserved.

anesthesiology.theclinics.com

Alongside these surgical advances, it is recognized that advanced anesthetic management of the HPB surgery patient has significantly contributed to improved outcomes. These advances have come predominantly through more appropriate preoperative patient selection, intraoperative techniques to prevent and manage blood loss, and postoperative enhanced recovery protocols with improved analgesic regimens.

The present article relates primarily to the management of patients undergoing hepatic resection. In this context, we address anesthetic and surgical considerations, including patient selection, alternative surgical management options, the reduction of operative blood loss, introduction of the components of postoperative enhanced recovery, and considerations related to postoperative liver dysfunction and failure.

HEPATIC RESECTION
Outcomes of Hepatic Resection

Hepatic resection is performed for a number of underlying pathologies, including benign or malignant primary tumors, secondary metastases (predominantly colorectal), and liver trauma. Surgical criteria for patient selection are important.[1] If hepatic malignancy is involved, operative resection is established as the only currently available modality of treatment with curative potential.

Patients with untreated but potentially resectable hepatic malignancy have been reported to have a median survival time of less than 6 months,[2] with virtually no 5-year survival. Surgical treatment for hepatocellular carcinoma prolongs 10-year survival to 15%.[3] Five-year survival after hepatic resection for metastases is 33%,[4] compared with 11% in those not undergoing operative resection. The aim of hepatic resection is to effect clear tumor margins, while ensuring adequate remaining residual liver to prevent postoperative hepatic insufficiency. The relevance of a clear resection margin is reflected in survival. For patients with tumor-free margins greater than 1 cm, a 5-year disease-free survival rate of 35% can be expected. Survival rates are 21% for patients for whom tumor margins are less than 1 cm, and no 5-year survivors can be expected when the margins are involved by tumor.[5]

Hepatic Regeneration

Residual liver volume after surgery is important to postoperative hepatic dysfunction.[6] The volume of liver that can be safely resected in humans is approximately 80%,[7] assuming good function in the remaining liver, although there are early reports of survival after resections of 90%.[8] The potential for these massive resections (or extensive ablations) relies on postoperative hepatic regeneration, which has a complex mechanism.[9] Under normal circumstances, the human liver initiates regeneration within 3 days and has reached its original size by 6 months,[10] although some studies have shown full restoration at 3 months. Rapid regeneration may allow complete functional recovery within 2 to 3 weeks.[11]

Preoperative Portal Vein Embolization

If there is a predicted risk of liver failure developing after a procedure, through need to remove large liver components, then the preemptive maneuvers of portal embolization of affected segments, some weeks before resection can stimulate regeneration in the proposed liver remnant, thereby enhancing postoperative liver function.[12–14] An increase of 40% to 60% in the size of the nonembolized liver can be anticipated in noncirrhotic livers.[15,16] Similarly, chemoembolization can be used in potentially unresectable hepatocellular carcinoma to reduce tumor mass and increase residual function to an extent that may permit definitive resection.

Alternatives/Adjuncts to Hepatic Resection

Because only approximately 10% to 20% of patients presenting with hepatic malignancy are suitable for resection, other types of less invasive HPB surgical techniques are used, with good success rates,[17] to achieve reduction of tumor mass and symptomatic control. Radiofrequency ablation,[17,18] cryoablation,[19,20] and the recently applied selective internal radiation therapy techniques[21,22] can be performed percutaneously, laparoscopically, or during open laparotomy. The percutaneous approach is usually indicated for palliation,[23] whereas laparoscopic ablation is selected for smaller, superficially located, or easily accessible tumors with intraoperative ultrasound guidance. Open surgical ablation is indicated for larger or deeply located malignancy and may be combined with hepatic resection where multiple tumors are present. Ablation probes inserted into the tumor center aim to locally destroy tumor mass through heat ($100°C$–$110°C$) or by cooling (with liquid nitrogen). Potential complications of these techniques include hemorrhage (including hepatic capsular rupture), biliary leak, and thrombocytopenia and myoglobinuria, which have been reported in more extensive procedures.

PREOPERATIVE CONSIDERATIONS

Perioperative management of HPB patients depends a complete understanding of the potential benefits, limitations, and perioperative risks of major surgical procedures, in the context of either coexisting disease states and/or preexisting liver disease.

Hepatic Resection in Patients Without Comorbidity

A significant component of metastatic (especially colorectal secondaries) HPB surgery is undertaken in otherwise fit patients. In these situations, prolonged preoperative assessment of anesthetic fitness is not required, even for extensive resections and where malignant disease is present, because this will lead to unacceptable delays in treatment. Surgery after preoperative neoadjuvant chemotherapy for colorectal metastases is often delayed by up to 4 weeks to allow for patient recovery and to reduce postoperative and surgical complications. However, there is no benefit in delaying surgery for longer than 4 weeks.[24]

Hepatic Resection, Age, and Comorbid Disease

Improvements in anesthetic and surgical techniques, which have been successful in improving outcomes, are already translating into more extensive HPB surgery being undertaken in older individuals with more comorbid diseases.[25,26] Advancing chronologic age should not be viewed as a surgical barrier and there are multiple series suggesting that resections for hepatocellular carcinoma and colorectal metastases can be performed safely in these patients.[25,27] Recent evidence suggests that cardiorespiratory fitness may have a more important influence on perioperative outcomes in HPB surgery than chronologic age per se.[28] Nevertheless, advancing age reduces liver size and blood flow, decreases drug metabolism (phase I), and increases the incidence of alcohol-induced cirrhosis through environmental exposure.[29] Prolonged exposure to environmental factors also leads to the development of covert forms of liver disease, reducing hepatic reserve and increasing susceptibility to hepatic ischemia–reperfusion injury during resection.[29] Importantly, steatohepatitis constitutes the third commonest liver disease in the United States and has been estimated to be present in 20% of the US population. The etiology may be secondary to alcohol intake or related primarily to diabetes and/or obesity in the form of nonalcoholic steatohepatitis. Even so, there may be a paradoxic protective benefit of steatohepatitis after liver resection for colorectal metastases.[30]

Hepatic Resection and Preexisting Liver Disease

Where preexisting liver disease is present, increased perioperative risk depends on the nature and severity of the disease and the extent of hepatic dysfunction. This condition requires more specific assessment. Cirrhotics have an increased incidence of surgical intervention for multiple reasons, including variceal bleeding and increased hepatoma formation. Patients with cirrhosis have insufficient hepatocyte function to meet the increased metabolic demands after partial hepatectomy,[31] and have significantly reduced levels of hepatic regeneration after liver resection, making them extremely vulnerable to posthepatectomy liver failure. Although chronic liver disease is not an absolute contraindication to resection, morbidity and mortality increases dramatically with worsening hepatic dysfunction. One severity scoring system is the Child–Pugh score (**Table 1**), which was originally used to assess chronic liver disease prognosis but has since been used for major surgery outcome. Child–Pugh class B or C (scores of 7–9 and 10–15, respectively) may exclude a patient from major resection. However, Child–Pugh class A (score of 5–6) patients should be considered for surgery and in these patients there is significant incentive toward optimizing preoperative medical care to improve the postoperative prognosis. However, in terms of risk prediction for hepatic surgery, none of the preexisting systems relating liver disease severity to perioperative outcome is ideal. The Child–Pugh scoring system has demonstrated an association with perioperative risk in patients undergoing esophageal transaction, nonshunt surgery, and abdominal surgery. The Model for End-Stage Liver Disease score may be important where there is existing cirrhosis[32] and hepatocellular carcinoma,[33] but should not be used in the context of elective hepatic resection with normal liver function.[34] Patients with cholangitis may also be at high risk of postoperative complications.[35] One risk prediction model suggests that renal impairment, bleeding, ascites, American Society of Anesthesiologists grade, histologic diagnosis of cirrhosis, and intraoperative hypotension are the most important perioperative factors related to postoperative outcome.[36] However, because newer operative procedures have evolved and the benefits of improved diagnostic facilities, including biochemical parameters, are absent from these predictive scoring systems, the applicability of these systems to newer HPB surgery risk prediction is uncertain.

Table 1 Child-Pugh scoring system			
Measure	1 Point	2 Points	3 Points
Total bilirubin μmol/L (mg/dL)	<34 (<2)	34–50 (2–3)	>50 (>3)
Serum albumin (g/dL)	>3.5	2.8–3.5	<2.8
PT/INR: http://en.wikipedia.org/wiki/ Prothrombin_time - International_ normalized_ratio	<1.7	1.71–2.30	>2.30
Ascites	None	Mild	Moderate to severe
Hepatic encephalopathy	None	Grade I-II (or suppressed with medication)	Grade III-IV (or refractory)

Clinically, the relevance of each preoperative severity marker to an individual's potential risk may be more practical. Nutritional status and albumin are important factors common to the postoperative recovery of all surgical patients and are not discussed further herein. More specific markers of liver disease severity include jaundice, coagulopathy, ascites, and encephalopathy.

Jaundice

The importance of preoperative jaundice is owing to its prominent association with perioperative renal impairment.[37–39] The mean incidence of postoperative renal impairment in surgical patients with jaundice is 8%, but may be as high 18%. Whereas the overall postoperative mortality rate in surgical patients with jaundice ranges from 0% to 27%, the mortality for jaundiced patients who go on to develop acute renal failure is estimated at 65%. Thus, development of postoperative renal failure is a poor prognostic sign. The etiology of postoperative renal failure in the setting of liver disease is multifactorial and includes central volume depletion, defective renal vascular reactivity, vasoactive mediator imbalance (in which local prostaglandins play a prominent role), and the effect of endotoxin. This makes the renal vasculature susceptible to renotoxic drugs such as nonsteroidal anti-inflammatory drugs and contrast media. Preoperative measures to prevent the onset of renal impairment have included adequate preoperative hydration, mannitol infusion, bile salts, and lactulose. However, none have demonstrated consistent benefit in adequate clinical trials. Preoperative percutaneous or endoscopic biliary drainage before major HPB surgery does not improve perioperative outcome consistently and may increase the incidence of cholangitis, known to be a poor prognostic factor for outcome. However, preoperative biliary drainage followed by portal vein embolization has been advocated as a beneficial strategy for major hepatectomy in perihilar cholangiocarcinoma.[40] Prolonged periods of preoperative drainage may allow for the resolution of jaundice, but does not lead to improved perioperative outcome. Therefore, biliary drainage should be limited to 2 weeks before surgery.[41]

Coagulopathy

Correction of coagulation before liver resection is essential where central neuraxial blockade is being considered. Vitamin K, fresh frozen plasma, or cryoprecipitate may be required to correct liver-related coagulopathy preoperatively. Reduction in platelet counts in these patients is common, but abnormalities in platelet function are often more relevant. Therefore, the preoperative administration of platelets is better guided by laboratory testing (eg, thromboelastogram) results than by clinical judgment.

Ascites

The development of ascites is a poor prognostic sign in cirrhosis and may adversely influence perioperative respiratory mechanics. Furthermore, ascites, secondary to splanchnic arteriolar vasodilatation, develops at the expense of circulating intravascular fluid. In conjunction with medical therapy, including diuresis and paracentesis, there is a real risk of significant intravascular hypovolemia. Attempts should be made to correct this state preoperatively and it is important to recognize that perioperative fluid limitation does not prevent the development of postoperative ascites.

Encephalopathy

Subclinical hepatic encephalopathy is present in 30% to 70% of cirrhotics and can be detected by subtle psychometric testing. Elective hepatic surgery should be deferred until the cause of preoperative encephalopathy is ascertained and effective treatment is provided. Preoperative lactulose may prevent encephalopathy from worsening, but treatment of the cause, for example, infection or hemorrhage, is more important. This is particularly relevant wherever postoperative encephalopathy develops de novo, because it is often difficult to distinguish between encephalopathy and drug intoxication. Drug-induced intoxication has a much better prognosis than spontaneous encephalopathy.

INTRAOPERATIVE CONSIDERATIONS

Excessive surgical blood loss is related to adverse short- and long-term postoperative outcomes after liver resection.[42] Because resting total hepatic blood flow represents about 25% of cardiac output (1200–1400 mL/min; ~100 mL/min/100 g), surgical transection of liver parenchyma carries a high risk of blood loss. Reduction of blood loss is therefore a major consideration during the intraoperative period. Advances in surgical technique, equipment, and anesthetic measures have all been useful in reducing blood loss and are detailed herein.

Surgical Vascular Occlusion

Hepatic vascular occlusion is used to reduce blood loss from the liver surface during surgical dissection (**Fig. 1**).[43,44] Although occlusion times of up to 60 minutes are considered safe in noncirrhotic livers, postoperative hepatic insufficiency and encephalopathy may occur with shorter durations.[45,46] In cirrhotic livers, 30 minutes is considered safe and possibly up to 60 minutes in early disease.[47]

Pringle maneuver

Pringle[48] first described a technique to prevent bleeding during hepatic trauma surgery by clamping the hepatoduodenal ligament and interrupting blood flow in both the hepatic artery and portal vein. The Pringle maneuver (PM) is generally well-tolerated haemodynamically,[49] even though it is associated with a 10% increase in mean arterial pressure, a 40% increase in systemic vascular resistance, and a 10% decrease in cardiac output. However, prolonged interruption of hepatic inflow (>1 hour in normal liver and >30 minutes in pathologic livers)[50] may cause ischemia/reperfusion injury to the remaining liver. Recent evidence suggests that the PM should be avoided in hepatectomy for malignancy owing to deleterious effects on tumor recurrence.[51]

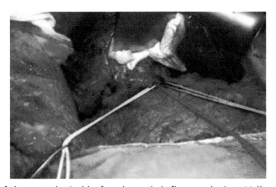

Fig. 1. Isolation of the portal triad before hepatic inflow occlusion. Yellow, bile duct; red 1, right hepatic artery; red 2, left hepatic artery; blue, portal vein.

Intermittent Pringle maneuver

An intermittent vascular occlusive technique (intermittent PM [IPM]) has been developed to reduce the risk of ischemia/reperfusion. This incorporates 15 to 20 minutes of interrupted liver blood flow, followed by a 5-minute period of reperfusion and incorporates the mechanism of organ preconditioning.[52,53] IPM reduces splanchnic congestion and decreases hepatic ischemia/reperfusion injury. A randomized, controlled trial concluded that a compromised liver better tolerates IPM than continuous PM,[52] but there is no significant benefit where normal parenchyma exists. However, disadvantages of IPM include increased blood loss from the transection surface during the unclamped period and prolongation of the transection phase. A recent European survey[54] suggests that IPM is the method of choice for hepatic resection, with a total ischemic time limited to 15 to 30 minutes.

Selective inflow occlusion

Selectively occluding the blood flow to the left or right hemiliver during resection may further reduce theoretically the risk of hepatic ischemic/reperfusion injury seen with IPM. However, meta-analysis has failed to show any significant improvement in outcome when compared with either PM or IPM, except for resections on cirrhotic livers.[55,56] This technique also requires extensive hilar dissection, which can make subsequent resection technically challenging.

Total vascular exclusion

Total vascular exclusion incorporates isolation of suprahepatic, subdiaphragmatic, and infrahepatic vena cava combined with the PM. Total vascular exclusion reduces bleeding, but carries with it significant per and postoperative morbidity ($\leq$50%) and mortality up to 10%[57,58] and there is no evidence for benefit over the PM.[56] The technique is usually restricted to cases where the tumor arises near to or involves either the retrohepatic vena cava or the confluence of hepatic veins and vena cava. Approximately 10% of patients will not tolerate the hemodynamic effects of vena caval occlusion and may require venovenous bypass.

Surgical Equipment Development

Developments in HPB surgical equipment have also assisted in reducing perioperative blood loss. The optimal device would aim to destroy liver parenchyma while achieving hemostasis. Unfortunately, no current equipment achieves both these goals and so combination equipment is used.[59]

Cavitron ultrasonic aspirator (CUSA) uses acoustic vibrational force, produced by saline, to promote liver parenchymal disruption (**Fig. 2**).[60,61] A newer device, the harmonic scalpel,[62,63] is a saline-linked radiofrequency sealer that delivers energy through saline dripping from the tip, causing coagulation via necrosis on the transection surface. The large hepatic vessels are left intact by these techniques and exposed vascular structures are separately ligated, stapled,[64] or controlled with diathermy. There is no definitive evidence for one technique, because clinical studies tend to include small patient numbers. Control of residual bleeding of the resected liver surface may be achieved by use of argon beam coagulation or the spray application of fibrin glue.[65,66]

Anesthetic Technique

Intraoperative

Anesthetic techniques during hepatic resection aim to reduce the need for vascular occlusion techniques by minimizing the potential for blood loss through optimum fluid

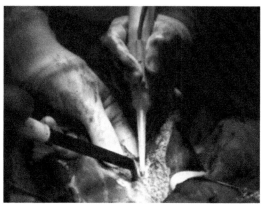

Fig. 2. Hepatic resection using combined Cavitron ultrasonic aspirator (CUSA) and diathermy techniques.

management and the avoidance of unnecessary blood transfusion through appropriate correction of coagulopathy.

Managing central venous pressure The reduction of hepatic venous congestion by careful control of central venous pressure (CVP) during hepatic resection has long been associated with a reduction in intraoperative blood loss.[67–69] CVP control is achieved by combining pharmacologic or epidural-based vasodilatation with the limitation of intravenous fluid given before resection. Jones and colleagues[68] found that the volume of blood loss during liver resection correlated with CVP, regardless of using inflow occlusion. A CVP of 5 cm H_2O or less resulted in a median blood loss of 200 mL and blood transfusions in only 5% of patients compared with a 1000-mL blood loss and 48% blood transfusions in patients with a CVP greater than 5 cm H_2O ($P = .0001$ and $P = .0008$, respectively). However, this study was performed in an era where advanced surgical dissection equipment was not available. A more recent Cochrane review[70] evidenced that a lower CVP reduced blood loss in comparison to control (mean difference, 419.35 mL; 95% CI, –575.06 to –263.63), but there was no difference in red blood cell transfusion requirements (standardized mean difference, –0.31; 95% CI, –0.65 to 0.03), intraoperative morbidity, or long-term survival benefits.[14] The avoidance of positive end-expiratory pressure (PEEP) has also been a mainstay of liver surgery since an increase in PEEP may increase CVP. However, a recent study[71] has shown that increasing PEEP from 5 to 10 cm H_2O, increased hepatic and portal venous pressure by only 1 mmHg. The requirement to reduce postoperative pulmonary complications after major upper abdominal surgery, means that further studies are required to define the effect of PEEP on surgical outcome.

Problems associated with reduced central venous pressure during hepatic resection Maintaining a low CVP may lead to cardiovascular instability, the potential for intraoperative hypovolemia, and susceptibility to reduce renal and hepatosplanchnic blood flow. Where there is ongoing blood loss, the risks of lowering the CVP and maintaining a controlled but potentially hypovolemic state must be weighed against the benefits for minimizing blood loss. More recently, the use of stroke volume variation methods has been suggested as an appropriate replacement for CVP monitoring.[72] However, more appropriately, the two measurements may be used in a synergistic combination to ensure reduced venous pressure (CVP), while maintaining normovolemia (stroke volume variation). Wherever low CVP practices are used in an attempt to reduce blood loss, there may be the requirement for supplementary vaso-constrictors (eg, phenyl ephedrine, vasopressin, or norepinephrine) to maintain systemic blood pressure for perfusion of other organs. However, vasoconstrictors may lead to splanchnic vasoconstriction and secondary hepatic ischemia. Nevertheless, in most reported series where a low CVP technique has been used, with or without the judicious use of vasoconstriction, there does not seem to be an increased incidence of organ (especially renal) failure. Another possible complication of low CVP techniques is air embolus.[73] Diligence in monitoring sudden changes in end-tidal CO_2 and in cauterizing open hepatic vessels is vital.

Management of coagulation The coagulopathy associated with liver disease can contribute significantly to the potential for perioperative bleeding. The liver is the site of production of all coagulation factors (excluding von Willebrand factor) and many coagulation inhibitors, fibrinolytic proteins, and their inhibitors. The liver is also responsible for the breakdown of many of the activated factors of coagulation and fibrinolysis. In addition, platelet abnormalities and thrombocytopenia secondary to cirrhosis and hypersplenism are common in liver disease. Hence, it is clear how a complete range of coagulation abnormalities from hypocoagulability, accelerated fibrinolysis, through to disseminated intravascular coagulation and hypercoagulable states associated with low protein C and S levels can be encountered perioperatively. The complex clotting abnormalities of liver disease are succinctly reviewed by Kang.[74] Preoperative assessment of coagulation is a mandatory part of the workup for major hepatic resection. However, the complex interactions of the numerous aspects of coagulation system often make for uncertain significance of single factor levels. Thromboelastography provides a method for assessing clot formation, coagulation processes, and fibrinolysis. It provides clinical information within 10 to 20 minutes and is therefore used as a point-of-contact guide to appropriate perioperative management of coagulopathy in major hepatic resections.

The natural choice for correcting coagulopathy in liver disease is fresh frozen plasma because it contains all the coagulation and inhibitory factors. However, its effects are relatively short lived and it has the disadvantages of a large volume load and potential cross-infection concerns. Cryoprecipitate is a good source of fibrinogen and tends to be administered for documented hypofibrinogenemia. Platelets transfused during major resections often have only a transient effect, because they undergo splenic sequestration. The antifibrinolytic agent, tranexamic acid has shown promise in reducing transfusion requirement in liver resection and can be used in hepatic surgery with anticipated high blood loss.[75–77] However, a Cochrane review was less supportive in their role during resection.[78] Newer agents such as activated factor VII have been used to good effect in liver failure with active hemorrhage,[79] but a role in elective liver resections remains uncertain.[80]

Other considerations for coagulopathy Because the liver is the site of citrate metabolism, it is important to ensure adequate serum calcium levels during severe coagulopathy and where large volumes of citrated blood products are being transfused. Because major liver resections are often prolonged, the infusion of large fluid volumes and an "open" abdomen provides an efficient heat sink. Invasive temperature monitoring (esophageal or rectal) and scrupulous attention to active warming of the patient and all infusions must be undertaken perioperatively. Even mild hypothermia can lead to increased blood loss, particularly through impairment in platelet function. Laboratory tests of coagulation are performed at 37°C, and may remain normal requiring adjustment where hypothermia exists.

POSTOPERATIVE CONSIDERATIONS

General postoperative complications of major abdominal surgery are also relevant to HPB surgery. In addition, the immediate complications more specific to patients undergoing major hepatic resection include on going coagulopathy and active bleeding, onset or exacerbation of liver failure with encephalopathy, renal impairment, and late biliary leak. For this reason, early postoperative care (12–24 hours) after liver resection should have the facility for the continuation of invasive hemodynamic monitoring and close observation of renal function. In most UK hospitals, this often necessitates critical care.

Nevertheless, enhanced recovery programs developing as the accepted standard for postoperative care in other areas of major surgery have been used in the context of liver resection surgery and have been associated with significant reductions in hospital length of stay and perioperative complications.[81]

Elements of the Enhanced Recovery program of specific relevance to HPB surgery include the following.

Preoperative Carbohydrate Loading

No study has directly studied the use of carbohydrate loading in patients undergoing liver resection. However, an enhanced recovery program in which carbohydrate loading was used showed a reduction in both length of stay and complications.[82]

Surgical Drains

Surgical practice has traditionally placed a drain in the subphrenic space close to the resection surface. The main proposed advantages are the prevention of subphrenic fluid collection, early identification of postoperative bleeding[83] and bile leak,[83,84] and prevention of ascitic fluid accumulation. However, the evidence that surgical drainage is conflicting. A Cochrane review of surgical drainage after liver resection surgery[85] found that bleeding and bile leakage that required emergency surgical or radiologic intervention was uncommon in the early postoperative period after hepatic resection and that prophylactic drainage did not help in the identification or management of these complications. Drainage did not influence mortality rates, and there was an increase in both chest complications and postoperative wound infections. In conclusion, there is no evidence to support routine drain use after liver resections.

Nasogastric Tubes/Oral Nutrition

Nasogastric tube placement and drainage of gastric contents have been routine in liver resection surgery. However, their routine use has been questioned. A randomized, controlled trial of 200 patients[86] concluded that nasogastric tube placement was associated with increase risk of atelectasis and pulmonary complications. Nasogastric tube placement did reduce vomiting rates, but 20% of patients experienced severe discomfort. Their routine use cannot be recommended in the majority of patients. Early oral nutrition after surgery has also been a goal for enhanced recovery programs and has been shown to be achievable after liver resection. Early oral intake allows for discontinuation of IV fluids and accelerated recovery. One study,[87] even though negative for its primary endpoint for the use of laxatives, showed that oral fluid intake can be resumed on the day of surgery in 94% of patients and reintroduction of diet was achieved in 37% on day 1 and in 78% by day 2.

Deep Venous Thrombosis Prophylaxis

Patients undergoing liver resection with prolonged surgery and with underlying metastatic cancer are at risk of postoperative venous thromboembolism. Successful liver resection, with acceptable retained liver function, often leads to a procoagulant postoperative state. Thromboelastogram monitoring also demonstrates a state of postoperative hypercoagulability after living donor hepatectomy.[88] Reduction in liver function leads to a decrease in both procoagulant and anticoagulant factors by up to 50%.[89] Therefore, venous thromboembolism may occur even in the presence of elevated standard measures of anticoagulation such as International Normalized Ratio and partial thromboplastin time.[90,91] In a retrospective review of 415 patients undergoing major hepatectomy, administration of pharmacologic thromboprophylaxis lowered the rate of venous thromboembolism but did not increase the rate of blood transfusion after hepatectomy.[92] On balance, it is recommended that pharmacologic thromboprophylaxis should be part of an enhanced recovery program unless there is an obvious contraindication.

Analgesia

The risks and benefits of any mode of analgesia need to be considered for each individual in deciding the best treatment of postoperative pain. Because this group of patients is at risk of renal impairment and coagulation defects, nonsteroidal antiinflammatory agents should be avoided wherever possible. Opiates that are metabolized in the liver and excreted renally have the potential disadvantage of accumulation with cerebral depressant effects in a population with a tendency to encephalopathy. Use of epidural techniques have been the preferred postoperative analgesic option, given the proposed benefits on postoperative recovery after major surgery and use of large surgical incisions during hepatic surgery. However, a major concern is the associated prolongation of prothrombin time that may develop during surgery. It is debatable whether this coagulopathy increases the risk of epidural hematoma, but it often delays epidural catheter removal and increases administration of corrective blood products.[93] Several studies have suggested that intrathecal opiates are a suitable alternative to epidural analgesia and have a number of advantages, especially in terms of embracing the enhanced recovery ethos.[94] A recent prospective, observational study[95] compared thoracic epidural with intrathecal morphine and fentanyl patient-controlled analgesia. Although CVP and blood loss were lower in the epidural group, in contrast, time to mobilization, fluid requirements, and length of stay were lower in the intrathecal morphine plus fentanyl patient-controlled analgesia group. Pain scores were not different in the first 5 postoperative days.

Postoperative Liver Dysfunction or Failure

In the event of acute liver failure arising after liver resection, attempts should be made to support the patient to allow sufficient time for regeneration of the remaining liver. The mainstay of this is ensuring optimal standards of intensive care management, including airway control, adequate hydration, inotropic and renal support as needed, control of coagulopathy and active bleeding and consideration of N-acetyl cysteine (NAC) infusion. Beneficial effects have been seen in systemic and cerebral hemodynamics in acute liver failure of other causes, an effect not related to stimulation of liver regeneration or hepatoprotection, but initially assigned to improvements in systemic oxygen delivery and oxygen extraction.[96] A later paper[97] refuted the effects of NAC on oxygen delivery and extraction in hepatic failure, suggesting instead that the microcirculatory effects also seen when NAC is used in sepsis may be a more important effect. A recent study,[98] however, has shown that the use of NAC does not reduce alanine aminotransferase levels, suggesting that it does not reduce hepatocellular injury. There was also a higher level of post-hepatic liver failure. Further studies are needed in patients at higher risk of major hepatic failure in those undergoing more extensive resections with a background of significant preoperative liver disease.

SUMMARY

HPB surgical outcome has improved with advancements in surgical technique, training, and equipment. In addition, perioperative management, including improved patient selection, preoperative venous embolization, and intraoperative maneuvers to reduce blood loss, have played an important role in postoperative outcome. Developing enhanced recovery programs that include intrathecal opiate analgesia and improved postoperative mobilization will undoubtedly lead to further improvements in future outcomes.

REFERENCES

1. Van Thiel DH, Wright HI, Fagiuoli S, et al. Preoperative evaluation of a patient for hepatic surgery. J Surg Oncol Suppl 1993;3:49–51.
2. Savage AP, Malt RA. Survival after hepatic resection for malignant tumours. Br J Surg 1992;79(10):1095–101.
3. Franssen B, Jibara G, Tabrizian P, et al. Actual 10-year survival following hepatectomy for hepatocellular carcinoma. HPB (Oxford) 2014;16(9):830–5.
4. Cummings LC, Payes JD, Cooper GS. Survival after hepatic resection in metastatic colorectal cancer. Cancer 2007;109(4):718–26.
5. Dhir M, Lyden ER, Wang A, et al. Influence of margins on overall survival after hepatic resection for colorectal metastasis: a meta-analysis. Ann Surg 2011;254(2): 234–42.
6. Schindl MJ, Redhead DN, Fearon KC, et al. The value of residual liver volume as a predictor of hepatic dysfunction and infection after major liver resection. Gut 2005;54(2):289–96.
7. Mullin EJ, Metcalfe MS, Maddern GJ. How much liver resection is too much? Am J Surg 2005;190(1):87–97.
8. Starzl TE, Putnam CW, Groth CG, et al. Alopecia, ascites, and incomplete regeneration after 85 to 90 per cent liver resection. Am J Surg 1975;129(5):587–90.
9. Kountouras J, Boura P, Lygidakis NJ. Liver regeneration after hepatectomy. Hepatogastroenterology 2001;48(38):556–62.
10. Gove CD, Hughes RD. Liver regeneration in relationship to acute liver failure. Gut 1991;(Suppl):S92–6.
11. Nagasue N. Liver resection for hepatocellular carcinoma: Indications, techniques, complications, and prognostic factors. J Hepatobiliary Pancreat Surg 1998;5(1):7–13.
12. Farges O, Belghiti J, Kianmanesh R, et al. Portal vein embolization before right hepatectomy: prospective clinical trial. Ann Surg 2003;237(2):208–17.
13. Ribero D, Abdalla EK, Madoff DC, et al. Portal vein embolization before major hepatectomy and its effects on regeneration, resectability and outcome. Br J Surg 2007;94(11):1386–94.
14. Abulkhir A, Limongelli P, Healey AJ, et al. Preoperative portal vein embolization for major liver resection. Ann Surg 2008;247(1):49–57.
15. van Lienden KP, van den Esschert JW, de Graaf W, et al. Portal vein embolization before liver resection: a systematic review. Cardiovasc Intervent Radiol 2013; 36(1):25–34.
16. Kawasaki S, Makuuchi M, Kakazu T, et al. Resection for multiple metastatic liver tumors after portal embolization. Surgery 1994;115(6):674–7.

17. Siperstein AE, Berber E, Ballem N, et al. Survival after radiofrequency ablation of colorectal liver metastases. Ann Surg 2007;246(4):559–67.
18. Peng ZW, Liu FR, Ye S, et al. Radiofrequency ablation versus open hepatic resection for elderly patients (>65 years) with very early or early hepatocellular carcinoma. Cancer 2013;119(21):3812–20.
19. Heniford BT, Arca MJ, Iannitti DA, et al. Laparoscopic cryoablation of hepatic metastases. Semin Surg Oncol 1998;15(3):194–201.
20. Ravikumar TS, Kane R, Cady B, et al. 5-year study of cryosurgery in the treatment of liver tumors. Arch Surg 1991;126(12):1520–3.
21. Pöpperl G, Helmberger T, Münzing W, et al. Selective internal radiation therapy with SIR-spheres® in patients with nonresectable liver tumors. Cancer Biother Radiopharm 2005;20(2):200–8.
22. Stubbs RS, Wickremesekera SK. Selective internal radiation therapy (SIRT): a new modality for treating patients with colorectal liver metastases. HPB (Oxford) 2004;6(3):133–9.
23. Howard JH, Tzeng CW, Smith JK, et al. Radiofrequency ablation for unresectable tumors of the liver. Am Surg 2008;74(7):594–600.
24. Welsh FK, Tilney HS, Tekkis PP, et al. Safe liver resection following chemotherapy for colorectal metastases is a matter of timing. Br J Cancer 2007;96(7):1037–42.
25. Schiergens TS, Stielow C, Schreiber S, et al. Liver resection in the elderly: significance of comorbidities and blood loss. J Gastrointest Surg 2014;18(6):1161–70.
26. Mastoraki A, Tsakali A, Papanikolaou IS, et al. Outcome following major hepatic resection in the elderly patients. Clin Res Hepatol Gastroenterol 2014;38:462–6. http://dx.doi.org/10.1016/j.clinre.2014.01.009.
27. Taniai N, Yoshida H, Yoshioka M, et al. Surgical outcomes and prognostic factors in elderly patients (75 years or older) with hepatocellular carcinoma who underwent hepatectomy. J Nippon Med Sch 2013;80(6):426–32.
28. Snowden CP, Prentis J, Jacques B, et al. Cardiorespiratory fitness predicts mortality and hospital length of stay after major elective surgery in older people. Ann Surg 2013;257(6):999–1004.
29. Prentis JM, Snowden CP. Ageing and Hepatic Function: Chapter 9, p(64–70). In: Dodds, Kumar, Veering, editors. Anaesthesia for the Elderly Patient. Oxford (United Kingdom): Oxford University Press; 2014.
30. Parkin E, O'Reilly DA, Adam R, et al. The effect of hepatic steatosis on survival following resection of colorectal liver metastases in patients without preoperative chemotherapy. HPB (Oxford) 2013;15(6):463–72.
31. Wu CC, Ho WL, Yeh DC, et al. Hepatic resection of hepatocellular carcinoma in cirrhotic livers: is it unjustified in impaired liver function? Surgery 1996;120(1):34–9.
32. Teh SH, Nagorney DM, Stevens SR, et al. Risk factors for mortality after surgery in patients with cirrhosis. Gastroenterology 2007;132(4):1261–9.
33. Cucchetti A, Ercolani G, Vivarelli M, et al. Impact of model for end-stage liver disease (MELD) score on prognosis after hepatectomy for hepatocellular carcinoma on cirrhosis. Liver Transpl 2006;12(6):966–71.
34. Schroeder RA, Marroquin CE, Bute BP, et al. Predictive indices of morbidity and mortality after liver resection. Ann Surg 2006;243(3):373–9.
35. Melendez J. Extended hepatic resection: a 6-year retrospective study of risk factors for perioperative mortality. J Am Coll Surg 2001;192(1):47–53.
36. Kim DH, Kim SH, Kim KS, et al. Predictors of mortality in cirrhotic patients undergoing extrahepatic surgery: comparison of Child-Turcotte-Pugh and model for end-stage liver disease-based indices. ANZ J Surg 2013. http://dx.doi.org/10.1111/ans.12198.

37. Uslu A, Cayci M, Nart A, et al. Renal failure in obstructive jaundice. Hepatogastroenterology 2005;52(61):52–4.
38. Betjes MG, Bajema I. The pathology of jaundice-related renal insufficiency: cholemic nephrosis revisited. J Nephrol 2006;19(2):229–33.
39. Padillo FJ, Cruz A, Briceño J, et al. Multivariate analysis of factors associated with renal dysfunction in patients with obstructive jaundice. Br J Surg 2005;92(11):1388–92.
40. Nimura Y. Preoperative biliary drainage before resection for cholangiocarcinoma (Pro). HPB (Oxford) 2008;10(2):130–3.
41. Son JH, Kim J, Lee SH, et al. The optimal duration of preoperative biliary drainage for periampullary tumors that cause severe obstructive jaundice. Am J Surg 2013; 206(1):40–6.
42. Jarnagin WR, Gonen M, Fong Y, et al. Improvement in perioperative outcome after hepatic resection: analysis of 1,803 consecutive cases over the past decade. Ann Surg 2002;236(4):397–406.
43. Otsubo T. Control of the inflow and outflow system during liver resection. J Hepatobiliary Pancreat Sci 2012;19(1):15–8.
44. Dixon E, Vollmer CM, Bathe OF, et al. Vascular occlusion to decrease blood loss during hepatic resection. Am J Surg 2005;190(1):75–86.
45. Bismuth H, Dennison AR. Segmental liver resection. Adv Surg 1993;26:189–208.
46. Delva E, Camus Y, Nordlinger B, et al. Vascular occlusions for liver resections. Operative management and tolerance to hepatic ischemia: 142 cases. Ann Surg 1989;209(2):211–8.
47. Nagasue N, Uchida M, Kubota H, et al. Cirrhotic livers can tolerate 30 minutes ischaemia at normal environmental temperature. Eur J Surg 1995;161(3):181–6.
48. Pringle JH. V. Notes on the arrest of hepatic hemorrhage due to trauma. Ann Surg 1908;48(4):541.
49. Lentschener C, Ozier Y. Anaesthesia for elective liver resection: some points should be revisited. Eur J Anaesthesiol 2002;19(11):780–8.
50. Smyrniotis VE, Kostopanagiotou GG, Contis JC, et al. Selective hepatic vascular exclusion versus Pringle maneuver in major liver resections: prospective study. World J Surg 2003;27(7):765–9.
51. Xiaobin F, Zipei L, Shuguo Z, et al. The Pringle manoeuvre should be avoided in hepatectomy for cancer patients due to its side effects on tumor recurrence and worse prognosis. Med Hypotheses 2009;72(4):398–401.
52. Petrowsky H, McCormack L, Trujillo M, et al. A prospective, randomized, controlled trial comparing intermittent portal triad clamping versus ischemic preconditioning with continuous clamping for major liver resection. Ann Surg 2006; 244(6):921–8.
53. Gomez D, Homer-Vanniasinkam S, Graham AM, et al. Role of ischaemic preconditioning in liver regeneration following major liver resection and transplantation. World J Gastroenterol 2007;13(5):657–70.
54. van der Bilt JD, Livestro DP, Borren A, et al. European survey on the application of vascular clamping in liver surgery. Dig Surg 2007;24(6):423–35. http://dx.doi.org/ 10.1159/000108325.
55. Wang HQ, Yang JY, Yan LN. Hemihepatic versus total hepatic inflow occlusion during hepatectomy: a systematic review and meta-analysis. World J Gastroenterol 2011;17(26):3158.
56. Gurusamy KS, Sheth H, Kumar Y, et al. Methods of vascular occlusion for elective liver resections. Cochrane Database Syst Rev 2009;(1):CD007632.
57. Edwards MJ, Bentley FR. Major hepatic resection under total vascular exclusion with extracorporeal venovenous bypass. Am Surg 1994;60(4):231–3.

58. Emond JC, Kelley SD, Heffron TG, et al. Surgical and anesthetic management of patients undergoing major hepatectomy using total vascular exclusion. Liver Transpl Surg 1996;2(2):91–8.

59. Aloia TA, Zorzi D, Abdalla EK, et al. Two-surgeon technique for hepatic parenchymal transection of the noncirrhotic liver using saline-linked cautery and ultrasonic dissection. Ann Surg 2005;242(2):172–7.

60. Fasulo F, Giori A, Fissi S, et al. Cavitron ultrasonic surgical aspirator (CUSA) in liver resection. Int Surg 1992;77(1):64–6.

61. Koo BN, Kil HK, Choi JS, et al. Hepatic resection by the Cavitron ultrasonic surgical aspirator increases the incidence and severity of venous air embolism. Anesth Analg 2005;101(4):966–70.

62. Sugo H, Mikami Y, Matsumoto F, et al. Hepatic resection using the harmonic scalpel. Surg Today 2000;30(10):959–62.

63. Aldrighetti L, Pulitanò C, Arru M, et al. "Technological" approach versus clamp crushing technique for hepatic parenchymal transection: a comparative study. J Gastrointest Surg 2006;10(7):974–9.

64. Kaneko H, Otsuka Y, Takagi S, et al. Hepatic resection using stapling devices. Am J Surg 2004;187(2):280–4.

65. de Boer MT, Klaase JM, Verhoef C, et al. Fibrin sealant for prevention of resection surface-related complications after liver resection: a randomized controlled trial. Ann Surg 2012;256(2):229–34.

66. Ding H, Yuan JQ, Zhou JH, et al. Systematic review and meta-analysis of application of fibrin sealant after liver resection. Curr Med Res Opin 2013;29(4): 387–94.

67. Chen H, Merchant NB, Didolkar MS. Hepatic resection using intermittent vascular inflow occlusion and low central venous pressure anesthesia improves morbidity and mortality. J Gastrointest Surg 2000;4(2):162–7.

68. Jones RM, Moulton CE, Hardy KJ. Central venous pressure and its effect on blood loss during liver resection. Br J Surg 1998;85(8):1058–60.

69. Li Z, Sun YM, Wu FX, et al. Controlled low central venous pressure reduces blood loss and transfusion requirements in hepatectomy. World J Gastroenterol 2014; 20(1):303–9.

70. Gurusamy KS, Li J, Sharma D, et al. Cardiopulmonary interventions to decrease blood loss and blood transfusion requirements for liver resection. Cochrane Database Syst Rev 2009;(4):CD007338.

71. Sand L, Rizell M, Houltz E, et al. Effect of patient position and PEEP on hepatic, portal and central venous pressures during liver resection. Acta Anaesthesiol Scand 2011;55(9):1106–12.

72. Dunki-Jacobs EM, Philips P, Scoggins CR, et al. Stroke volume variation in hepatic resection: a replacement for standard central venous pressure monitoring. Ann Surg Oncol 2014;21(2):473–8.

73. Hatano Y, Murakawa M, Segawa H, et al. Venous air embolism during hepatic resection. Anesthesiology 1990;73(6):1282–5.

74. Kang Y. Coagulopathies in hepatic disease. Liver Transpl 2000;6(4 Suppl 1): S72–5.

75. Boylan JF, Klinck JR, Sandler AN, et al. Tranexamic acid reduces blood loss, transfusion requirements, and coagulation factor use in primary orthotopic liver transplantation. Anesthesiology 1996;85(5):1043–8.

76. Wu CC, Ho WM, Cheng SB, et al. Perioperative parenteral tranexamic acid in liver tumor resection: a prospective randomized trial toward a "blood transfusion-"free hepatectomy. Ann Surg 2006;243(2):173–80.

77. Ortmann E, Besser MW, Klein AA. Antifibrinolytic agents in current anaesthetic practice. Br J Anaesth 2013;111(4):549–63.

78. Gurusamy KS, Li J, Sharma D, et al. Pharmacological interventions to decrease blood loss and blood transfusion requirements for liver resection. Cochrane Database Syst Rev 2009;(4):CD008085.

79. White B, McHale J, Ravi N, et al. Successful use of recombinant FVIIa (Novoseven) in the management of intractable post-surgical intra-abdominal haemorrhage. Br J Haematol 1999;107(3):677–8.

80. Chavez-Tapia NC, Alfaro-Lara R, Tellez-Avila F, et al. Prophylactic activated recombinant factor VII in liver resection and liver transplantation: systematic review and meta-analysis. PLoS One 2011;6(7):e22581.

81. Schultz NA, Larsen PN, Klarskov B, et al. Evaluation of a fast-track programme for patients undergoing liver resection. Br J Surg 2013;100(1):138–43.

82. Jones C, Kelliher L, Dickinson M, et al. Randomized clinical trial on enhanced recovery versus standard care following open liver resection. Br J Surg 2013; 100(8):1015–24.

83. Bona S, Gavelli A, Huguet C. The role of abdominal drainage after major hepatic resection. Am J Surg 1994;167(6):593–5.

84. Sarr MG, Parikh KJ, Minken SL, et al. Closed-suction versus Penrose drainage after cholecystectomy. A prospective, randomized evaluation. Am J Surg 1987; 153(4):394–8.

85. Gurusamy KS, Samraj K, Davidson BR. Routine abdominal drainage for uncomplicated liver resection. Cochrane Database Syst Rev 2007;(3):CD006232.

86. Pessaux P, Regimbeau JM, Dondéro F, et al. Randomized clinical trial evaluating the need for routine nasogastric decompression after elective hepatic resection. Br J Surg 2007;94(3):297–303.

87. Hendry PO, van Dam RM, Bukkems SF, et al. Randomized clinical trial of laxatives and oral nutritional supplements within an enhanced recovery after surgery protocol following liver resection. Br J Surg 2010;97(8):1198–206.

88. Cerutti E, Stratta C, Romagnoli R, et al. Thromboelastogram monitoring in the perioperative period of hepatectomy for adult living liver donation. Liver Transpl 2004;10(2):289–94.

89. Bezeaud A, Denninger MH, Dondero F, et al. Hypercoagulability after partial liver resection. Thromb Haemost 2007;98(6):1252–6.

90. Senzolo M, Sartori MT, Lisman T. Should we give thromboprophylaxis to patients with liver cirrhosis and coagulopathy? HPB (Oxford) 2009;11(6):459–64.

91. Lesmana CR, Inggriani S, Cahyadinata L, et al. Deep vein thrombosis in patients with advanced liver cirrhosis: a rare condition? Hepatol Int 2010;4(1): 433–8.

92. Reddy SK, Turley RS, Barbas AS, et al. Post-operative pharmacologic thromboprophylaxis after major hepatectomy: does peripheral venous thromboembolism prevention outweigh bleeding risks? J Gastrointest Surg 2011;15(9): 1602–10.

93. Tzimas P, Prout J, Papadopoulos G, et al. Epidural anaesthesia and analgesia for liver resection. Anaesthesia 2013;68(6):628–35.

94. Sakowska M, Docherty E, Linscott D, et al. A change in practice from epidural to intrathecal morphine analgesia for hepato-pancreato-biliary surgery. World J Surg 2009;33(9):1802–8.

95. Kasivisvanathan R, Abbassi-Ghadi N, Prout J, et al. A prospective cohort study of intrathecal versus epidural analgesia for patients undergoing hepatic resection. HPB (Oxford) 2014;16(8):768–75.

96. Harrison PM, Wendon JA, Gimson AE, et al. Improvement by acetylcysteine of hemodynamics and oxygen transport in fulminant hepatic failure. N Engl J Med 1991;324(26):1852–7.
97. Walsh TS, Hopton P, Philips BJ, et al. The effect of N-acetylcysteine on oxygen transport and uptake in patients with fulminant hepatic failure. Hepatology 1998; 27(5):1332–40.
98. Robinson SM, Saif R, Sen G, et al. N-acetylcysteine administration does not improve patient outcome after liver resection. HPB (Oxford) 2013;15(6):457–62.

Anesthesia for Esophagectomy

Adam Carney, MA, MB BChir, MRCP, FRCA[a],*, Matt Dickinson, MBBS, MSc, FRCA, FFICM[b]

KEYWORDS

- Esophagectomy • Esophageal cancer • Anesthesia • Perioperative management
- Enhanced Recovery • Perioperative complications

KEY POINTS

- Esophagectomy remains a high-risk operation with significant perioperative morbidity and mortality.
- Patients should be appropriately selected for surgery, and offered an evidence-based risk assessment for their postoperative outcome to allow informed, shared decision making.
- Perioperative management is complex, and in many areas evidence is limited and needs to be carefully translated. However, close attention to detail in many areas of perioperative management should improve postoperative outcome.
- An enhanced recovery pathway for esophagectomy should be implemented as standard practice.

INTRODUCTION

Esophageal cancer is the eighth most common cancer worldwide and the sixth most common cause of cancer death. In 2011 there were 7603 deaths from esophageal cancer in the United Kingdom, accounting for 5% of all deaths from cancer.[1]

Esophageal cancer presents as either squamous cell carcinoma or adenocarcinoma. Until relatively recently, squamous cell carcinoma accounted for most esophageal cancers worldwide; however, most new cases in the Western world are now adenocarcinoma.[2] The incidence of adenocarcinoma has increased 4-fold over the past 25 years, and it is the most rapidly increasing cancer in the United States.[2,3]

Risk factors for adenocarcinoma include gastroesophageal reflux disease (GERD), Barrett esophagus, obesity, smoking, and a diet low in fruit.[2,4] Alcohol and smoking are established risk factors for squamous cell carcinoma.[2]

Dr A. Carney has received travel expenses from the EBPOM group (Evidence Based PeriOperative Medicine). Dr M. Dickinson has no disclosures.

[a] Department of Anaesthesia, Nottingham University Hospitals NHS Trust, City Campus, Hucknall Road, Nottingham NG5 1PB, UK; [b] Department of Anaesthesia, Perioperative Medicine and Pain, Royal Surrey County Hospital NHS Foundation Trust, Egerton Road, Guildford, Surrey GU2 7XX, UK
* Corresponding author.
E-mail address: adam.carney@nuh.nhs.uk

Anesthesiology Clin 33 (2015) 143–163
http://dx.doi.org/10.1016/j.anclin.2014.11.009
1932-2275/15/$ – see front matter © 2015 Elsevier Inc. All rights reserved.

anesthesiology.theclinics.com

Overall 5-year survival from esophageal cancer is between 15% and 25%,[5] but only 25% to 30% of patients are potentially curable at presentation.[6]

Esophagectomy (often alongside neoadjuvant chemotherapy) is the gold-standard curative treatment for localized esophageal cancer.[7] More than 5000 esophagectomies are performed in the United States and United Kingdom each year. The operation is an invasive and complex procedure carrying a high postoperative morbidity and mortality.[8] Overall postoperative mortality remains around 8%, although rates in high-volume centers (>50 operations per year) are typically less than 5%.[9–11] Both volume and standard of care seem to influence mortality, as 5-year survival after surgery is quoted at between 25% and 50%,[7,10] with the best 5-year survival figures appearing to come from university hospitals (49.2%, compared with 27.3% for nonteaching hospitals).[12] There is some evidence that anesthetic expertise influences outcome,[10] but a relationship has not been established between anesthetic volume and outcome.

Significant postoperative complications can occur in up to 60% of esophagectomies,[13] with respiratory complications occurring in 25% of cases, cardiovascular in 12%, and anastomotic leak in 16%. Major pulmonary complications cause 50% of postoperative deaths.[14]

Improvement in outcome may be achieved by appropriate risk assessment and patient selection, choice of surgical technique, and optimization of perioperative patient care. Two recent reviews of anesthetic management for esophagectomy have focused on perioperative areas such as pulmonary morbidity, ventilatory management, thoracic epidural analgesia, intraoperative fluid management, the esophagogastric anastomosis and conduit perfusion, vasopressor therapy, anastomotic leak, cardiac arrhythmias, and venous thromboembolism.[15,16] It is unlikely that any single perioperative intervention alone will show benefit in outcome; however, an approach addressing several factors, and standardizing care (essentially an Enhanced Recovery After Surgery [ERAS] package) may demonstrate a significant impact.[15] ERAS in colorectal surgery has halved complication rates and reduced length of stay by 3 days.[17] Given the high risk and complexity of esophagectomy, it seems likely that standardized ERAS protocols in high-volume centers should help decrease both morbidity and mortality following esophagectomy.[9,15]

This review addresses preoperative assessment and patient selection, perioperative care (focusing on pulmonary prehabilitation, ventilation strategies, goal-directed fluid therapy [GDFT], analgesia, and cardiovascular complications), minimally invasive surgery, and current evidence for ERAS in esophagectomy.

PREOPERATIVE ASSESSMENT AND PATIENT SELECTION

Esophagectomy is a high-risk procedure because of the invasive nature of the operation (with both abdomen and thorax being breached) and the preoperative pathophysiologic status of the patient.[18] Although patients with potentially resectable disease should be offered surgery, it should not be undertaken on patients unable to survive the physiologic insult of the operation.

The changing epidemiology of esophageal cancer means the profile of comorbidities among patients is changing. Obesity, GERD, and ischemic heart disease are all increasing while patients are also getting older. Thirty percent of candidates for potentially curative surgery are American Society of Anesthesiologists (ASA) grade III or IV.[19,20]

Accurately predicting which patients will develop complications is not easy. The following have been shown to be risk factors for morbidity and/or mortality after esophagectomy.[5,10,13]

- Poor cardiopulmonary function (smoking, reduced vital capacity, low preoperative arterial oxygen tension)
- Poor cardiorespiratory function
- Age
- Tumor stage
- Diabetes mellitus
- Cardiac dysfunction
- Impaired general health
- Hepatic dysfunction

One retrospective analysis found general health, cardiac function, hepatic function, and respiratory function to be the major influences on postoperative mortality.[21] A prospective scoring system was subsequently developed which, when applied prospectively to aid patient selection, decreased the postoperative mortality from 9.4% to 1.6%.[22]

Other more generic scoring systems, such as POSSUM and P-POSSUM, have been used in general surgery to estimate postoperative mortality for an individual patient.[23–25] A dedicated scoring system to predict postoperative mortality specifically for esophagogastric surgery (O-POSSUM) has also been developed, although it has not been consistently shown to be any more accurate a predictor of postoperative mortality than P-POSSUM,[20,26–28] often overpredicting mortality.[29,30] More recently, frailty scores have been used to predict morbidity and mortality, and may be an important area to pursue when assessing and selecting patients for esophagectomy, especially as the population ages.[31]

The ARISCAT score was developed to provide a predictive index for the development of postoperative pulmonary complications (PPCs). The resulting risk index is based on the following 7 objectives: age, preoperative blood oxygen saturation (Spo_2), presence of recent respiratory infection, presence of preoperative anemia, location of surgical incision, duration of surgery, and whether the surgery was undertaken as an emergency procedure.[32] The score has recently been adopted as a standard by the European Society of Anesthesiologists/European Society of Intensive Care Medicine joint task force on perioperative outcome measures.[33] Most esophagectomy patients will fall into the calculated ARISCAT high-risk category.

Although predictive scores are a good starting point for appropriate patient selection, often more accurate assessment is subsequently required. Oxygen consumption increases 50% in the immediate postoperative period,[34,35] so prospective operative patients need to be able to increase their cardiac output and O_2 delivery. Patients who are unable to meet this metabolic demand, thought to equate to 4 metabolic equivalents, are at increased perioperative risk.[36,37]

There are various ways of assessing cardiopulmonary fitness, including the Duke Activity Status Index (DASI),[38] the Shuttle Walk Test (SWT),[39,40] and Cardiopulmonary Exercise Testing (CPET).[41] Older and colleagues[41] first defined an anaerobic threshold (AT) of 11 mL/min/kg as a clear correlation between preoperative functional reserve and operative risk, and the Improving Surgical Outcomes Group[42] recommend CPET before high-risk surgery.

Evidence for CPET results improving the outcome in esophagectomy is limited. One recent study has shown a correlation between AT and the development of cardiopulmonary complications (CPCs), with CPCs occurring in 42% of patients with an AT of less than 9 mL/min/kg compared with 29% of patients with an AT of greater than 9 mL/min/kg but less than 11 mL/min/kg, and 20% of patients with an AT of greater than 11 mL/min/kg.[43] Both peak (Vo_{2peak})[44] and maximum (Vo_{2max})[45] oxygen uptake have also been shown to correlate with CPCs, with one study concluding that a Vo_{2max} of 800 mL/min/m^2 allows esophagectomy to be safely performed.[45] Snowden and colleagues[46] showed that an anaerobic threshold of less than 10.1 mL/kg/min was an independent predictor of increased postoperative complications in major surgery. Based on these 3 articles,[43,45,46] the following CPET values are proposed as predictive of significant postoperative complications in esophagectomy.

- AT less than 10.1 mL/kg/min
- Vo_{2max} less than 800 mL/min/m^2

Murray and colleagues[36] compared an incremental SWT with CPET in patients about to have an esophagogastrectomy, and showed that distance achieved in an SWT correlated well with measures of O_2 uptake obtained through formal CPET. Of 43 patients who walked farther than 340 m during a formal SWT, none died during the first 30 postoperative days, but of 8 patients who walked less than 340 m, 5 of 8 died and 2 of the 8 were still on intensive care at 30 days.

Struthers and colleagues[47] found that although both DASI and SWT are sensitive and specific predictors of Vo_{2peak} greater than 15 mL/kg/min and AT of greater than 11 mL O_2/kg/min, many patients with a poor SWT or DASI had satisfactory CPET results. The investigators concluded that CPET is therefore probably the only test that provides an objective measure of cardiopulmonary fitness.[47]

A combination of cardiopulmonary function assessment (using CPET or SWT) and frailty assessment,[48] combined with predictive morbidity scores, may prove to be a valid way of pursuing informed, shared decision making[49] regarding patient suitability for esophagectomy, although further research is needed to refine this approach.

PERIOPERATIVE ISSUES

Pulmonary complications are the most common cause of postoperative morbidity and mortality in patients following esophagectomy. The occurrence of pulmonary complications is seen in up to 10% to 25% of patients, resulting in a mortality of up to 50%.[50,51] Perioperative risk factors include age, an independent prognosticator for morbidity,[52] a low preoperative body mass index, a history of cigarette smoking and preexisting pulmonary dysfunction, the experience of the surgeon, the duration of both the operation and one-lung ventilation (OLV), and the occurrence of an anastomotic leak.[53] Various strategies have been developed to reduce the incidence of these complications, outlined herein.

Preoptimization

The period of time preceding surgery presents an opportunity to ensure that patients are in the best possible condition, by addressing modifiable risk factors and optimizing preexisting comorbidities. This concept is now being recognized as "prehabilitation." Areas of interest include identification and treatment of anemia, optimizing nutrition, smoking cessation, optimizing medical therapies, and preoperative physiotherapy.[54] There is a paucity of evidence specifically relating to esophageal surgery; however, 3 areas that have been studied in thoracic patients provide evidence that may be transitioned to the esophagectomy population: smoking cessation, optimization of chronic obstructive pulmonary disease (COPD), and preoperative pulmonary rehabilitation.[55]

The United Kingdom National Institute for Health and Clinical Excellence (NICE) recommends that all smokers should be offered nicotine replacement to help stop smoking,[56] as smoking is associated with a higher likelihood of 30-day mortality and serious postoperative complications.[57]

COPD is common in patients with esophageal cancer, and data suggest that the use of long-acting β-agonists, combined with inhaled steroids, may reduce postoperative complications.[58,59] Evidence from patients undergoing lung resection for lung cancer suggests that the combination of optimized medical treatment combined with an intensive preoperative physical therapy program may result in improved lung function and exercise capacity in patients with COPD.[60,61]

Preoperative inspiratory muscle training has been shown in one study to improve respiratory function, but not outcome, in patients undergoing esophagectomy.[62] However, this study may have been underpowered, as reductions in pulmonary complications were demonstrated by a large randomized controlled trial in high-risk cardiac patients.[63]

It is biologically plausible that the non–lipid-decreasing effects of HMG-CoA (3-hydroxy-3-methyl-glutaryl coenzyme A) reductase inhibitors (statins) may modify many of the underlying processes that lead to the development of acute respiratory distress syndrome (ARDS) in surgical patients. These effects include the potential to reduce vascular permeability and inflammatory cytokines, increase the levels of anti-inflammatory cytokines, and promote the repair of damaged endothelium.[64] In a recent proof-of-concept randomized, placebo-controlled trial, patients undergoing esophagectomy were allocated to either 80 mg simvastatin or placebo in the perioperative period. Pretreatment with simvastatin decreased biomarkers of inflammation and reduced epithelial and systemic endothelial injury. However, there was no statistically significant difference between the groups for the development of acute lung injury.[65] There remains clinical equipoise, illustrated by a large retrospective cohort study that evaluated the association between preoperative statin therapy and the development of postoperative ARDS in patients undergoing elective high-risk thoracic and aortic vascular surgery.[64] Of 1845 patients, 722 were receiving preoperative statin therapy, with no statistically significant differences between the groups for the development of ARDS, mortality, length of stay in hospital, or ventilator-free days.

Ventilation Strategies

Esophagectomy elicits a marked systemic inflammatory response syndrome, and a relationship between local and systemic inflammatory mediators has been described. These mediators include proinflammatory and anti-inflammatory mediators such as interleukin (IL)-6, IL-8, and IL-10.[66] OLV is the standard technique used to facilitate the surgical procedure in both open and minimally invasive approaches. Pulmonary damage can be caused by retraction of the collapsed lung during surgery and by reinsufflation at the end of surgery following resection of the tumor. In addition, both volutrauma and atelectrauma should be avoided, and adoption of the principles of the ARDSNet trial[67] is advocated. These principles include maintaining inspiratory plateau pressure below 35 cm H_2O by reducing tidal volume to as low as 5 to 6 mL/kg, and optimizing positive end-expiratory pressure (PEEP) to a setting above the lower inflection point.[68,69] Recent studies have looked at the optimal levels of PEEP in open abdominal surgery. The large, multicenter, PROVHILO randomized controlled trial found that there was no difference in the development of PPCs between patients receiving levels of PEEP set at 12 cm H_2O, combined with recruitment maneuvers, and those receiving a low level of PEEP (<2 cm H_2O) without recruitment maneuvers during anesthesia for open abdominal surgery. However, there were more episodes of intraoperative hypotension requiring vasoactive drugs in patients receiving the higher level of PEEP.[70] The recent IMPROVE trial also compared 2 ventilation strategies in anesthetized patients undergoing major abdominal surgery. One group received a tidal volume of 10 to 12 mL/kg of predicted body weight, with no PEEP or recruitment maneuvers, while the other group received a lung-protective strategy with tidal volumes of 6 to 8 mL/kg of predicted body weight, a PEEP of 6 to 8 cm H_2O and recruitment maneuvers repeated every 30 minutes of 30 cm H_2O for 30 seconds. The group receiving the lung-protective strategy had significantly fewer major pulmonary and extrapulmonary complications in the first 7 days after surgery.[71] Although these studies did not look specifically at patients receiving OLV, others have shown that during OLV improvements in oxygenation and lung mechanics can be observed after a recruitment maneuver combined with PEEP values of up to 10 cm H_2O.[72]

While there seems to be benefit in optimizing PEEP to the dependent, ventilated lung, there is also evidence that the application of continuous positive airway pressure (CPAP) to the collapsed lung reduces pulmonary damage, hypoxia, and consequent inflammation. Significantly lower concentrations of IL-1α, IL-1β, IL-8, IL-10, tumor necrosis factor α, macrophage inflammatory protein 1α, and pulmonary and activation-regulated chemokine were found in bronchoalveolar lavage fluid of collapsed lungs that had 5 cm H_2O CPAP applied, compared with those with no CPAP. There were, however, no differences in systemic concentrations of these mediators.[66]

There is conflicting evidence regarding the optimal ventilation mode for OLV. Tugrul and colleagues[73] found that pressure control ventilation (PCV) improved oxygenation in comparison with volume control ventilation (VCV), with the higher observed pulmonary shunt in the VCV group being attributable to higher plateau pressures. This finding contrasts with those of Unzueta and colleagues,[74] who found no improvement in oxygenation while using PCV during OLV, in comparison with VCV. However, they did observe lower peak airway pressures.

There is evidence that both sevoflurane and desflurane, when compared with propofol, produce a beneficial local immunomodulatory effect in patients undergoing OLV for thoracic surgery, significantly reducing inflammatory mediators and improving clinical outcomes.[75,76]

Avoidance of Postoperative Pulmonary Complications

The occurrence of passive reflux in patients following esophagectomy, caused by denervation of the stomach and excision of the lower esophageal sphincter, predisposes patients to the development of PPCs. Routine decompression of the gastric conduit can provide protection against aspiration and distension of the anastomosis. Although performing a pyloroplasty may reduce the incidence of gastric outflow obstruction and speed up gastric emptying, its contribution to reducing aspiration has yet to be established,[77] and some investigators recommend omitting the procedure because it may favor biliary reflux esophagitis.[78] Early extubation following surgery avoids the complications associated with mechanical ventilation, has been shown to be safe, is not associated with increased respiratory morbidity, and reduces length of stay in the intensive care unit.[79–81] Adoption of the 5 components of the Institute for Health Improvement Ventilator Bundle, adapted for postoperative esophagectomy patients, is good practice even in nonventilated patients. These 5 components are: the use of profiling beds, allowing the thorax to be kept upright at all times, and elevation of the head of the bed; daily sedation holds and assessment of readiness to extubate; peptic ulcer disease prophylaxis; deep venous ulcer prophylaxis; and daily oral care with chlorhexidine (and, in the United Kingdom version, supraglottic aspiration).[82]

Perioperative Fluid Management

Accurate fluid management is a key component of perioperative anesthesia during thoracic surgery.[83] Too little fluid could compromise perfusion of vital organs and surgical anastomoses, but fluid overload could lead to pulmonary edema and subsequent acute lung injury (ALI) (which carries a mortality rate of <50%),[52,84,85] or anastomotic edema and, therefore, leak.[86] Patients who have such postoperative complications but survive to hospital discharge have reduced long-term survival.[87,88] It is therefore crucial that intraoperative fluid management is optimized for each individual patient undergoing esophagectomy, to maximize perfusion pressure and oxygen delivery to vital organs and the gut mucosa.[89]

Many studies advocate restrictive rather than liberal fluid management in gastrointestinal (GI) surgery, showing better GI recovery time and reduced morbidity (especially pulmonary).[90–93] Three studies that have reviewed fluid management in esophagectomy (2 as part of a multimodal anesthesia regime) have found that restricting intraoperative fluids reduced postoperative morbidity and potentially shortened the recovery period.[81,93,94] It should be noted, however, that fluid restriction often means avoidance of fluid excess (eg, <4 L of crystalloid).[86]

GDFT (defined as the monitoring of hemodynamic parameters and rational fluid administration based on information obtained, to optimize tissue perfusion)[84] has been shown to shorten length of stay in hospital and decrease postoperative morbidity in major lower GI surgery.[95–97] GDFT should be used to target fluid boluses to maximize cardiac output while avoiding fluid excess. GDFT has potential benefits for esophagectomy with theoretic prevention of splanchnic (and thus anastomotic) vasoconstriction,[89,98,99] and the avoidance of fluid overload and subsequent ALI.

No studies assessing the impact of GDFT on outcome in esophagectomy have been published; however, 5 meta-analyses and 1 review of major abdominal surgery all demonstrate fewer complications and shorter stay with GDFT.[99–103]

Three of the meta-analyses showed that a greater volume of fluid was administered when GDFT was used, but a fourth found greater benefit with GDFT than with a non-GDFT "liberal" fluid strategy.[99] GDFT has been studied in 16 patients undergoing esophagectomy as part of a study assessing GDFT and pulmonary fluid overload in thoracic surgery requiring OLV. Goal-directed fluid was guided by stroke volume (SV) variation (SVV), and the investigators concluded that SVV-guided fluid management did not result in pulmonary fluid overload.[104] SVV is traditionally used during positive pressure ventilation, with a closed chest, and tidal volumes of 8 mL/kg. During thoracotomy the intrathoracic pressure changes that cause a drop in preload, leading to SVV, are not consistent; therefore SVV, as a sole observation, is of limited value. SVV has been shown to be predictive of postoperative intravascular hypovolemia in esophagectomy,[105] and a low intraoperative stroke volume index may represent a risk factor for acute kidney injury in the early postoperative period.[106]

The OPTIMISE trial is the largest single study thus far of GDFT in major GI surgery, and patients having upper GI operations constituted 224 of the 734 enrolled patients.[103] Although statistical outcome showed no difference in postoperative complications between the 2 groups, there was a trend toward fewer complications in the GDFT intervention group, and there was also no difference in total amount of fluid given between the 2 groups.

Overall, this evidence would suggest that GDFT should lead to a more individualized approach to achieving the correct amount of fluid, need not result in excessive fluid administration, and is likely to reduce complications and possibly, therefore, mortality in esophagectomy.

Although further research is required in esophagectomy patients, the authors' approach to perioperative fluid optimization would be:

- Abdominal phase: optimize SV
- Thoracic phase: maintain SV (avoiding aggressive fluid loading)

- Early postoperative phase (I): optimize SV for 12 hours
- Postoperative phase (II): aim to restrict total daily fluid intake to less than 30 mL/kg

Cardiovascular Issues

In the successive annual National Oesophagogastric Cancer Audits that are undertaken in England and Wales it has been found that, after pneumonia and anastomotic leak, the third most frequent complication in the early postoperative period is supraventricular arrhythmia. Over the last 20 years, reported incidences of atrial fibrillation after esophagectomy have trended downward from 64% to 5%. Although this might be due to patient selection, modern surgical and anesthetic techniques, or arrhythmia prophylaxis, it is possible that variation in study design and single-center reports bias these data.[107–109] The development of an arrhythmia is important, as it is associated with morbidity and a 20% relative increase in mortality risk.[110,111] However, it is uncertain as to what extent arrhythmia is an independent risk factor for adverse outcomes. Arrhythmia may be directly related to the extent of intrathoracic dissection and pericardial irritation.[107] Arrhythmia is also associated with age, preexisting cardiac disease, blood loss, infection, and anastomotic leak. Arrhythmia may therefore be the cardiac manifestation of other pathologic processes. Whether atrial fibrillation is a marker or mediator of adverse outcomes in patients after esophagectomy remains uncertain. That atrial fibrillation per se could produce morbidity and mortality in this context is plausible, and if it proves to be the case then it is important because the clinical value of preoperative and intraoperative adverse outcome indicators may be supplemented by this specific postoperative predictor. Indeed, in the context of esophagectomy, postoperative complications may be more important predictors of survival than preoperative health.[87]

The use of the potential prophylactic properties of magnesium sulfate, digoxin, β-adrenergic receptor blockade, diltiazem, and amiodarone has been proposed.[107,108,112–115] A meta-analysis supports the use of calcium-channel blockers and β-blockers in the general thoracic surgical population[111]; however, following the publication of the POISE trial and a further meta-analysis, the use of β-blockade in patients undergoing low-risk or intermediate-risk noncardiac surgery is not supported.[116,117] Although there is no evidence that prophylactic digoxin is effective at reducing the incidence of supraventricular arrhythmias in esophagectomy patients,[112] a prophylactic infusion of amiodarone has been shown to significantly reduce the incidence of atrial fibrillation in patients undergoing transthoracic esophagectomy.[118]

Historically there have been concerns raised that the use of vasopressors may impair gastric conduit blood flow locally, and splanchnic blood flow more generally, following work done in animal models subjected to hemorrhage.[119] These investigators concede that their experimental conditions of acute hemorrhagic hypovolemia, corrected solely by the use of norepinephrine, require further investigation to evaluate the clinical significance. Under normovolemic conditions, whereby the gastric conduit has microvascular stunning and is pressure passive, the use of vasopressors have be found to have no adverse effect on gastric microvascular flow[120] and may actually improve it.[121] No association between the use of phenylephrine or ephedrine and the rate of postoperative anastomotic leak has been found.[122] Using vasopressors to increase the mean arterial blood pressure to greater than 70 mm Hg has not been shown to have a beneficial effect on the microcirculation.[120] However, the meta-analysis that was incorporated into the recent OPTIMISE trial, which compared the use of cardiac output–guided hemodynamic therapy using fluids and dopexamine with usual care, found a reduction in complication rates.[103] The findings of a meta-regression analysis also suggest that dopexamine infusion at low dose, providing mild inotropic and vasodilatory effects, is associated with improved outcomes following major surgery.[123]

Thoracic Epidural Analgesia Versus Paravertebral Analgesia

Postoperative pain after esophagectomy can be difficult to manage. Both abdominal and thoracic components of the operation cause wound and visceral pain, and the practice of inserting an intercostal chest drain (necessary if lymphadenectomy has been performed) only adds to the range of dermatomes for which analgesia needs to be considered.

Thoracic epidural analgesia (TEA) has been shown to offer many benefits in esophagectomy, providing gold-standard analgesia,[124,125] reducing respiratory complications,[126–128] and reducing the incidence of post-thoracotomy pain.[129,130] TEA has also been associated with decreased incidence of anastomotic leakage,[68] possibly resulting from improved microcirculation in the gastric conduit.[131] TEA has therefore been central to multimodal standardized perioperative care pathways, which have shown improved outcomes.[78–81,128,132]

However, TEA is not necessarily a panacea, as the incidence of failure may be as high as 12%,[133] there are significant risks with insertion, and hypotension can cause problems such as reduction in splanchnic blood flow and, therefore, a decrease in oxygen flux at the gastric anastomosis.[132,134,135] There is evidence, however, that either adrenaline or phenylephrine infusions titrated to restore mean arterial pressure will increase flux at the anastomosis.[132,134]

Several recent reviews and meta-analyses have shown that paravertebral blockade with a continuous infusion via a catheter provides pain relief comparable with that achieved by epidural analgesia, and is associated with fewer complications, in thoracotomy.[136–138] Paravertebral blockade has been described in esophagectomy,[139] and is standard practice in some United Kingdom hospitals for minimally invasive esophagectomy. Local data show excellent analgesia comparable with epidural analgesia, and shorter stays in the intensive therapy unit; however, further studies looking at outcomes are needed.

Chronic Postsurgical Pain

Pain that continues after the surgical wound has healed is known as chronic postsurgical pain, and may last for 3 to 6 months after surgery.[140] It is particularly problematic following thoracotomy, with an estimated incidence of chronic pain occurring in 25% to 60% of patients. Of these patients, 10% will experience severe, disabling pain (>5 out of a pain score of 10).[141–144] Risk factors for developing chronic postsurgical pain include psychosocial conditions such as anxiety, depression, malignant disease, social network, and social status. Elderly patients have a lower risk, but women have an increased risk.[145]

During thoracotomy, rib retraction causes extensive nerve damage to the intercostal nerves,[146] as do pericostal sutures placed when closing the wound. The use of intracostal sutures, placed by drilling small holes in the lower rib, has been shown to reduce this nerve impingement and chronic postsurgical pain.[147]

In addition to the established techniques of multimodal analgesia, combining regional or neuraxial anesthetic techniques, there is a growing interest in the use of other adjuncts to reduce the occurrence of acute and chronic postsurgical pain. However, none of these have specifically studied the effect in patients undergoing esophagectomy. The use of systemic magnesium and ketamine has been the subject of recent meta-analyses. Systemic magnesium was found to reduce postoperative pain and opioid consumption, and the investigators recommended considering its use to reduce postoperative pain.[148] Similarly, intravenous ketamine was found to be a useful adjunct for postoperative analgesia.[149] Finally, it is now accepted that the use of gabapentinoids is effective in reducing immediate postoperative pain and opioid consumption, and the currently available data support the conclusion that they may prevent chronic postsurgical pain, although further studies are required to confirm this.[150]

MINIMALLY INVASIVE ESOPHAGECTOMY

Minimally invasive esophagectomy (MIE) techniques involve either completely endoscopic resection, via thoracoscopic and laparoscopic approaches, or hybrid approaches whereby one part of the procedure is performed endoscopically. Advocates of the technique claim that the physiologic stress and pain are less, as are lengths of stay in hospital. Findlay and colleagues[9] undertook a review of the current published evidence supporting MIE that included 4 reviews and 3 meta-analyses. These studies have been criticized for being nonrandomized and of poor quality, but the investigators concluded that MIE was associated with lower blood loss, shorter hospital stay, and reduced total morbidity (but no difference in 30-day mortality), and was at least comparable with open surgery.[151] A single randomized controlled trial found that MIE reduced blood loss, respiratory complications, and length of stay, and provided a better quality of life at 6 weeks without any difference in node harvest.[152] In the context of the available evidence MIE has been recommended, provided the appropriate expertise is available.[9]

The anesthetic challenges of MIE include prolonged surgery, often in the prone position, the subsequent increased difficulties of lung isolation and OLV in the prone position, and complications relating to extraperitoneal CO_2 (pneumothorax, pneumomediastinum, and surgical emphysema).[153]

ENHANCED RECOVERY IN ESOPHAGECTOMY

ERAS is a concept advocating best practice in perioperative care, focusing on optimal recovery and discharge for patients.[154] The classic components comprise 5 elements:

1. Preoperative assessment, planning, and preparation before admission
2. Reducing the physiologic stress of the operation
3. A structured approach to immediate postoperative and perioperative management, including pain relief
4. Early mobilization
5. Early enteral feeding

ERAS has been shown to decrease complications and shorten length of stay in hospital, with most studies providing evidence in colorectal surgery.[17] The relatively high morbidity and mortality associated with esophagectomy would suggest that significant gains could be made by applying ERAS or standardized perioperative care pathways to esophagectomy; however, not all standard ERAS elements are necessarily applicable to esophagectomy.[155]

Evidence suggests that surgical treatment of esophageal cancer is possible with moderate morbidity and low mortality,[80] and that ERAS in esophagectomy can reduce anastomotic leak, pulmonary complications, and length of stay.[156] An ERAS program needs to be more than just a formalized pathway, it needs to focus on optimizing clinical aspects or perioperative care.[157] Although most patients with esophageal carcinoma can tolerate an enhanced recovery pathway, those younger than 65 years or who have no comorbidities have the best results.[158]

Findlay and colleagues[9] have recently published a systematic review of 6 published studies and have produced evidence-based guidelines on ERAS for esophagectomy. Their key points are summarized as follows.

- Length of stay can be reduced to a median of 8 days
- Morbidity (especially pulmonary) can be reduced
- Mortality can be reduced

Findlay and colleagues[9] conclude that key components of ERAS for esophagectomy should include the following components.

Preoperative Management

Counseling
- Focused preoperative counseling is an independent predictor of ERAS success.
- Multimodal counseling targeted to the patient's own expectations is advised.

Carbohydrate Loading
- Carbohydrate loading attenuates catabolism-induced neuroendocrine surgical stress response, insulin resistance, hyperglycemia, and muscle breakdown. It can also reduce nausea and vomiting, and expedite hospital discharge.
- Carbohydrate drinks 2 to 3 hours before surgery are advised.

Preoperative Hemoglobin Optimization
- Anemia in esophageal cancer is common, increasing transfusion requirements and subsequent morbidity and mortality.
- Preoperative iron for 2 to 3 weeks can improve hemoglobin and reduce transfusion (Colorectal).
- Preoperative oral iron for iron deficiency anemia is recommended.

Intraoperative Management

Preemptive Analgesia
- Pain after esophagectomy is multifactorial, involving somatic and visceral afferents from the abdomen, thorax, and neck.
- Nonsteroidal anti-inflammatories predispose to anastomotic leakage in colorectal surgery.
- Preemptive analgesia with epidural is recommended.

Minimally Invasive Esophagectomy
- MIE probably causes less morbidity, fewer anastomotic leaks, less blood loss, and shorter stay.
- MIE is recommended with appropriate expertise.

Perioperative Fluid Therapy
- Avoidance of fluid excess decreases pulmonary complications.
- GDFT could prevent splanchnic (and therefore anastomotic) vasoconstriction.
- The use of a "balanced" rather than "liberal" or "restricted" fluid protocol is recommended.
- GDFT is recommended.

Postoperative Management

Chest Drains
- Chest drains can worsen pain, ventilation, and mobilization.
- Use of chest drains should be minimized.

- One chest drain is as effective as two.
- Chest drains can be removed when draining 200 mL/d.

Gastric Conduit Decompression
- Conduit decompression via a nasogastric tube is recommended.

Nutritional Support
- Early enteral feeding is recommended.

Oral Intake
- The optimal timing of oral intake after esophagectomy is unclear.

Analgesia
- TEA remains the gold standard in open esophagectomy.
- Paravertebral block provides equivalent analgesia for thoracotomy, with fewer pulmonary complications and side effects.

Urinary Catheter
- Urinary catheters should be removed as soon as practical when not required for monitoring.
- Removal on postoperative day 1 reduces urinary tract infections and has a recatheterization rate of 10%.

Venous Thromboembolism (VTE) Prophylaxis
- The risk of VTE is high (7%) after esophagectomy.
- All patients should receive combined pharmacologic and mechanical prophylaxis while in hospital unless contraindicated.

Early Mobilization
- Early mobilization is recommended.

SUMMARY

Esophagectomy is a complex operation with significant morbidity and mortality, requiring anesthetic and surgical expertise and careful attention to detail. Although each individual anesthetic improvement or part of an ERAS program may not individually change outcome, the overall perioperative management can be seen as the "aggregation of marginal gains"[159] (a phrase synonymous with Sir Dave Brailsford, the manager of Team Sky, a British professional cycling team), and should help decrease postoperative complications.

REFERENCES

1. Oesophageal cancer incidence statistics. Cancer research UK website. 2014. Available at: http://www.cancerresearchuk.org/cancer-info/cancerstats/types/oesophagus/incidence/uk-oesophageal-cancer-incidence-statistics. Accessed September 9, 2014.
2. Holmes RS, Vaughan TL. Epidemiology and pathogenesis of esophageal cancer. Semin Radiat Oncol 2007;17(1):2–9.
3. Pohl H, Sirovich B, Welch HG. Esophageal adenocarcinoma incidence: are we reaching the peak? Cancer Epidemiol Biomarkers Prev 2010;19(6):1468–70.

4. Anderson L, Watson RG, Murphy SJ, et al. Risk factors for Barrett's oesophagus and oesophageal adenocarcinoma: results from the FINBAR study. World J Gastroenterol 2007;13(10):1585–94.
5. Pennefather SH. Anaesthesia for oesophagectomy. Curr Opin Anaesthesiol 2007;20(1):15–20.
6. Bussières JS. Open or minimally invasive esophagectomy: are the outcomes different? Curr Opin Anaesthesiol 2009;22(1):56–60.
7. Mariette C, Piessen G, Triboulet JP. Therapeutic strategies in oesophageal carcinoma: role of surgery and other modalities. Lancet Oncol 2007;8(6):545–53.
8. Markar SR, Karthikesalingam A, Thrumurthy S, et al. Volume-outcome relationship in surgery for esophageal malignancy: systematic review and meta-analysis 2000-2011. J Gastrointest Surg 2012;16(5):1055–63.
9. Findlay JM, Gillies RS, Millo J, et al. Enhanced recovery for esophagectomy: a systematic review and evidence-based guidelines. Ann Surg 2014;259(3): 413–31.
10. Sherry KM, Smith FG. Anaesthesia for oesophagectomy. BJA CEPD Reviews 2003;3(3):87–90.
11. Migliore M, Choong CK, Lim E, et al. A surgeon's case volume of oesophagectomy for cancer strongly influences the operative mortality rate. Eur J Cardiothorac Surg 2007;32(2):375–80.
12. Verhoef C, van de Weyer R, Schaapveld M, et al. Better survival in patients with esophageal cancer after surgical treatment in university hospitals: a plea for performance by surgical oncologists. Ann Surg Oncol 2007;14(5):1678–87.
13. McCulloch P, Ward J, Tekkis PP, ASCOT Group of Surgeons, British Oesophago-Gastric Cancer Group. Mortality and morbidity in gastro-oesophageal cancer surgery: initial results of ASCOT multicentre prospective cohort study. BMJ 2003;327(7425):1192–7.
14. Briez N, Piessen G, Torres F, et al. Effects of hybrid minimally invasive oesophagectomy on major postoperative pulmonary complications. Br J Surg 2012; 99(11):1547–53.
15. Ng JM. Perioperative anesthetic management for esophagectomy. Anesthesiol Clin 2008;26(2):293–304.
16. Jaeger JM, Collins SR, Blank RS. Anesthetic management for esophageal resection. Anesthesiol Clin 2012;30(4):731–47.
17. Spanjersberg WR, Reurings J, Keus F, et al. Fast track surgery versus conventional recovery strategies for colorectal surgery. Cochrane Database Syst Rev 2011;(2):CD007635. http://dx.doi.org/10.1002/14651858.CD007635.pub2.
18. Congedo E, Aceto P, Petrucci R, et al. Preoperative anesthetic evaluation and preparation in patients requiring esophageal surgery for cancer. Rays 2005; 30(4):341–5.
19. Lerut T, Nafteux P, Moons J, et al. Quality in the surgical treatment of cancer of the esophagus and gastroesophageal junction. Eur J Surg Oncol 2005;31(6): 587–94.
20. Filip B, Hutanu I, Radu I, et al. Assessment of different prognostic scores for early postoperative outcomes after esophagectomy. Chirurgia (Bucur) 2014; 109(4):480–5.
21. Bartels H, Stein HJ, Siewert JR. Preoperative risk analysis and postoperative mortality of oesophagectomy for resectable oesophageal cancer. Br J Surg 1998;85(6):840–4.
22. Bartels H, Stein HJ, Siewert JR. Risk analysis in esophageal surgery. Recent Results Cancer Res 2000;155:89–96.

23. Copeland GP, Jones D, Walters M. POSSUM: a scoring system for surgical audit. Br J Surg 1991;78(3):355–60.
24. Prytherch DR, Whiteley MS, Higgins B, et al. POSSUM and Portsmouth POS-SUM for predicting mortality. Physiological and operative severity score for the enumeration of mortality and morbidity. Br J Surg 1998;85(9):1217–20.
25. Neary WD, Heather BP, Earnshaw JJ. The physiological and operative severity score for the enumeration of mortality and morbidity (POSSUM). Br J Surg 2003; 90(2):157–65.
26. Nagabhushan JS, Srinath S, Weir F, et al. Comparison of P-POSSUM and O-POSSUM in predicting mortality after oesophagogastric resections. Postgrad Med J 2007;83(979):355–8.
27. Dutta S, Al-Mrabt NM, Fullarton GM, et al. A comparison of POSSUM and GPS models in the prediction of postoperative outcome in patients undergoing oesophago-gastric cancer resection. Ann Surg Oncol 2011;18(10):2808–17. .
28. Lai F, Kwan TL, Yuen WC, et al. Evaluation of various POSSUM models for pre-dicting mortality in patients undergoing elective oesophagectomy for carci-noma. Br J Surg 2007;94(9):1172–8.
29. Bosch DJ, Pultrum BB, de Bock GH, et al. Comparison of different risk-adjustment models in assessing short-term surgical outcome after transthoracic esophagec-tomy in patients with esophageal cancer. Am J Surg 2011;202(3):303–9.
30. Lagarde SM, Maris AK, de Castro SM, et al. Evaluation of O-POSSUM in predict-ing in-hospital mortality after resection for oesophageal cancer. Br J Surg 2007; 94(12):1521–6.
31. Hodari A, Hammoud ZT, Borgi JF, et al. Assessment of morbidity and mortality after esophagectomy using a modified frailty index. Ann Thorac Surg 2013; 96(4):1240–5.
32. Canet J, Gallart L, Gomar C, et al, ARISCAT Group. Prediction of postoperative pulmonary complications in a population-based surgical cohort. Anesthesiology 2010;113(6):1338–50.
33. Jammer I, Wickboldt N, Sander M, et al. Standards for definitions and use of outcome measures for clinical effectiveness research in perioperative medicine: European Perioperative Clinical Outcome (EPCO) definitions: a statement from the ESA-ESICM joint taskforce on perioperative outcome measures. Eur J Anaesthesiol 2014. [Epub ahead of print].
34. Older P, Smith R. Experience with the preoperative invasive measurement of haemodynamic, respiratory and renal function in 100 elderly patients scheduled for major abdominal surgery. Anaesth Intensive Care 1988;16(4):389–95.
35. Kusano C, Baba M, Takao S, et al. Oxygen delivery as a factor in the develop-ment of fatal postoperative complications after oesophagectomy. Br J Surg 1997;84(2):252–7.
36. Murray P, Whiting P, Hutchinson SP, et al. Preoperative shuttle walking testing and outcome after oesophagogastrectomy. Br J Anaesth 2007;99(6):809–11.
37. Eagle KA, Berger PB, Calkins H, et al. ACC/AHA guideline update for perioper-ative cardiovascular evaluation for noncardiac surgery—executive summary. A report of the American College of Cardiology/American Heart Association Task Force on Practice Guidelines (Committee to Update the 1996 Guidelines on Perioperative Cardiovascular Evaluation for Noncardiac Surgery). Anesth Analg 2002;94(5):1052–64.
38. Hlatky MA, Boineau RE, Higginbotham MB, et al. A brief self-administered ques-tionnaire to determine functional capacity (the Duke Activity Status Index). Am J Cardiol 1989;64(10):651–4.

39. Singh SJ, Morgan MD, Scott S, et al. Development of a shuttle walking test of disability in patients with chronic airways obstruction. Thorax 1992;47(12): 1019–24.
40. Morales FJ, Martínez A, Méndez M, et al. A shuttle walk test for assessment of functional capacity in chronic heart failure. Am Heart J 1999;138(2 Pt 1):291–8.
41. Older P, Smith R, Courtney P, et al. Preoperative evaluation of cardiac failure and ischemia in elderly patients by cardiopulmonary exercise testing. Chest 1993; 104(3):701–4.
42. Modernising care for patients undergoing major surgery. Improving patient outcomes and Increasing clinical efficiency. Available at: http://www.reducinglengthofstay.org.uk/isog.html. Accessed September 9, 2014.
43. Moyes LH, McCaffer CJ, Carter RC, et al. Cardiopulmonary exercise testing as a predictor of complications in oesophagogastric cancer surgery. Ann R Coll Surg Engl 2013;95(2):125–30.
44. Forshaw MJ, Strauss DC, Davies AR, et al. Is cardiopulmonary exercise testing a useful test before esophagectomy? Ann Thorac Surg 2008;85(1):294–9.
45. Nagamatsu Y, Shima I, Yamana H, et al. Preoperative evaluation of cardiopulmonary reserve with the use of expired gas analysis during exercise testing in patients with squamous cell carcinoma of the thoracic esophagus. J Thorac Cardiovasc Surg 2001;121(6):1064–8.
46. Snowden CP, Prentis JM, Anderson HL, et al. Submaximal cardiopulmonary exercise testing predicts complications and hospital length of stay in patients undergoing major elective surgery. Ann Surg 2010;251(3):535–41.
47. Struthers R, Erasmus P, Holmes K, et al. Assessing fitness for surgery: a comparison of questionnaire, incremental shuttle walk, and cardiopulmonary exercise testing in general surgical patients. Br J Anaesth 2008;101(6):774–80.
48. Rockwood K, Song X, MacKnight C, et al. A global clinical measure of fitness and frailty in elderly people. CMAJ 2005;173(5):489–95.
49. Weston WW. Informed and shared decision-making: the crux of patient-centered care. CMAJ 2001;165(4):438–9.
50. Law S, Wong KH, Kwok KF, et al. Predictive factors for postoperative pulmonary complications and mortality after esophagectomy for cancer. Ann Surg 2004; 240(5):791.
51. Ferguson MK, Durkin AE. Preoperative prediction of the risk of pulmonary complications after esophagectomy for cancer. J Thorac Cardiovasc Surg 2002; 123(4):661–9.
52. McKevith JM, Pennefather SH. Respiratory complications after oesophageal surgery. Curr Opin Anaesthesiol 2010;23(1):34–40.
53. Tandon S, Batchelor A, Bullock R, et al. Perioperative risk factors for acute lung injury after elective oesophagectomy. Br J Anaesth 2001;86(5):633–8.
54. Durrand JW, Batterham AM, Danjoux GR. Pre-habilitation (i): aggregation of marginal gains. Anaesthesia 2014;69(5):403–6.
55. Jones NL, Edmonds L, Ghosh S, et al. A review of enhanced recovery for thoracic anaesthesia and surgery. Anaesthesia 2013;68(2):179–89.
56. Killoran A, Crombie H, White P, et al. NICE public health guidance update. J Public Health (Oxf) 2010;32:451–3.
57. Turan A, Mascha EJ, Roberman D, et al. Smoking and perioperative outcomes. Anesthesiology 2011;114(4):837–46.
58. Ueda K, Tanaka T, Hayashi M, et al. Role of inhaled tiotropium on the perioperative outcomes of patients with lung cancer and chronic obstructive pulmonary disease. J Thorac Cardiovasc Surg 2010;58:38–42.

59. Bolukbas S, Eberlein M, Eckhoff J, et al. Short-term effects of inhalative tiotropium/formoterol/budenoside versus tiotropium/formoterol in patients with newly diagnosed chronic obstructive pulmonary disease requiring surgery for lung cancer: a prospective randomized trial. Eur J Cardiothorac Surg 2011; 39:995–1000.

60. Nagarajan K, Bennett A, Agostini P, et al. Is preoperative physiotherapy/pulmonary rehabilitation beneficial in lung resection patients? Interact Cardiovasc Thorac Surg 2011;13(3):300–2.

61. Benzo R, Wigle D, Novotny P, et al. Preoperative pulmonary rehabilitation before lung cancer resection: results from two randomized studies. Lung Cancer 2011; 74(3):441–5.

62. Dettling DS, Schaaf M, Blom RL, et al. Feasibility and effectiveness of preoperative inspiratory muscle training in patients undergoing oesophagectomy: a pilot study. Physiother Res Int 2013;18(1):16–26.

63. Hulzebos EH, Helders PJ, Favié NJ, et al. Preoperative intensive inspiratory muscle training to prevent postoperative pulmonary complications in high-risk patients undergoing CABG surgery: a randomized clinical trial. JAMA 2006; 296(15):1851–7.

64. Yadav H, Lingineni RK, Slivinski, et al. Preoperative statin administration does not protect against early postoperative acute respiratory distress syndrome: a retrospective cohort study. Anesth Analg 2014;119(4):891–8.

65. Shyamsundar M, McAuley DF, Shields MO, et al. Effect of simvastatin on physiological and biological outcomes in patients undergoing esophagectomy: a randomized placebo-controlled trial. Ann Surg 2014;259(1):26–31.

66. Verhage RJ, Boone J, Rijkers GT, et al. Reduced local immune response with continuous positive airway pressure during one-lung ventilation for oesophagectomy. Br J Anaesth 2014;112(5):920–8.

67. Ventilation with lower tidal volumes as compared with traditional tidal volumes for acute lung injury and the acute respiratory distress syndrome. The Acute Respiratory Distress Syndrome Network. N Engl J Med 2000; 342(18):1301–8.

68. Michelet P, D'Journo XB, Roch A, et al. Protective ventilation influences systemic inflammation after esophagectomy: a randomized controlled study. Anesthesiology 2006;105(5):911–9.

69. Slinger PD, Kruger M, McRae K, et al. Relation of the static compliance curve and positive end-expiratory pressure to oxygenation during one-lung ventilation. Anesthesiology 2001;95(5):1096–102.

70. The PROVE Network Investigators for the Clinical Trial Network of the European Society of Anaesthesiology. High versus low positive end-expiratory pressure during general anaesthesia for open abdominal surgery (PROVHILO trial): a multicentre randomised controlled trial. Lancet 2014;384:495–503.

71. Futier E, Constantin JM, Paugam-Burtz C, et al, IMPROVE Study Group. A trial of intraoperative low-tidal-volume ventilation in abdominal surgery. N Engl J Med 2013;369(5):428–37.

72. Ferrando C, Mugarra A, Gutierrez A, et al. Setting individualized positive end-expiratory pressure level with a positive end-expiratory pressure decrement trial after a recruitment maneuver improves oxygenation and lung mechanics during one-lung ventilation. Anesth Analg 2014;118(3):657–65.

73. Tugrul M, Camci E, Karadeniz H, et al. Comparison of volume controlled with pressure controlled ventilation during one-lung anaesthesia. Br J Anaesth 1997;79(3):306–10.

74. Unzueta MC, Casas JI, Moral MV. Pressure-controlled versus volume-controlled ventilation during one-lung ventilation for thoracic surgery. Anesth Analg 2007; 104(5):1029–33.
75. De Conno E, Steurer MP, Wittlinger M, et al. Anesthetic-induced improvement of the inflammatory response to one-lung ventilation. Anesthesiology 2009;110(6): 1316–26.
76. Schilling T, Kozian A, Kretzschmar M, et al. Effects of propofol and desflurane anaesthesia on the alveolar inflammatory response to one-lung ventilation. Br J Anaesth 2007;99(3):368–75.
77. Khan O, Manners J, Rengarajan A, et al. Does pyloroplasty following esophagectomy improve early clinical outcomes? Interact Cardiovasc Thorac Surg 2007;6(2):247–50.
78. Palmes D, Weilinghoff M, Colombo-Benkmann M, et al. Effect of pyloric drainage procedures on gastric passage and bile reflux after esophagectomy with gastric conduit reconstruction. Langenbecks Arch Surg 2007;392(2):135–41.
79. Brodner G, Pogatzki E, Van Aken H, et al. A multimodal approach to control postoperative pathophysiology and rehabilitation in patients undergoing abdominothoracic esophagectomy. Anesth Analg 1998;86(2):228–34.
80. Low DE, Kunz S, Schembre D, et al. Esophagectomy—it's not just about mortality anymore: standardized perioperative clinical pathways improve outcomes in patients with esophageal cancer. J Gastrointest Surg 2007;11(11):1395–402.
81. Neal JM, Wilcox RT, Allen HW, et al. Near-total esophagectomy: the influence of standardized multimodal management and intraoperative fluid restriction. Reg Anesth Pain Med 2003;28(4):328–34.
82. Resar R, Pronovost P, Haraden C, et al. Using a bundle approach to improve ventilator care processes and reduce ventilator-associated pneumonia. Jt Comm J Qual Patient Saf 2005;31(5):243–8.
83. Slinger PD. Perioperative fluid management for thoracic surgery: the puzzle of postpneumonectomy pulmonary edema. J Cardiothorac Vasc Anesth 1995; 9(4):442–51.
84. Chau EH, Slinger P. Perioperative fluid management for pulmonary resection surgery and esophagectomy. Semin Cardiothorac Vasc Anesth 2014;18(1): 36–44.
85. Ca sado D, López F, Martí R. Perioperative fluid management and major respiratory complications in patients undergoing esophagectomy. Dis Esophagus 2010;23(7):523–8.
86. Marjanovic G, Villain C, Juettner E, et al. Impact of different crystalloid volume regimes on intestinal anastomotic stability. Ann Surg 2009;249(2):181–5.
87. Khuri SF, Henderson WG, DePalma RG, et al. Determinants of long-term survival after major surgery and the adverse effect of postoperative complications. Ann Surg 2005;242(3):326–41.
88. Head J, Ferrie JE, Alexanderson K, et al. Whitehall II prospective cohort study. Diagnosis-specific sickness absence as a predictor of mortality: the Whitehall II prospective cohort study. BMJ 2008;337:a1469.
89. Ng JM. Update on anesthetic management for esophagectomy. Curr Opin Anaesthesiol 2011;24(1):37–43.
90. Lobo DN, Bostock KA, Neal KR, et al. Effect of salt and water balance on recovery of gastrointestinal function after elective colonic resection: a randomised controlled trial. Lancet 2002;359(9320):1812–8.
91. Brandstrup B, Tønnesen H, Beier-Holgersen R, et al. Effects of intravenous fluid restriction on postoperative complications: comparison of two perioperative fluid

regimens: a randomized assessor-blinded multicenter trial. Ann Surg 2003; 238(5):641–8.

92. Nisanevich V, Felsenstein I, Almogy G, et al. Effect of intraoperative fluid management on outcome after intraabdominal surgery. Anesthesiology 2005; 103(1):25–32.

93. Kita T, Mammoto T, Kishi Y. Fluid management and postoperative respiratory disturbances in patients with transthoracic esophagectomy for carcinoma. J Clin Anesth 2002;14(4):252–6.

94. Buise M, Van Bommel J, Mehra M, et al. Pulmonary morbidity following esophagectomy is decreased after introduction of a multimodal anesthetic regimen. Acta Anaesthesiol Belg 2008;59(4):257–61.

95. Noblett SE, Snowden CP, Shenton BK, et al. Randomized clinical trial assessing the effect of Doppler-optimized fluid management on outcome after elective colorectal resection. Br J Surg 2006;93(9):1069–76.

96. Wakeling HG, McFall MR, Jenkins CS, et al. Intraoperative oesophageal Doppler guided fluid management shortens postoperative hospital stay after major bowel surgery. Br J Anaesth 2005;95(5):634–42.

97. Benes J, Chytra I, Altmann P, et al. Intraoperative fluid optimization using stroke volume variation in high risk surgical patients: results of prospective randomized study. Crit Care 2010;14(3):R118.

98. Giglio MT, Marucci M, Testini M, et al. Goal-directed haemodynamic therapy and gastrointestinal complications in major surgery: a meta-analysis of randomized controlled trials. Br J Anaesth 2009;103(5):637–46.

99. Kimberger O, Arnberger M, Brandt S, et al. Goal-directed colloid administration improves the microcirculation of healthy and perianastomotic colon. Anesthesiology 2009;110(3):496–504.

100. Walsh SR, Tang T, Bass S, et al. Doppler-guided intra-operative fluid management during major abdominal surgery: systematic review and meta-analysis. Int J Clin Pract 2008;62(3):466–70.

101. Abbas SM, Hill AG. Systematic review of the literature for the use of oesophageal Doppler monitor for fluid replacement in major abdominal surgery. Anaesthesia 2008;63(1):44–51.

102. Corcoran T, Rhodes JE, Clarke S, et al. Perioperative fluid management strategies in major surgery: a stratified meta-analysis. Anesth Analg 2012;114(3):640–51.

103. Pearse RM, Harrison DA, MacDonald N, et al, OPTIMISE Study Group. Effect of a perioperative, cardiac output-guided hemodynamic therapy algorithm on outcomes following major gastrointestinal surgery: a randomized clinical trial and systematic review. JAMA 2014;311(21):2181–90.

104. Haas S, Eichhorn V, Hasbach T, et al. Goal-directed fluid therapy using stroke volume variation does not result in pulmonary fluid overload in thoracic surgery requiring one-lung ventilation. Crit Care Res Pract 2012;2012:687018.

105. Kobayashi M, Koh M, Irinoda T, et al. Stroke volume variation as a predictor of intravascular volume depression and possible hypotension during the early postoperative period after esophagectomy. Ann Surg Oncol 2009;16(5):1371–7.

106. Sugasawa Y, Hayashida M, Yamaguchi K, et al. Usefulness of stroke volume index obtained with the FloTrac/Vigileo system for the prediction of acute kidney injury after radical esophagectomy. Ann Surg Oncol 2013;20(12):3992–8.

107. Saran T, Perkins GD, Javed MA, et al. Does the prophylactic administration of magnesium sulphate to patients undergoing thoracotomy prevent postoperative supraventricular arrhythmias? A randomized controlled trial. Br J Anaesth 2011; 106(6):785–91.

108. Ritchie AJ, Whiteside M, Tolan M, et al. Cardiac dysrhythmia in total thoracic oe-sophagectomy. A prospective study. Eur J Cardiothorac Surg 1993;7(8):420–2.
109. Mowat IR, Dickinson MC. Prophylactic magnesium sulphate and postoperative supraventricular arrhythmias in patients undergoing thoracotomy. Br J Anaesth 2011;107(6):1005.
110. Murthy SC, Law S, Whooley BP, et al. Atrial fibrillation after esophagectomy is a marker for postoperative morbidity and mortality. J Thorac Cardiovasc Surg 2003;126(4):1162–7.
111. Sedrakyan A, Treasure T, Browne J, et al. Pharmacologic prophylaxis for post-operative atrial tachyarrhythmia in general thoracic surgery: evidence from ran-domized clinical trials. J Thorac Cardiovasc Surg 2005;129(5):997–1005.
112. Ritchie AJ, Tolan M, Whiteside M, et al. Prophylactic digitalization fails to control dysrhythmia in thoracic esophageal operations. Ann Thorac Surg 1993;55(1): 86–8.
113. Jakobsen CJ, Bille S, Ahlburg P, et al. Perioperative metoprolol reduces the fre-quency of atrial fibrillation after thoracotomy for lung resection. J Cardiothorac Vasc Anesth 1997;11:746–51.
114. Terzi A, Furlan G, Chiavacci P, et al. Prevention of atrial tachyarrhythmias after non-cardiac thoracic surgery by infusion of magnesium sulfate. Thorac Cardio-vasc Surg 1996;44(6):300.
115. Fernando HC, Jaklitsch MT, Walsh GL, et al. The Society of Thoracic Surgeons practice guideline on the prophylaxis and management of atrial fibrillation asso-ciated with general thoracic surgery: Executive summary. Ann Thorac Surg 2011;92:1144–52.
116. Devereaux PJ, Yang H, Yusuf S, et al. Effects of extended-release metoprolol succinate in patients undergoing non-cardiac surgery (POISE trial): a rando-mised controlled trial. Lancet 2008;371(9627):1839–47.
117. Bangalore S, Wetterslev J, Pranesh S, et al. Perioperative β blockers in pa-tients having non-cardiac surgery: a meta-analysis. Lancet 2008;372(9654): 1962–76.
118. Tisdale JE, Wroblewski HA, Wall DS, et al. A randomized, controlled study of amiodarone for prevention of atrial fibrillation after transthoracic esophagec-tomy. J Thorac Cardiovasc Surg 2010;140(1):45–51.
119. Theodorou D, Drimousis PG, Larentzakis A, et al. The effects of vasopressors on perfusion of gastric graft after esophagectomy. An experimental study. J Gastrointest Surg 2008;12(9):1497–501.
120. Klijn E, Niehof S, De Jonge J, et al. The effect of perfusion pressure on gastric tissue blood flow in an experimental gastric tube model. Anesth Analg 2010; 110(2):541–6.
121. Van Bommel J, De Jonge J, Buise MP, et al. The effects of intravenous nitroglyc-erine and norepinephrine on gastric microvascular perfusion in an experimental model of gastric tube reconstruction. Surgery 2010;148(1):71–7.
122. Zakrison T, Nascimento BA Jr, Tremblay LN, et al. Perioperative vasopressors are associated with an increased risk of gastrointestinal anastomotic leakage. World J Surg 2007;31(8):1627–34.
123. Pearse RM, Belsey JD, Cole JN, et al. Effect of dopexamine infusion on mortality following major surgery: individual patient data meta-regression analysis of pub-lished clinical trials. Crit Care Med 2008;36(4):1323–9.
124. Flisberg P, Törnebrandt K, Walther B, et al. Pain relief after esophagectomy: thoracic epidural analgesia is better than parenteral opioids. J Cardiothorac Vasc Anesth 2001;15(3):282–7.

125. Rudin A, Flisberg P, Johansson J, et al. Thoracic epidural analgesia or intravenous morphine analgesia after thoracoabdominal esophagectomy: a prospective follow-up of 201 patients. J Cardiothorac Vasc Anesth 2005;19(3):350–7.
126. Ballantyne JC, Carr DB, deFerranti S, et al. The comparative effects of postoperative analgesic therapies on pulmonary outcome: cumulative meta-analyses of randomized, controlled trials. Anesth Analg 1998;86(3):598–612.
127. Watson A, Allen PR. Influence of thoracic epidural analgesia on outcome after resection for esophageal cancer. Surgery 1994;115(4):429–32.
128. Whooley BP, Law S, Murthy SC, et al. Analysis of reduced death and complication rates after esophageal resection. Ann Surg 2001;233(3):338–44.
129. Katz J, Jackson M, Kavanagh BP, et al. Acute pain after thoracic surgery predicts long-term post-thoracotomy pain. Clin J Pain 1996;12(1):50–5.
130. Sentürk M, Ozcan PE, Talu GK, et al. The effects of three different analgesia techniques on long-term postthoracotomy pain. Anesth Analg 2002;94(1): 11–5.
131. Lázár G, Kaszaki J, Abrahám S, et al. Thoracic epidural anesthesia improves the gastric microcirculation during experimental gastric tube formation. Surgery 2003;134(5):799–805.
132. Pathak D, Pennefather SH, Russell GN, et al. Phenylephrine infusion improves blood flow to the stomach during oesophagectomy in the presence of a thoracic epidural analgesia. Eur J Cardiothorac Surg 2013;44(1):130–3.
133. Hansdottir V, Philip J, Olsen MF, et al. Thoracic epidural versus intravenous patient-controlled analgesia after cardiac surgery: a randomized controlled trial on length of hospital stay and patient-perceived quality of recovery. Anesthesiology 2006;104(1):142–51.
134. Al-Rawi OY, Pennefather SH, Page RD, et al. The effect of thoracic epidural bupivacaine and an intravenous adrenaline infusion on gastric tube blood flow during esophagectomy. Anesth Analg 2008;106(3):884–7, Table of contents.
135. Richards ER, Kabir SI, McNaught CE, et al. Effect of thoracic epidural anaesthesia on splanchnic blood flow. Br J Surg 2013;100(3):316–21.
136. Davies RG, Myles PS, Graham JM. A comparison of the analgesic efficacy and side-effects of paravertebral vs epidural blockade for thoracotomy—a systematic review and meta-analysis of randomized trials. Br J Anaesth 2006;96(4): 418–26.
137. Baidya DK, Khanna P, Maitra S. Analgesic efficacy and safety of thoracic paravertebral and epidural analgesia for thoracic surgery: a systematic review and meta-analysis. Interact Cardiovasc Thorac Surg 2014;18(5):626–35.
138. Ding X, Jin S, Niu X, et al. A comparison of the analgesia efficacy and side effects of paravertebral compared with epidural blockade for thoracotomy: an updated meta-analysis. PLoS One 2014;9(5):e96233. http://dx.doi.org/10.1371/journal.pone.0096233.
139. Sabanathan S, Shah R, Tsiamis A, et al. Oesophagogastrectomy in the elderly high risk patients: role of effective regional analgesia and early mobilisation. J Cardiovasc Surg (Torino) 1999;40(1):153–6.
140. Merskey H, Bogduk H, editors. Classification of chronic pain: descriptions of chronic pain syndromes and definitions of pain terms. Seattle (WA): IASP Press; 1994.
141. Gotoda Y, Kambara N, Sakai T, et al. The morbidity, time course and predictive factors for persistent post-thoracotomy pain. Eur J Pain 2001;5(1):89–96.
142. Gottschalk A, Cohen SP, Yang S, et al. Preventing and treating pain after thoracic surgery. Anesthesiology 2006;104(3):594–600.

143. Kalso E, Perttunen K, Kaasinen S. Pain after thoracic surgery. Acta Anaesthesiol Scand 1992;36(1):96–100.
144. Perttunen K, Tasmuth T, Kalso E. Chronic pain after thoracic surgery: a follow-up study. Acta Anaesthesiol Scand 1999;43(5):563–7.
145. Wildgaard K, Ravn J, Kehlet H. Chronic post-thoracotomy pain: a critical review of pathogenic mechanisms and strategies for prevention. Eur J Cardiothorac Surg 2009;36(1):170–80.
146. Kehlet H, Jensen TS, Woolf CJ. Persistent postsurgical pain: risk factors and prevention. Lancet 2006;367(9522):1618–25.
147. Cerfolio RJ, Price TN, Bryant AS, et al. Intracostal sutures decrease the pain of thoracotomy. Ann Thorac Surg 2003;76(2):407–12.
148. De Oliveira GS, Castro-Alves LJ, Khan JH, et al. Perioperative systemic magnesium to minimize postoperative pain: a meta-analysis of randomized controlled trials. Anesthesiology 2013;119(1):178–90.
149. Laskowski K, Stirling A, McKay WP, et al. A systematic review of intravenous ketamine for postoperative analgesia. Can J Anaesth 2011;58(10):911–23.
150. Schmidt PC, Ruchelli G, Mackey SC, et al. Perioperative gabapentinoids: choice of agent, dose, timing, and effects on chronic postsurgical pain. Anesthesiology 2013;119(5):1215–21.
151. Nagpal K, Ahmed K, Vats A, et al. Is minimally invasive surgery beneficial in the management of esophageal cancer? A meta-analysis. Surg Endosc 2010;24(7): 1621–9.
152. Biere SS, van Berge Henegouwen MI, Maas KW, et al. Minimally invasive versus open oesophagectomy for patients with oesophageal cancer: a multicentre, open-label, randomised controlled trial. Lancet 2012;379(9829):1887–92.
153. Rucklidge M, Sanders D, Martin A. Anaesthesia for minimally invasive oesophagectomy. Cont Educ Anaesth Crit Care Pain 2010;10(2):43–8.
154. Paton F, Chambers D, Wilson P, et al. Effectiveness and implementation of enhanced recovery after surgery programmes: a rapid evidence synthesis. BMJ Open 2014;4(7):e005015. http://dx.doi.org/10.1136/bmjopen-2014-005015.
155. Lassen K, Soop M, Nygren J, et al, Enhanced Recovery After Surgery (ERAS) Group. Consensus review of optimal perioperative care in colorectal surgery: Enhanced Recovery After Surgery (ERAS) Group recommendations. Arch Surg 2009;144(10):961–9.
156. Markar SR, Karthikesalingam A, Low DE. Enhanced recovery pathways lead to an improvement in postoperative outcomes following esophagectomy: systematic review and pooled analysis. Dis Esophagus 2014. http://dx.doi.org/10.1111/dote.12214.
157. Findlay JM, Tustian E, Millo J, et al. The effect of formalizing enhanced recovery after esophagectomy with a protocol. Dis Esophagus 2014. [Epub ahead of print].
158. Jiang K, Cheng L, Wang JJ, et al. Fast track clinical pathway implications in esophagogastrectomy. World J Gastroenterol 2009;15(4):496–501.
159. Available at: http://www.teamsky.com/article/0,27290,17547_5792058,00.html#ZXHacb6DmyK8g5AO.97. Accessed September 9, 2014.

Anesthesia for Major Urologic Surgery

James O.B. Cockcroft, MB ChB, FRCA[a],*, Colin B. Berry, MBBS, FRCA[a],
John S. McGrath, BMBS, FRCS, MD[b], Mark O. Daugherty, MBBCh, FRCA[a]

KEYWORDS

- Enhanced recovery • Shared decision making • Surgical approach • Robot assisted
- Laparoscopic • Prostatectomy • Cystectomy • Robotic prostatectomy

KEY POINTS

- Anesthesia for major urology surgery has changed greatly with the advent of laparoscopic and robot-assisted surgical techniques.
- Enhanced recovery pathways are now established in complex major urologic surgery and are reducing lengths of stay and postoperative complications. This model is extremely important to deliver optimal health care from the decision to operate to the return to normal patient function.
- Anesthetic considerations differ between established robotic surgical centers and those still perfecting the older approach (operative times much greater).
- The success of enhanced recovery pathways in urologic surgery depends upon preoperative assessment, preparation and compliance with all the perioperative elements. Attention to detail and fastidious preparation are the keys to successful anesthesia and outcomes in robotic surgery.

PATIENT POPULATION

The mean age for patients undergoing cystectomy is 60 years. This age is typical of the population of men undergoing major urologic surgery. The patients affected are an elderly cohort, usually with multiple significant comorbidities. They often have a malignancy, associated renal dysfunction, and present a challenge to the anesthetist in the perioperative setting.

ENHANCED RECOVERY CARE PATHWAY

Most surgical pathways in the United Kingdom are now based on the principles of enhanced recovery.[1,2] This care pathway begins when the patient is still at home, before surgery, and does not end until the patient has returned to the presurgery functional status.

[a] Department of Anaesthesia, Royal Devon and Exeter NHS Foundation Trust, Barrack Road, Exeter, Devon EX2 5DW, UK; [b] Department of Urology and Exeter Health Services Research Unit, Royal Devon and Exeter NHS Foundation Trust, Barrack Road, Exeter, Devon EX2 5DW, UK
* Corresponding author.
E-mail address: jimcockcroft@hotmail.com

Anesthesiology Clin 33 (2015) 165–172
http://dx.doi.org/10.1016/j.anclin.2014.11.010   anesthesiology.theclinics.com

The preassessment process follows and places the emphasis on the shared decision making that underpins this approach to perioperative care. This process covers various generic issues but may also involve individual risk stratification, cardiopulmonary exercise testing, perioperative management of anticoagulants, and assessment of postoperative high dependency requirements. The patient's health status is also optimized by management of anemia, glycemic control, and treatment of hypertension, as well as dietary, weight, and smoking-cessation advice before surgery.

A consultant-led, multidisciplinary decision can be made as to which procedure and approach is required for each patient.

Major urologic surgery has 2 main categories:

- Upper tract surgery: simple or radical nephrectomy, radical nephroureterectomy, nephron-sparing surgery
- Pelvic surgery: radical cystectomy with urinary diversion and radical prostatectomy

The surgical approach to these procedures differs greatly and there has been rapid adoption of minimally invasive surgery in recent years, particularly with the advent of robot-assisted surgery. The procedure as well as the approach therefore influence the anesthetic techniques recommended.

The authors' unit has been a designated cancer center since 2005 and undertakes approximately 300 robotic pelvic cases per year.[3] All cystectomies and prostatectomies are now completed robotically, and the unit has been a national leader in enhanced recovery with one of the shortest lengths of stay in the United Kingdom for radical pelvic surgery.

This unit has ceased using intraoperative cell salvage for cystectomies, because the blood transfusion requirement in robotics has been minimal, decreasing length of stay and cost.

Latest advances include the introduction of day-case robotically assisted laparoscopic prostatectomy.

All patients requiring radical cystectomy undergo preoperative cardiopulmonary exercise testing, and this allows risk stratification for the planned level of dependency in the postoperative period. The high-dependency setting is only used in those patients identified as high risk.

Most radical nephrectomies and nephron-sparing surgery are now performed by laparoscopic or robotically assisted laparoscopic approach. Open renal surgery is reserved for tumors involving the inferior vena cava or large, centrally placed tumors requiring partial nephrectomy for which a laparoscopic approach is not feasible.

SPECIFIC ANESTHETIC CONSIDERATIONS FOR OPEN PROCEDURES

- Blood loss: use of intraoperative cell salvage, transfusion requirements[3]
- Pain relief: preemptive, intraoperative, and postoperative (multimodal)
- Regional anesthesia: rectus sheath catheters[4] (placed by the anesthetist using ultrasonography), resulting in earlier mobilization than thoracic epidural anesthesia
- Heat loss: forced-air warmers, fluid warming devices

SPECIFIC CONSIDERATIONS FOR LAPAROSCOPIC PROCEDURES

- Pneumoperitoneum: cardiovascular stability, hypercarbia, postoperative pain
- Potential for concealed bleeding

As with any laparoscopic surgery, issues with ventilation, maintenance of normocapnia, and cardiovascular stability can occur during any urologic procedure involving pneumoperitoneum. Because of the prolonged nature of the surgery in urology, problems with hypercarbia, vagally mediated bradycardia, and postoperative shoulder tip pain are more common.

It is also important to understand that significant surgical bleeding can be masked when operating laparoscopically, and can be much more difficult to control, should it occur.

ROBOT-ASSISTED SURGERY

Robotic surgery is gaining dominance over the conventional laparoscopic approach for most pelvic procedures and nephron-sparing surgery.[5] The surgeon operates from a nonsterile, seated control unit that is separate from the robot. The operating arms are positioned between the legs of the patient and a steep head-down (Trendelenburg) lithotomy position is required to prevent abdominal contents from obscuring the view of the pelvis. Four operating arms attached to intra-abdominal ports extend over the patient. These ports remain in place for the duration of the procedure and the instruments, inserted via the ports, are manipulated by the magnified movements of the surgeon in the control unit (**Fig. 1**).

Differences from traditional laparoscopic surgery:
- Emergency access to patient: a plan to disengage instruments, remove the trocars, and unlock the robot, before leveling the patient, must be decided, communicated, and rehearsed for any airway emergency or cardiac arrest scenario.
- Muscle relaxation: maintenance of neuromuscular block and complete avoidance of patient movement is mandatory while the fixed trocars are in place, to avoid potential tissue injury.

Specific Considerations for Robot-assisted Surgery

Complications/concerns with robot-assisted surgery[6]:
Prolonged lithotomy position predisposes to:
- Lower (and rarely upper) extremity nerve injury (particularly femoral nerve)
- Pressure areas and compartment syndrome of the lower limbs
Prolonged Trendelenburg[7] predisposes to:
- Ocular injury including corneal abrasions and ischemic optic neuropathy caused by high intraocular pressures[8–10]
- Laryngeal (and facial) edema and respiratory distress

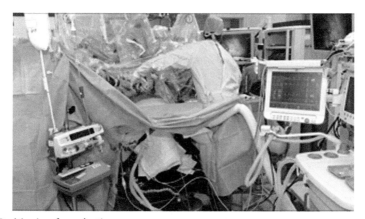

Fig. 1. Positioning for robotics.

- Risk of cerebral edema, as well as increased intracranial pressure, due to reduction in cerebral venous return due to the high intra-abdominal pressures and head-down position
- Decreased functional residual capacity and decreased pulmonary compliance causing increased ventilatory pressures and increased atelectasis

Prolonged pneumoperitoneum predisposes to:

- Carbon dioxide subcutaneous emphysema (up to 4% of cases)
- Carbon dioxide air embolism is also possible[11,12]

NEPHRECTOMY

Most patients undergoing nephrectomy are presenting with renal cancer. These patients must be screened for other comorbidities or mass lesions and invasion into any other tissues, in order to plan not only the appropriate surgical procedure and postoperative management plan but also the choice of anesthetic. They have often been identified via screening and present asymptomatically, but can be a complex cohort of patients, who must be managed by an experienced team.

These patients are positioned laterally (operative side up) for the procedure in most cases, although in recent times the breaking of the table has not been widely used.

ANESTHETIC TEMPLATE

A template for the anesthetic management of robot-assisted prostatectomy is detailed later. Significant differences in anesthetic and surgical management of patients undergoing other major urologic procedures is also outlined for completeness.

ROBOT-ASSISTED SURGERY

Duration: approximately 3 to 4 hours (surgical time, 2–3 hours)
Incision: multiple robotic-arm trocars with surgical instruments attached
Positioning: steep head-down lithotomy (approximately 27°), arms wrapped by sides

Recommended Techniques

Preoperative visit

- Consent for spinal under general anesthetic: performed at end of operation if prostate has been difficult to dissect and the bladder is thin walled, which would increase the likelihood of postoperative bladder spasm, which is otherwise difficult to treat (shared decision making between surgeon and anesthetist)
- Warn patient about sore throat, due to the endotracheal tube, facial edema, catheter insertion, lower abdominal (and sometimes penile) pain, and the need for early mobilization

PREMEDICATION

- Drugs to reduce gastric acid and increase gastric emptying (eg, omeprazole 40 mg by mouth and metoclopramide 10 mg by mouth)
- Addition of preemptive analgesia after consent is obtained (eg, oxycodone 15 mg by mouth)

ANESTHETIC ROOM

- Thromboembolic stockings (if not contraindicated)

- All invasive lines on 1 side (opposite side to robot assistant; usually the left) for less interference during procedure (normally a 16G intravenous cannula and 20G arterial cannula)
- Anesthetize patient on the surgical table, lying directly on gel pad, with gel head support
- General anesthesia, endotracheal tube (taped not tied to avoid cerebral venous congestion), positive pressure ventilation (optimal positive end-expiratory pressure)
- Orogastric tube (for gastric deflation) and oral temperature probe
- Saline-soaked ribbon gauze throat pack (to protect against gastric contents re-fluxing up lacrimal ducts and causing corneal burns)
- Eye protection with lubricating ointment, tape, and padding
- Padded right-angled bar placed just caudad to the patient's chin to protect head from surgical instruments
- Arms wrapped by patient's sides, which limits intraoperative access: plan lines appropriately and attach patient identification to forehead after routine safety checks
- Arterial transducer on board fixed at the level of the shoulder

INTRAOPERATIVE

- Forced-air warmer to upper chest and fluid warmer
- Bolsters under knees (**Fig. 2**), gel pads under ankles, and calf pumps
- Steep head-down position (try for 27°, depending on patient body habitus and ventilatory pressures); some centers use shoulder bolsters
- Preincision surgical antibiotic prophylaxis as per local protocol
- IV dexamethasone to decrease inflammation and swelling
- Consider antisialagogue of choice - not routinely used (eg, IV glycopyrrolate 200 mg, which decreases secretions and the chance of bradyarrhythmias with pneumoperitoneum and remifentanil infusion)
- Buscopan reduces bladder spasm in recovery (can increase heart rate)
- Remifentanil infusion with volatile maintenance in oxygen/air mix is used most commonly
- With careful attention to airway pressures, a second dose of muscle relaxant is rarely required

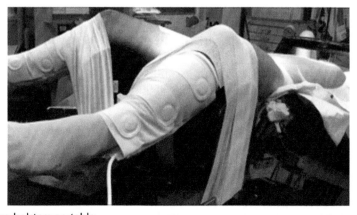

Fig. 2. Leg bolsters on table.

FLUID THERAPY

- Limit fluid therapy during procedure while lower renal tract is disrupted. For most surgery this requires less than 800 mL. Then administer up to 1200 mL (approximately) of crystalloid once urethra is reconnected by the surgeon (communicate closely): total 2000 mL
- Blood loss is usually less than 300 mL

SURGICAL CONCLUSION

- Administer antiemetic and analgesics (eg, IV ondansetron 4 mg, IV paracetamol 1 g, IV nonsteroidal antiinflammatory drug [NSAID] of choice, and IV oxycodone); often give small dose of furosemide to stimulate diuresis
- As soon as robot is disengaged, flatten patient out and perform recruitment maneuvers to the lungs
- Consider spinal after discussion with surgeon before emergence (if bladder spasm is a problem, spinal is advised): no opiate, aim to cover 3 hours after surgery
- Sit patient up as soon as surgery is complete: slow wake up over 10 to 15 minutes while remifentanil action wears off (this period reduces cerebral edema and risk of agitation and confusion postoperatively)
- Ensure normocapnia and cuff leak before extubation

POSTOPERATIVE PRESCRIPTION

- Postoperative pain is normally only mild to moderate
- Regular multimodal analgesia, antiemetic, and venous thromboembolic prophylaxis (eg, oxycodone 10–15 mg by mouth twice a day, paracetamol 1 g by mouth 4 times a day, NSAID of choice unless contra-indicated, metoclopramide 10 mg by mouth 3 times a day, and subcutaneous venous thromboembolism prophylaxis as per local protocol)
- As required: short-acting opiate and Buscopan for gastrointestinal/bladder spasm

Key Points

- Prolonged head-down position and pneumoperitoneum
- Limited patient access (**Fig. 3**)
- Avoid any patient movement during robotic instrumentation
- Sit up before extubation and demonstrate cuff leak

COMMON SURGICAL PROCEDURES AND IMPLICATIONS FOR THE ANESTHETIST
Radical Cystectomy (Robotic)

As for robot-assisted prostatectomy, except:
- Patient leveled to 15° for the ileal conduit or orthotopic neobladder (using a lower-midline (subumbilical) incision)
- Rectus sheath catheters for analgesia
- Seventy-two hours of oxycodone twice a day postoperatively for analgesia
- Increased duration of surgery
- Increased risk of complications of position and pneumoperitoneum

Radical Cystectomy (Open)

As mentioned for open procedures:
- Intraoperative cell salvage is used routinely

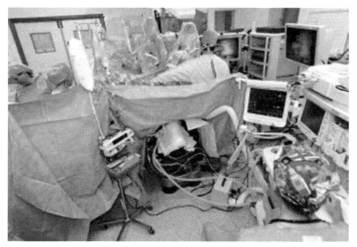

Fig. 3. Limited access to the patient for the anesthetist.

- Lower-midline (subumbilical) incision
- Rectus sheath catheters cover incisional pain (often placed under sterile conditions by anesthetist using ultrasonography, before surgical start); used for 5 days
- Opiates cover visceral pain for first 24 to 36 hours
- Blood transfusion can be required (usually in the postoperative days)
- Fluid management should be designed to maintain normovolemia and zero balance
- Complications secondary to pneumoperitoneum are no longer a concern

Mu receptor antagonists (eg, alvimopan) are used in some centers for open cystectomy. They have a limited ability to cross the blood-brain barrier so do not antagonize the analgesic effects of opioids but reduce peripheral effects such as ileus.

Radical Prostatectomy (Open)

- Lower-midline (subumbilical) incision
- Rectus sheath catheters (less visceral pain than cystectomy)
- Early food and fluids well tolerated
- Mobile within hours after surgery

Radical Nephrectomy

- Often completed using a laparoscopic approach, but requires a small incision at the end of the procedure to remove the kidney (surgical local anesthetic only required to port sites and wounds)
- Patient positioned laterally on the operating table
- Patient-controlled analgesia effective postoperatively
- If planned as an open procedure, consider epidural or wound-infiltration catheters

Partial Nephrectomy

- Usually completed via the laparoscopic approach (surgical local only)
- Patient positioned laterally on the operating table

SUMMARY OF ANESTHETIC MANAGEMENT

- There should be collaboration between the anesthesia or perioperative medicine team and the surgical team from the time a decision to operate is made. This collaboration ensures optimal management of comorbidities, shared decision making, and the management of risk.
- Early assessment of risk helps to determine the level of care patients receive postoperatively, which allows effective resource planning.
- Patients are less likely to need high-dependency care and blood transfusion than previously, when traditional approaches to major urologic surgery were used.
- The routine application of excellent standards of all aspects of anesthetic care applies to this specialist area.
- This operating environment is complex and differs from traditional practice in many ways. The anesthetic team need specific training and regular experience to make their best contributions to good patient outcomes.
- Specific scenarios (such as undocking) must be rehearsed to enable access to, and treatment of, patients in an emergency.
- Outcome and quality improvements can only be made if robust data are collected and regularly reviewed.

REFERENCES

1. NHS Enhanced Recovery Partnership. Enhanced recovery: consensus statement. NHS Improving Quality 2012/13.
2. Cerantola Y, Valerio M, Persson B, et al. Guidelines for perioperative care after radical cystectomy for bladder cancer: Enhanced Recovery After Surgery (ERAS) society recommendations. Clin Nutr 2013;32:879–87.
3. Dutton TJ, Daugherty MO, Mason RG, et al. Implementation of the Exeter enhanced recovery programme for patients undergoing radical cystectomy. BJU Int 2014;113(5):719–25.
4. Dutton TJ, McGrath JS, Daugherty MO. Use of rectus sheath catheters for pain relief in patients undergoing major pelvic urological surgery. BJU Int 2014;113(2):246–53.
5. O'Hara J. Anesthesia for select urologic procedures. ASA Refresher Courses in Anesthesiology 2011;39(1):115–9.
6. Gainsburg DM. Anesthetic concerns for robotic-assisted laparoscopic radical prostatectomy. Minerva Anestesiol 2012;78(5):596–604.
7. Phong SV, Koh LK. Anaesthesia for robotic-assisted radical prostatectomy: considerations for laparoscopy in the Trendelenburg position. Anaesth Intensive Care 2007;35:281–5.
8. Weber ED, Colyer MH, Lesser RL, et al. Posterior ischemic optic neuropathy after minimally invasive prostatectomy. J Neuroophthalmol 2007;27:285–7.
9. Awad H, Santilli S, Ohr M, et al. The effects of steep Trendelenburg positioning on intraocular pressure during robotic radical prostatectomy. Anesth Analg 2009; 109:473–8.
10. Kalmar AF, Foubert L, Hendricks JF, et al. Influence of steep Trendelenburg position and CO_2 pneumoperitoneum on cardiovascular, cerebrovascular, and respiratory homeostasis during robotic prostatectomy. Br J Anaesth 2010;104:433–9.
11. Hong JY, Kim WO, Kil HK. Detection of subclinical CO_2 embolism by transesophageal echocardiography during laparoscopic radical prostatectomy. Urology 2010;75:581–4.
12. Smith J, Pruthi RS, McGrath JS. Enhanced recovery programmes for patients undergoing radical cystectomy. Nat Rev Urol 2014;11:437–44.

Evidence-Based Anesthesia for Major Gynecologic Surgery

Jeanette R. Bauchat, MD[a],
Ashraf S. Habib, MBBCh, MSc, MHSc, FRCA[b],*

KEYWORDS

- Enhanced recovery • ERAS • Gynecologic surgery • Fast track

KEY POINTS

- Studies on enhanced recovery after major gynecologic surgery are limited but seem to have similar outcome benefits to populations who have had colorectal surgery.
- Effective regional anesthetic techniques used in gynecologic surgery include spinal anesthesia, epidural analgesia, transversus abdominis plane blocks, local anesthetic wound infusions, and intraperitoneal instillation catheters.
- Effective nonopioid analgesics known to reduce opioid consumption after gynecologic surgery include pregabalin, gabapentin, nonsteroidal antiinflammatory drugs, cyclooxygenase 2 inhibitors, and paracetamol.
- A multimodal antiemetic strategy to reduce the baseline risk of postoperative nausea and vomiting in conjunction with combination antiemetic therapy is imperative in this high-risk population.
- Randomized controlled trials of the ideal fluid management strategies in this surgical population are needed.

INTRODUCTION

The last 2 decades have seen significant changes in the surgical approach to gynecologic surgery. Minimally invasive surgeries have been more commonly performed and have been associated with comparable long-term outcomes compared with open surgery.[1] Although operative time is longer with minimally invasive surgery, hospital stay is significantly shorter, and analgesic and antiemetic needs are significantly reduced compared with open surgery.[1,2] However, there has been little attention to optimizing other surgical and anesthetic elements of the perioperative care of these patients.

The authors have no conflicts of interest.
[a] Northwestern University, Feinberg School of Medicine, 250 East Huron Street, F5-704, Chicago, IL 60611, USA; [b] Duke University Medical Center, Box 3094, Durham, NC 27710, USA
* Corresponding author.
E-mail address: ashraf.habib@duke.edu

The concepts and practices of enhanced recovery after surgery (ERAS) are well established for colorectal surgery but until recently have not been applied to gynecologic surgery. High-quality meta-analyses have shown the effectiveness of ERAS principles in reducing hospital length of stay and overall complications but not necessarily surgical complications.[3,4] Studies that assess fast-tracking or enhanced recovery after major gynecologic surgery typically apply the ERAS guidelines derived from colorectal surgery, because there are no specific guidelines for enhanced recovery after major gynecologic surgery. In this article, major gynecologic surgery refers to the surgeries listed in **Box 1**.

Some general concepts of the ERAS protocol apply to all surgical patient populations (**Box 2**).[5] The means by which individual components of the ERAS protocol are achieved may differ, depending on the patient population and type of surgery. For example, unlike colorectal surgery, gynecologic surgery patients are all women. It is well established that women differ significantly from men from a pharmacokinetic and pharmacodynamic standpoint, which may influence the optimal anesthetic drug choice and antiemetic or analgesic strategies in ERAS protocols for gynecologic surgery compared with colorectal surgeries.[6]

This article focuses on meta-analyses, randomized controlled trials (RCTs), and large prospective impact studies conducted in the gynecologic surgery population investigating aspects of the ERAS protocol over which anesthesiologists exercise the most influence. The best evidence is presented for 4 specific aspects of the ERAS protocol: anesthetic choice, nonopioid multimodal pain management, postoperative nausea and vomiting (PONV) prevention strategies, and fluid management. This article concludes with the general ERAS principles applied to this specific patient population, because anesthesiologists should be aware of all the ERAS interventions as we become leaders of the perioperative surgical home.

ENHANCED RECOVERY AFTER MAJOR GYNECOLOGIC SURGERY

The first descriptive study exploring ERAS principles in major gynecologic surgery was conducted 10 years ago.[7] The benefits of implementation of ERAS principles in the gynecologic surgery population were explored in 1 RCT,[8] but mostly in preintervention and postintervention studies. Studies assessing impact of ERAS protocol implementation on outcomes for major gynecologic surgeries are summarized in **Table 1**. All of those studies reported a reduction in the duration of hospital stay, in addition to other

---

Box 1
Major gynecologic surgeries included in this article

Laparotomy for malignant gynecologic cancers

    Hysterectomy, lymphadenectomy, omentectomy

    Complex cytoreductive surgery

Urogynecologic pelvic organ prolapse surgery

Total or partial abdominal hysterectomy

Vaginal hysterectomy

Abdominal myomectomy

Salpingo-oophorectomy

Ovarian cystectomy

Box 2
Common aspects to all ERAS protocols

- Preoperative care
  - Optimize preoperative care for specific diseases (eg, adjusting insulin or antihypertensive medications before surgery)
  - Preoperative counseling
- Intraoperative care
  - Optimizing prophylactic antibiotic administration
  - Use of regional anesthesia intraoperatively
  - Use of minimally invasive surgery when feasible
  - Maintenance of intraoperative normothermia
  - Optimize fluid management
  - Nausea and vomiting prophylaxis
  - Optimize oxygen delivery
- Postoperative care
  - Optimize sleep
  - Ileus prevention (ie, early feeding, avoid nasogastric tube, early mobilization)
  - Minimize drains, tubes, and catheters
  - Opioid-sparing multimodal pain management
  - Continue home medications
  - Postoperative discharge planning
  - Thromboembolic prophylaxis (ie, pneumatic compression devices, anticoagulation)

---

improvements. However, there was tremendous variation in the ERAS interventions used and how each intervention was standardized. For instance, few studies attempted to standardize intraoperative anesthetic technique.[8–11] The opioid-sparing analgesic protocol varied from no standardization,[12] to nerve blocks,[13] multimodal nonopioid oral analgesics,[9] or different neuraxial analgesic techniques.[8–11] Administration of prophylactic antiemetics was standardized in 5 of those 8 studies, but they differed markedly in the type and number of agents used.[8,9,11,13,14] Intraoperative fluid administration was clearly standardized in only 1 study.[8]

REGIONAL ANESTHETIC TECHNIQUES FOR ENHANCED RECOVERY AFTER MAJOR GYNECOLOGIC SURGERY

Opioid-sparing analgesic regimens are believed to be an integral part of an ERAS protocol, because opioids have been implicated in immunosuppression, postoperative hyperalgesia, PONV, paralytic ileus, and delay of early mobilization as a result of sedation.[15–17] A variety of regional techniques, including neuraxial and peripheral nerve blocks may be used to provide postoperative analgesia, reducing opioid consumption and blunting the surgical stress response.[18]

There are no RCTs delineating the ideal intraoperative anesthetic protocol to support ERAS principles, even in guidelines already established for colorectal surgery. Nonetheless, intraoperative neuraxial anesthesia has been implemented in multiple

Table 1
Summary of studies using enhanced recovery principles for major gynecologic surgeries

Reference, Surgery Type	Study Type	Number of Patients	Implemented ERAS Interventions	Summary of ERAS Outcomes
Kroon et al,[8] 2010 Abdominal hysterectomy	RCT	Control (N = 26) ERAS (N = 27)	**Control** Preoperative: Paracetamol and NSAID or COX-2 inhibitor Intraoperative: General anesthesia N₂O + volatile agent PONV prophylaxis ondansetron Postoperative: Paracetamol + morphine PCA — **ERAS Protocol** Preoperative: Carbohydrate drink ≤2 h before surgery Paracetamol and NSAID or COX 2 inhibitor Intraoperative: Spinal anesthesia bupivacaine + morphine 100 µg PONV prophylaxis betamethasone + droperidol + ondansetron IV fluid restricted 500 mL/h Postoperative: IV fluids stopped with oral intake Paracetamol + NSAID	Shorter recovery room length of stay (median 180 vs 237 min) Lower rate of PONV on day 1 (11% vs 50%) Shorter time to oral intake (median 4 vs 5 h) Shorter duration of indwelling urinary catheter (median 9 vs 22 h) Reduced length of hospital stay (median 2 vs 3 d)
DeGroot et al,[135] 2014 Gynecologic cancer surgery	Nonrandomized prospective pre and post intervention	Pre (N = 38) Post (N = 77)	Preoperative: Counseling (not specified) Carbohydrate drink Avoidance of bowel preparations Intraoperative: Avoidance of long-acting anesthetic (not specified) Avoidance of opioids Thoracic epidural analgesia Avoidance of NG tubes Postoperative: Oral fluids day of surgery Normal diet POD 1 Early mobilization >3 times POD 1	Reduced length of hospital stay (median 5 vs 7 d) Increased rate of early feeding (oral fluids on POD 0 increased from 0% to 94%; normal diet on POD 1 increased from 0% to 58%) Reduced time to functional recovery[a] (median 3 d vs 6 d)

Kalogera et al,[9] 2013 Laparotomy gynecologic cancer surgery Urogynecologic organ prolapse surgery	Retrospective cohort pre and post intervention	Pre (N = 235) Post (N = 241)	*Preoperative:* Carbohydrate loading drink Fluids ≤4 h before surgery No bowel preparation Preoperative acetaminophen, COX-2 inhibitor, or gabapentin *Intraoperative:* Triple-agent antiemetic prophylaxis Minimize crystalloid, administer colloid if needed *Laparotomy analgesic medications:* Ketorolac or ketamine LA wound infiltration *Pelvic organ prolapse analgesic medications:* Spinal anesthesia + hydromorphone Ketorolac *Postoperative:* Postoperative fluids 40 mL/h X 24 h or until oral intake Early food intake POD 0 + nutritional supplement Early mobilization (out of bed night of surgery) Scheduled nonopioid analgesics: ketorolac or tramadol, paracetamol, oral hydromorphone as needed	Lower fluid administration (1 L less with no intraoperative hypotension) Reduced opioid usage (80% reduction over 48 h) Higher PONV rate (nausea 55.6% vs 38.5%; vomiting 17.3% vs 2.6%) Faster return of bowel function (1 d earlier) Reduced hospital length of stay by 4 d Cost savings ($7600 per patient) High patient satisfaction

(continued on next page)

Table 1
(continued)

Reference, Surgery Type	Study Type	Number of Patients	Implemented ERAS Interventions	Summary of ERAS Outcomes
Wijk et al,[14] 2014 Abdominal hysterectomy[b]	Retrospective pre and post intervention	Pre (N = 120) Post (N = 85)	**Preoperative:** Counseling regarding ERAS protocol; Malnourished patients given nutritional supplement; Carbohydrate drink 2 h before surgery; Preoperative paracetamol; Preoperative oral antibiotic. **Intraoperative:** Maintain normothermia with forced air and warm IV fluids; Standard antiemetic regimen: droperidol, dexamethasone, in addition, for high-risk patients, rescue treatment with ondansetron then metoclopramide. **Postoperative:** Standardized nonopioid analgesics: scheduled diclofenac and paracetamol; IV fluids stopped with oral intake, normal diet 2 h after surgery; Early mobilization (2 h after surgery); Routine thromboprophylaxis; Clear discharge criteria (eat normally, independent mobilization, oral analgesics, no bowel obstruction)	Rate of target length of stay (2 d) increased (53% vs 73%); Target length of stay correlated with increasing number of ERAS protocol parameter compliance; Reduced hospital length of stay (median 2.6 vs 2.3 d)
Sjetne et al,[12] 2014 Abdominal hysterectomy[b] Urogynecologic organ prolapse surgery	Nonrandomized prospective pre, immediately post, and 1 y post intervention	Pre (N = 35) Post (N = 45) 1 y Post (N = 45)	**Preoperative:** Counseling regarding ERAS protocol. **Intraoperative:** None specified. **Postoperative:** IV and urinary catheter removed in recovery room; Normal diet within hours (not specified) after surgery; Stopped routine postoperative enemas; Mobilization within hours after surgery; Oral analgesics started immediately	Reduced hospital length of stay (median days pre 4.7, post 3.4, 1 y post 3.4); Reduced nursing workload (patient contact minutes Pre 86 min, post 70.9 min, 1 y post 72.7 min)

Study	Design	N	Intervention	Outcomes
Yoong et al,[13] 2014 Vaginal hysterectomy	Retrospective case-matched pre and post intervention	Pre (N = 50) Post (N = 50)	Preoperative: Family support assessment Counseling regarding surgery (1 h audiovisual session/ discussion) Intraoperative: Surgical approach: avoid laparoscopy or abdominal incisions Regional anesthesia with pudendal and uterosacral nerve blocks Maintain intraoperative normothermia >36° Standardized antiemetic protocol: dexamethasone + ondansetron, rescue agent cyclizine Postoperative: No routine vaginal packing No routine urinary catheter Early feeding Early mobilization Hired RN discharge planner Standardized assessment algorithm to evaluate discharge readiness	Reduced hospital length of stay (median 22 h vs 45.5 h) Increase number of women discharged in <24 h (78% vs 15.6%) Reduced rate of vaginal packing (82.2% vs 52%) Reduced rate of urinary catheter use (96% vs 84.4%) Cost savings ($159.45 per patient)
Dickson et al,[10] 2012 Abdominal hysterectomy[c]	Retrospective case-matched pre and post intervention	Pre (N = 100) Post (N = 100)	Preoperative: Counseling regarding ERAS protocol Intraoperative: Spinal anesthesia with intrathecal morphine (60–100 µg) Postoperative: Early mobilization (day of surgery) Normal diet (day of surgery)	Increased use of spinal anesthesia (5% vs 83%) Reduced length of hospital stay (median 3 d vs 1 d)

(continued on next page)

Table 1
(continued)

Reference, Surgery Type	Study Type	Number of Patients	Implemented ERAS Interventions	Summary of ERAS Outcomes
Marx et al,[11] 2006 Laparotomy gynecologic cancer surgery	Retrospective pre and post intervention	Pre (N = 72) Post (N = 69)	Preoperative: No premedication Preoperative paracetamol No bowel preparation Thromboprophylaxis Intraoperative: Routine use of epidural anesthesia Antiemetic prophylaxis (dexamethasone + ondansetron) Routine antibiotic prophylaxis Postoperative: Routine use of epidural analgesia Food and nutritional supplements 4 h after surgery Magnesia (promotility agents) Early mobilization day or surgery and standardized mobilization Schedule to remove urinary and epidural catheter	Reduced hospital length of stay (median 6 d vs 5 d) Reduced severe complications (12.5% vs 1.4%)

Abbreviations: IV, intravenous; LA, local anesthetic; NG, nasogastric; NSAID, nonsteroidal antiinflammatory drug; PCA, patient controlled analgesia; POD, postoperative day; RN, registered nurse.
a Functional recovery score is based on: resumption of normal oral and food intake, independent mobilization, and pain controlled on oral analgesics.
b Malignant and benign indication.
c Benign indication.
Data from Refs.[8–14,135]

fast-track protocols because of proven benefits on attenuating the physiologic surgical stress response and showing opioid-sparing effects.[18] **Table 2**[18–28] summarizes the potential benefits of neuraxial anesthesia on ERAS protocol goals, as shown by several meta-analyses and RCTs. Despite the known benefits of regional anesthesia, there are few RCTs comparing general anesthesia alone with either regional anesthesia alone or a combination of general anesthesia with regional anesthesia in major gynecologic surgery.

Spinal Anesthesia

Most studies using regional anesthesia as a sole anesthetic are conducted in open abdominal hysterectomies or pelvic organ prolapse surgery under spinal anesthesia. **Table 3**[29–33] summarizes the RCTs that compare regional anesthesia as a sole technique or in combination with general anesthesia with general anesthesia alone on ERAS outcomes. Most of these studies show a clear benefit of spinal anesthesia compared with general anesthesia for reducing postoperative opioid consumption, likely because of the addition of intrathecal morphine to the spinal injectate.[29,30,32,33] Spinal anesthesia also seems to be more cost effective, in part because of shorter recovery room length of stays.[31,32] The effect of spinal anesthesia on hospital length of stay was mixed,[29,32] but the evidence favors spinal anesthesia for hysterectomies to enhance recovery in the immediate postoperative period.

Combined General and Epidural Anesthesia

Epidural anesthesia and analgesia is typically used as an adjuvant to general anesthesia and as a primary modality for postoperative pain management in hysterectomies and laparotomies for complex gynecologic cancer surgeries. There are few RCTs examining the impact of epidural analgesia on ERAS principles in this population. **Table 4**[34–38] summarizes RCTs comparing epidural analgesia for intraoperative

Table 2	
Potential positive impact of neuraxial anesthetic techniques on enhanced recovery principles	
ERAS Principle	**Positive Impact of Regional Anesthesia**
Attenuation of physiologic surgical stress response	Reduced endocrine and metabolic response to surgery[18] Thoracic epidurals reduced the incidence of myocardial infarction[19]
Reduction of inflammation	Reduced inflammatory markers[20]
Maintenance of normothermia	Inhibits physiologic demand of shivering[21]
Nausea and vomiting prophylaxis	Less nausea and vomiting than opioids if local anesthetics are used alone[22]
Optimization of oxygen delivery	Improve oxygen delivery[23] Reduced pulmonary complications[24]
Opioid-sparing multimodal pain management	Reduces opioid consumption[25] Excellent analgesia[22,26] Reduce chronic pain[27]
Optimization of sleep	Excellent analgesia[22,26]
Ileus prevention/early feeding	Promote gastric motility[22]
Early mobilization	Thoracic epidural can promote early mobilization as a result of excellent pain control[22]
Thromboembolic prophylaxis	Reduced deep vein thrombosis and pulmonary embolism[32]

Table 3
Summary of RCTs showing the impact of spinal anesthesia on ERAS outcomes

Type of Surgery	Study	Anesthetic Technique (Number of Patients)	Anesthetic Medication Administered	Other ERAS Interventions	ERAS Outcomes
Vaginal hysterectomy[a] ± urogynecologic pelvic organ prolapse surgery	Sprung et al,[29] 2006	Spinal anesthesia (N = 45) / General anesthesia (N = 44)	IT: bupivacaine + clonidine + morphine (≤200 µg) S: midazolam + propofol I: thiopental + fentanyl M: isoflurane + N_2O + morphine	Ketorolac 30 mg once	Favors spinal: Reduced morphine request rate in recovery room (70% vs 11%) Reduced morphine use in first 12 h (median 7.9 vs 14.8 mg) More patients with no pain at postoperative wk 2 (69% vs 48%) No difference: Request for antiemetic medications Hospital length of stay Functional status at 12 wk[b]
Abdominal hysterectomy[a]	Castro-Alves et al,[30] 2011	Spinal anesthesia (N = 34) / General anesthesia (N = 34)	IT: Bupivacaine + fentanyl + morphine (60 µg) S: Midazolam I: propofol + fentanyl M: isoflurane + fentanyl	Scheduled ketoprofen and metamizole Standardized antiemetic regimen (dexamethasone + ondansetron, rescue: metoclopramide)	Favors spinal: Higher quality of recovery scores at 24 h[c] (median difference of 17) Lower pain scores at rest and coughing at 24 h (4 vs 0 and 5 vs 2, respectively) Reduced morphine use in PACU (6 vs 0 mg) Reduced incidence of nausea (32% vs 12%)
Abdominal hysterectomy[a]	Borendal Wodlin et al,[31] 2011	Spinal anesthesia (N = 82) / General anesthesia (N = 80)	IT: bupivacaine + morphine (200 µg) I and M: propofol + fentanyl	Counseling regarding surgical procedure Preoperative paracetamol Postoperative scheduled paracetamol and NSAID (not specified) Early mobilization Early feeding	Favors spinal: More cost-effective ($969 savings per patient) Shorter recovery room length of stay (median 282 vs 234 min) Improved HRQoL scores[d]

Abdominal hysterectomy[e]	Massicotte et al,[32] 2009	Spinal anesthesia (N = 20) General anesthesia (N = 20)	IT: bupivacaine + fentanyl + morphine (150 µg) S: midazolam I: propofol + sufentanil M: desflurane + sufentanil	No premedication Postoperative scheduled indomethacin	Favors spinal: Reduced morphine use in first 48 h (median 19 vs 81 mg) Shorter recovery room length of stay (median 52 vs 73 min) Lower pain scores until the eighteenth hour (~30–50 lower VAS on a 100 VAS scale) Shorter hospital length of stay (median 2.2 vs 3.3 d) No difference: Nausea/vomiting
Abdominal hysterectomy[a]	Vaida et al,[33] 2000	Spinal and general anesthesia (N = 15) General anesthesia (N = 15)	IT: bupivacaine I: midazolam M: isoflurane + N$_2$O I: midazolam M: isoflurane + N$_2$O	None	Favors spinal: Longer time to first request of analgesia (median 48 vs 9 min) Reduced opioid use in recovery room and from 2–24 h (median 32 vs 40.5 mg)

Abbreviations: HRQoL, health-related quality of life; I, induction; IT, intrathecal; M, maintenance; N$_2$O, nitrous oxide; PACU, postanesthesia care unit; S, sedation; VAS, visual analog scale.

[a] Benign indication.

[b] Functional status as measured by the validated Short Form 36 health survey, which includes patient-perceived physical and social functioning, physical and emotional activity limitations, mental health, vitality, and general health assessment.

[c] Quality of recovery (QoR) score QoR-40 assesses physical comfort, physical independence, emotional state, psychological support, and pain. A 10-point difference in score reflects a 15% improvement in QoR.

[d] HRQoL assesses mobility, self-care, ability to undertake usual activities, pain/discomfort, anxiety/depression. A score of 0 indicates death, 1 indicates full health.

[e] Malignant and benign indication.

Data from Refs.[29–33]

Table 4
Summary of RCTs showing the impact of epidural anesthesia on ERAS outcomes

Type of Surgery	Study	Anesthetic Technique (Number of Patients)	Anesthetic Medication Administered	Other ERAS Interventions	ERAS Outcomes
Gynecologic cancer surgery	Ferguson et al,[34] 2009	Preincision epidural anesthesia + general anesthesia (N = 67) General anesthesia (N = 68)	PreE: bupivacaine + morphine for 24 h I and M: not specified I and M: not specified	Scheduled ketorolac for 48 h Early mobilization POD 1 Early feeding POD 1 Thromboembolic prophylaxis	Favors epidural: Lower mean pain scores at rest POD 1 (VAS 3.3 vs 4.3) Lower mean pain scores at rest on POD 2, 3, 4 (VAS 5.5, 5.0, 4.7 vs 6.7, 5.5, 5.7, respectively) Higher patient satisfaction No difference: Combined postoperative complications Nausea/vomiting Hospital length of stay
Major gynecologic surgery[a]	Katz et al,[35] 2003	Preincision epidural anesthesia + general anesthesia (N = 45) Postincision epidural injection + general anesthesia (N = 49) Sham epidural + general anesthesia (N = 47)	PreE: lidocaine + epinephrine + fentanyl 1 dose PostE: saline I: thiopental M: N$_2$O + isoflurane PreE: saline PostE: lidocaine + epinephrine + fentanyl 1 dose I: thiopental M: N$_2$O + isofluran PreE: saline PostE: saline I: thiopental + fentanyl M: N$_2$O + isoflurane	None specified	Favors preincision then postincision epidural over control: Cumulative 24 h morphine use lowest in preincision epidural (preE 57 mg vs postE 59 mg vs control 72 mg) Cumulative 48 h morphine use lowest in preincision epidural (preE 90 mg vs postE 95 mg vs control 113 mg)

Abdominal hysterectomy[b]	Jorgensen et al,[36] 2001	Preincision epidural injection + general anesthesia (N = 20); Postincision epidural injection + general anesthesia (N = 20); General anesthesia (N = 20)	PreE: lidocaine; PostE: bupivacaine for 24 h; I and M: see below; PreE: saline; PostE: bupivacaine for 24 h; I and M: see below; I: propofol + alfentanil + fentanyl; M: propofol + fentanyl	Scheduled paracetamol for 48 h and ketorolac for 72 h; Early feeding; Discharge planning	Favor preincision epidural (no differences between postE or control groups): Reduced pain scores during rest, coughing and movement for 24 h (VAS lower by 30 than other 2 groups); Reduced requests for morphine (60%–70% fewer requests than other 2 groups); Shorter time to first flatus; No difference: Nausea/vomiting; Time to first defecation; Readiness for discharge
Abdominal hysterectomy[b]	Chinachoti et al,[37] 2002	Preincision and postincision epidural + general anesthesia; Preincision epidural + general anesthesia	PreE: ropivacaine; PostE: ropivacaine for 24 h; PreE: ropivacaine; PostE: saline for 24 h	Ketorolac for 24 h	Favors continuing postoperative epidural: Lower pain scores at rest (difference of ~30 VAS, AUCM pain difference −11); Lower pain scores during coughing (difference of ~30 VAS, AUCM pain difference −11); Equivalent: Time to first mobilization

(continued on next page)

Table 4
(continued)

Type of Surgery	Study	Anesthetic Technique (Number of Patients)	Anesthetic Medication Administered	Other ERAS Interventions	ERAS Outcomes
Abdominal hysterectomy[c]	Wattwil et al,[38] 1989	Preincision epidural + general anesthesia (N = 20)	PreE: bupivacaine for 26–30 h I: thiopental M: isoflurane + N₂O	None specified	Favors epidural: Reduced pain scores (VAS mean 1.9 vs 4.4) Shorter time to first flatus (mean 31 vs 58 h) Shorter time to first defecation (mean 70 vs 103 h) Lower postoperative blood glucose at 3, 6, 9 h No difference: Hospital length of stay
		General anesthesia (N = 20)	I: thiopental M: isoflurane + N₂O		

Abbreviations: AUCM, area under the curve measurement; I, induction; M, maintenance; N₂O, nitrous oxide; POD, postoperative day; PostE, epidural injection after incision or procedure; PreE, epidural injection before incision; VAS, visual analog scale.

[a] Abdominal hysterectomy (malignant and benign indication, midline and horizontal incisions), myomectomy, salpingo-oophorectomy, ovarian cystectomy.

[b] Indication not specified.

[c] Malignant and benign indication.

Data from Refs.[34–38]

and postoperative pain management with an opioid-based analgesic regimen alone after general anesthesia. Overall, these studies confirm the superiority of epidural analgesia compared with patient-controlled opioid analgesia for postoperative pain management after major gynecologic surgery.[34–38] Two studies reported improved gastrointestinal function.[36,38] However, none of these studies reported that epidurals could shorten the hospital length of stay despite improved pain control, reduced opioid consumption, and faster return of gastrointestinal function.[34,36,38] This finding highlights the importance of incorporating other ERAS principles to optimize patient outcomes.

Impact of epidural infusion medications on outcomes with epidural analgesia
A Cochrane database review including 22 studies[22] concluded that epidural analgesia promotes faster return of bowel function compared with intravenous (IV) opioids, but there were not enough studies to ascertain whether epidural local anesthetic alone promotes faster return of bowel compared with epidural local anesthetic with opioid. Two RCTs[39,40] reported slower uptake of paracetamol (an indirect measure of gastric motility) in volunteers and patients receiving epidural morphine or fentanyl, with no effect on gastric motility in those receiving local anesthetic alone. In 1 RCT in major gynecologic surgery,[41] the incidence of PONV was lower and the hospital length of stay shorter with epidural bupivacaine + fentanyl compared with epidural bupivacaine + morphine, with no difference in return of bowel function. Four studies in the gynecologic surgery population[36,38,42,43] reported faster return of bowel function in patients receiving epidural local anesthetic alone compared with a combination of local anesthetic with opioids. Although the meta-analysis[22] reported that a combination of local anesthetic and opioid provides better postoperative pain control than local anesthetic alone, both groups had very low postoperative pain scores, and it may be beneficial to avoid epidural opioids (morphine in particular) to promote faster return of bowel function and add them into the epidural solution only if there is inadequate analgesia.

Impact of epidural anesthesia on survival in gynecologic cancer surgery
Retrospective and nonrandomized prospective trials report conflicting evidence of beneficial[44–47] or detrimental effect[48,49] of epidural analgesia with regards to tumor spread and survival in gynecologic oncology surgeries. Most retrospective trials,[50–52] but not all,[53] report possible survival benefit in women receiving epidural analgesia for gynecologic malignancies. Some studies[15,54] suggest that epidurals may inhibit tumor spread and growth because of intrinsic tumor suppression properties of local anesthetics and minimizing opioid-induced and surgically induced immunosuppression. On the other hand, an RCT in women undergoing surgery for ovarian cancer[55] reported that patients receiving combined epidural and general anesthesia showed higher antitumorigenic cytokines and natural killer cell cytotoxicity than women receiving general anesthesia alone.

Other Regional Anesthetic Techniques Combined with General Anesthesia

Transversus abdominis plane block
Transversus abdominis plane (TAP) block can be used for Pfannenstiel or midline incisions. A meta-analysis of 5 studies[56] reported reduction in 24-hour pain scores and opioid consumption (reduced morphine equivalents by 5–19 mg) in patients who received a TAP block compared with no block for major open gynecologic surgery. In a meta-analysis of 10 studies in all-type laparoscopic surgery,[57] 3 of which were gynecologic, TAP blocks were shown to be effective in reducing postoperative pain scores and opioid consumption, particularly when administered preoperatively. The TAP block has shown conflicting data with regard to improvement in quality of

recovery scores or opioid consumption after laparoscopic gynecologic surgery, but in line with the conclusions of the meta-analysis, it may be that the timing of TAP block administration was the difference between benefit (preoperative)[58] and no benefit (postoperative).[59]

One prospective, case-matched study in laparoscopic colorectal surgery incorporated TAP blocks into an established ERAS protocol, enabling further reduction of postoperative pain, opioid consumption, and hospital length of stay (median of 3 d vs 2 d).[60] The benefits of TAP blocks should be further studied in RCTs to assess their value as a part of ERAS protocols in gynecologic surgery.

Local anesthetic wound infusion

A large systematic review of 45 RCTs[61] reported that surgical wound catheter infiltration with local anesthetic provides effective postoperative analgesia, reducing overall pain scores and minimizing opioid consumption compared with an opioid-based analgesic technique. Although there were positive results for the subcategory of gynecology-urology procedures, cesarean sections and prostatectomies comprised 50% of these studies. A summary of studies in gynecologic surgery alone is presented in **Table 5**. For major gynecologic surgery, the benefits of subcutaneous local anesthetic wound infiltration were seen only with larger-volume (9 mL) intermittent boluses[62] but not lower-volume (2 mL) continuous local anesthetic infusions.[63,64] The location of the catheter is important to provide effective analgesia, because even higher-volume local anesthetic infiltration below the muscle layers did not provide effective analgesia as subcutaneous and intraperitoneal infiltration catheters.[62,65,66] Subcutaneous infiltration provided better patient satisfaction and lower pain scores and opioid consumption when compared directly with intraperitoneal infiltration.[65,67]

Local anesthetic wound infiltration

RCTs using incisional and deep would infiltration with local anesthetic before skin closure did not reduce opioid consumption in patients undergoing hysterectomy.[68,69] RCTs studying preincisional local anesthetic infiltration reported a minimal reduction in opioid consumption in hysterectomies[70] and no opioid-sparing effect in laparotomies for gynecologic cancer.[71] Neither preincisional nor postincisional local anesthetic wound infiltration was effective in reducing pain scores or opioid consumption for laparoscopic gynecologic surgery.[72] Only 1 study in highly motivated patients undergoing pelvic organ prolapse surgery[73] reported that this surgery could be performed under local anesthetic infiltration alone, and compared with general anesthesia, this technique was more cost effective, but no benefit was seen in opioid use, PONV, or hospital length of stay. Taken together, these trials show little to no effect of local anesthetic wound infiltration for gynecologic surgeries.

Intraperitoneal local anesthetics

The analgesic effect of intraperitoneal administration of a single dose of local anesthetics intraoperatively in patients undergoing open abdominal hysterectomy has yielded conflicting results.[74,75] However, a meta-analysis has confirmed the analgesic efficacy of continuous infusion of intraperitoneal local anesthetics.[76] Up to 40% opioid-sparing effects were reported with this technique after open abdominal hysterectomy,[77] with better efficacy using a patient-controlled technique compared with a continuous infusion.[78] Opioid-sparing effects of intraperitoneal lidocaine were greater compared with IV lidocaine after abdominal hysterectomy.[79]

OTHER OPIOID-SPARING MULTIMODAL ANALGESIC STRATEGIES FOR MAJOR GYNECOLOGIC SURGERY

γ-Aminobutyric Acid Analogs

In a recent meta-analysis of 6 RCTs,[80] preoperatively administered pregabalin reduced 24-hour morphine consumption (weighted mean difference −8.5 mg [95% confidence interval (CI), −5.71 to −11.29]) and postoperative pain scores compared with controls after major gynecologic surgery. There was a significant reduction in PONV with pregabalin at the expense of increased dizziness.[80] The dose range was 100 to 300 mg once or repeated every 8 to 12 hours.[80] A recent meta-analysis[81] suggested that for acute pain outcomes, there does not seem to be a significant benefit from repeated doses of pregabalin compared with a single dose administered before surgery and that analgesia was comparable with doses ranging from 100 to 300 mg.

In a meta-analysis of 14 RCTs using preoperative gabapentin for abdominal hysterectomy,[82] overall 24-hour morphine consumption was reduced from 24.3 to 55.9 mg to 13.2 to 42.7 mg, with a standardized mean difference of −0.67 (95% CI −1.2 to −0.07). When gabapentin was used preoperatively and postoperatively, the 24-hour morphine consumption was reduced from 25.7 to 80 mg to 20.3 to 55 mg, with a standardized mean difference of −1.45 (95% CI −1.79 to −1.11).[82] Most studies administered gabapentin 1 to 2 hours preoperatively in a single dose of 1200 mg or with smaller doses of 100 to 400 mg administered every 6 to 8 hours.[82] Dose-ranging studies in other patient populations suggest that the minimum effective dose of preoperative gabapentin is 600 mg.[83] PONV was also reduced in the gabapentin group, with no increased incidence of somnolence or dizziness compared with the control group.[82] Similar to pregabalin, combined preoperative and postoperative doses of gabapentin did not confer advantages compared with preoperative-only administration.[82] The potential side effects of these 2 drugs reported in meta-analyses of their perioperative use include sedation and visual disturbances.[81]

Arachidonic Acid Metabolism Inhibitors

Arachidonic acid is converted into prostaglandins via 2 cyclooxygenase (COX-1 and COX-2) pathways.[84] The uterus expresses both COX-1 and COX-2 at different levels throughout the menstrual cycle, making these ideal medications for use in gynecologic surgeries.[84]

In a meta-analysis of nonsteroidal antiinflammatory drugs (NSAIDs) and COX-2 inhibitors in all types of surgery, morphine-sparing effects of those agents were comparable with an approximate average reduction of 10 mg of morphine in 24 hours compared with placebo,[85] but the reduction in opioid-related side effects such as nausea was seen only with NSAIDs. The opioid-sparing effect of these agents ranged from 22% to 50 % in different studies in patients undergoing gynecologic surgery.[86–96] Although increased risk of bleeding is a theoretical concern with perioperative use of NSAIDs, a recent meta-analysis[97] suggested that perioperative ketorolac does not increase risk of bleeding.

Paracetamol (Acetaminophen) and Propacetamol

The IV formulation of paracetamol has been available in Europe since 2001 and was approved in the United States in 2010. Systematic reviews[85,98] show that both paracetamol and propacetamol reduce opioid consumption by 30%, which is equally efficacious to NSAIDs in the postoperative period for all-type surgery. Most studies in the gynecologic surgery population report an opioid-sparing effect of 30% to 40% with a 1-g to 2-g once-daily or twice-daily dosing regimen.[99–101] These agents have been

Table 5
Summary of the effects of wound infiltration catheters using local anesthetics on ERAS principles in major gynecologic surgery

Type of Surgery	Study	Group Allocation (Number of patients)	Wound Infiltration Catheter	Other ERAS Interventions	ERAS Outcomes
Laparotomy for gynecologic cancer[a]	Kushner et al,[64] 2005	LA catheter group (N = 40) Control catheter group (N = 40)	Location: subcutaneous Infusion: continuous bupivacaine 0.5% or saline at 2 mL/h	None specified	No difference: Pain scores Opioid consumption Time to first defecation Hospital length of stay
Abdominal hysterectomy[b]	Leong et al,[63] 2002	LA catheter group (N = 26) Control group: no catheter (N = 26)	Location: subcutaneous Infusion: continuous bupivacaine 0.5% at 2 mL/h	None specified	No difference: Pain scores Opioid consumption
Abdominal hysterectomy[c]	Zohar et al,[62] 2001	LA catheter group (N = 18) Control catheter group (N = 18)	Location: subcutaneous Infusion: PCA Bupivacaine 0.25% or saline ≤9 mL/h	Multimodal analgesia regimen	Favors subcutaneous instillation with LA: Reduced pain scores (VAS ~20 lower) Reduced morphine consumption in recovery room (mean 6 vs 12 mg) Reduced meperidine consumption overall (mean 29 vs 95 mg) Lower incidence of nausea (antiemetic treatment 44% vs 100%) Higher patient satisfaction (78% vs 39% rated analgesia good or excellent) Shorter hospital length of stay (6 vs 7 d)

Abdominal hysterectomy[b]	Kristensen et al,[66] 1999	LA catheter group (N = 22) Control catheter group (N = 19)	Location: bilateral catheters on each side of the incision, below muscle layer, above peritoneum Infusion: bupivacaine 0.25% or saline 15 mL each catheter every 4 h	None specified	No difference: Pain scores Opioid consumption
Abdominal hysterectomy[b]	Gupta et al,[65] 2004	LA catheter group (N = 20) Control catheter group (N = 20)	Location: intraperitoneal supracervical area Infusion: levobupivacaine 0.25% or saline at 5 mL/h	None specified	Favors intraperitoneal instillation with LA: Lower pain scores first 2 h (VAS ~20 lower) Reduced ketobemidone consumption at 4–24 h (mean 19 vs 31 mg) Reduced incidence of nausea (15% vs 50%) No difference: Hospital length of stay Time to mobilization

Abbreviations: LA, local anesthetic; PCA, patient-controlled analgesia.
[a] Malignant and benign indication.
[b] Benign indication.
[c] Indication not specified.
Data from Refs.[62–66]

compared directly with NSAIDs in the gynecologic surgery patient population, with equal efficacy to ketorolac[102] but slightly less efficacy compared with diclofenac.[87,103] A recent systematic review[104] also reported a reduction in PONV with the use of IV paracetamol. Additional opioid-sparing effects and PONV reduction are obtained when combining NSAIDs with paracetamol than either drug alone.[103,105]

Lidocaine Infusion

Meta-analyses and systematic reviews[106,107] reported that IV lidocaine infusions reduced postoperative pain, decreased opioid consumption, led to faster return of bowel function, and shortened hospital length of stay in abdominal surgeries. However, studies of patients undergoing open or laparoscopic hysterectomy have not shown benefits in reducing pain scores, opioid consumption, improving quality of recovery, or shortening hospital stays,[108–110] except for some reduction in inflammatory mediators and pain scores in the early postoperative period in 1 study.[110] The lack of analgesic benefit may be because the lidocaine infusions were used only in the intraoperative period in these trials. Although many studies of other abdominal surgeries continued the lidocaine infusion in the postoperative period, some studies also reported benefit after administration only in the intraoperative period.[106]

Ketamine Infusion

A meta-analysis of 70 studies[111] concluded that ketamine infusions improve postoperative analgesia and reduce opioid consumption, particularly in upper abdominal, thoracic, and major orthopedic procedures. Studies of ketamine use in women undergoing gynecologic surgery have yielded conflicting results. In an RCT in patients undergoing hysterectomy, an intraoperative ketamine infusion reduced morphine consumption by 35%, improved pain scores at 8 to 12 hours after surgery, and improved patient satisfaction with analgesia but did not promote faster return of bowel function or faster ambulation or reduce hospital length of stay.[112] Another RCT in a gynecologic surgery patient population[113] found that a preincision bolus followed by an intraoperative infusion or a bolus of ketamine at wound closure was more effective at reducing pain scores and morphine consumption (by 50%) than 1 preincision dose of ketamine. In patients undergoing myomectomies or hysterectomies for fibroids, no difference in pain scores or opioid consumption was found after a preincision bolus and intraoperative and postoperative infusion of ketamine.[108] The ketamine infusion dosing regimens varied greatly between studies, with initial dosing of 0.3 mg/kg to 0.5 mg/kg and a continuous infusion of 50 µg to 600 µg/kg/h intraoperatively only or up to 24 hours postoperatively.[108,112,113] It is unclear whether ketamine would provide routine benefit to gynecologic surgery patients or its use should be limited to certain patients, such as those with chronic pain conditions who are on long-term opioids.

REDUCING POSTOPERATIVE NAUSEA AND VOMITING AFTER MAJOR GYNECOLOGIC SURGERY

The Apfel simplified risk score for prediction of PONV includes 4 factors: female gender, history of PONV or motion sickness, nonsmoking status, and need for postoperative opioids.[114] Most women in the United States (82%) are nonsmokers, and major gynecologic surgery requires postoperative opioids, so this patient population typically has starting PONV risk of 60% according to the Apfel score.[115] Furthermore, although it has been debated whether the type of surgery is a risk factor for PONV, a meta-analysis of risk factors[116] reported that gynecologic surgery is an independent risk factor for PONV.

The Society for Ambulatory Anesthesia consensus guidelines for PONV recommend combination antiemetic therapy in this high-risk patient population and adoption of strategies to reduce the baseline risk of PONV.[117]

STRATEGIES TO REDUCE THE BASELINE RISK OF POSTOPERATIVE NAUSEA AND VOMITING

Avoid General Anesthesia by Using Regional Anesthesia

The use of regional anesthesia has been associated with up to 9-fold reduction in the incidence of PONV.[118] However, the influence of neuraxial analgesia on PONV is variable, depending on the technique used and the type of epidural medications administered. Compared with general anesthesia with an opioid-based analgesic technique, spinal anesthesia reduces PONV only if no or low-dose (60 μg) intrathecal morphine is used.[33,119]

Most studies using epidural analgesia for major gynecologic surgery combine this technique with general anesthesia, and this might not reduce PONV. Callesen and colleagues[119] compared PONV rates between an opioid-free combined spinal-epidural (CSE) technique (local anesthetic alone) and a general anesthetic group with epidural analgesia (local anesthetic and opioid) in patients undergoing hysterectomy. The cumulative 72-hour incidence of PONV was 50% in the CSE group and 100% in the combined general anesthetic with epidural group.[119] However, the need for supplementary opioids was higher in the CSE group.

Avoid Inhaled Agents and Nitrous Oxide if General Anesthesia Is Used

Inhaled agents increase the risk of PONV, particularly in the early postoperative period.[120] Nitrous oxide is associated with increased risk of PONV, particularly in women.[121] Total IV anesthesia with propofol is associated with a reduction in the risk of PONV, particularly in the first 6 hours after surgery, with a number needed to treat of 5.[122]

Minimize Intraoperative and Postoperative Opioids

Opioid-sparing techniques are an integral part of ERAS protocols, because they not only reduce PONV but also affect other opioid-related side effects that can affect patients' recovery and delay discharge, such as sedation and postoperative ileus. Despite the opioid-sparing effects of these interventions, their effects on reducing PONV are not consistent. A reduction in the risk of PONV was reported with intraperitoneal local anesthetic instillation catheters[77,79] but not with TAP blocks or subcutaneous infiltration catheters.[56,62,65] The γ-aminobutyric acid analogs show consistent reduction in PONV.[80,82] A meta-analysis including all types of surgery[123] reported a reduction in PONV with NSAIDs but not with COX-2 inhibitors. In a systematic review of 30 RCTs, IV paracetamol provided better analgesia and reduced PONV, despite no reduction in opioid consumption.[98,104]

Adequate Hydration

Intraoperative fluid management and its effects on ERAS principles, including PONV, seem to be highly dependent on the surgery, more specifically the length and extent of surgical damage. A systematic review of 80 studies[124] concluded that in minor and moderate ambulatory surgeries, including laparoscopic gynecologic surgeries, PONV could be reduced in patients receiving more liberal regimens (1–2 L of fluid). In 1 RCT in women with 2 to 4 risk factors for PONV having laparoscopic gynecologic surgery,[125] the liberal fluid group (3 mL/kg/h of fasting) had lower rates of PONV (59% vs 87%) than the restrictive group (2 mL/kg/h of fasting). Lower PONV rates were also

Table 6
Summary of goal-directed fluid therapy on ERAS outcomes for major gynecologic surgery

Reference, Surgery Type	Study Type	Description of Fluid Management (Number of Patients)	Other ERAS Interventions	Summary of ERAS Outcomes
McKenny et al,[131] 2013 Laparotomy gynecologic cancer surgery	RCT	**Intervention (N = 51)** SV measurement via esophageal Doppler US Algorithm: HES administered 3 mL/kg X1 SV >10% response, give another 3 mL/kg, until SV responds <10%, SV <10% response, repeat SV measurement 15 min. **Control (N = 50)** Fluid management at the anesthesiologist's discretion for: Urine output <0.5 mL/kg/h Unspecified increase in heart rate Unspecified decrease in SBP Unspecified decrease in CVP Replacement of estimated intraoperative losses	No ERAS protocol in the gynecologic surgery population at this institution	No reduction in hospital length of stay No difference in postoperative morbidity score No difference in gastrointestinal recovery
Chattopadhyay et al,[132] 2013 Laparotomy gynecologic cancer surgery	Prospective observational study	**Intervention** Advanced stage (N = 44) Early stage (N = 35) SV measurement via esophageal Doppler US No algorithm specified **Control** Advanced stage (N = 62) Early stage (N = 57) Hemodynamic-based fluid management Not specified	No ERAS protocol specified	Favors goal-directed therapy in advanced-stage disease only: Goal-directed fluid therapy associated with earlier postoperative recovery[a] (OR 2.8) Less PONV in goal-directed therapy (9% vs 24%)

| Gan et al,[133] 2002 Mixed major abdominal surgery[b] | RCT | Control (N = 50) Bolus 5 mL/kg LR followed by 5 mL/kg/h infusion during surgery | Intervention (N = 50) Bolus 5 mL/kg LR followed by 5 mL/kg/h infusion during surgery Algorithm: 200 mL HES if FTc[c] <0.35 s If SV > or = by the fluid challenge and FTc <0.35 s: fluid challenge was repeated If SV >10% and FTc >0.35 s, fluid challenge repeated until no further increase in SV occurred If FTc >0.40 s and = SV, further fluid was not given until SV decreased by 10% of the last value | No ERAS protocol specified | Favors goal-directed therapy: Shorter length of hospital stay in goal-directed therapy (median 5 vs 7 d) Faster oral intake (3 vs 4.7 d) Less PONV requiring antiemetic therapy (14% vs 36%) |

Abbreviations: CVP, central venous pressure; FTc, corrected flow time; HES, hydroxyethyl starch; LR, lactated Ringer; OR, odds ratio; SBP, systolic blood pressure; SV, stroke volume; US, ultrasonography.

[a] Early postoperative recovery defined as ≥2 of the following: mobilization on the first postoperative day, oral diet resumption on postoperative day 1; and return of bowel function on postoperative day 4 or earlier.

[b] Major elective general, urologic, or gynecologic surgery with anticipated blood loss >500 mL.

[c] FTc: aortic systolic flow time corrected for heart rate: index of systemic vascular resistance that is sensitive to changes in left ventricular preload.

Data from Refs.[131–133]

reported[126] in patients undergoing either laparoscopic gynecologic procedure or a cholecystectomy in a liberal fluid management group 15 mL/kg bolus (23%) versus the conservative fluid management group 2 mg/kg bolus (73%). A meta-analysis including 15 studies, 11 of which included patients undergoing gynecologic surgery, reported that compared with conservative fluid regimens, administration of supplemental IV crystalloids reduced the risk of early postoperative nausea (relative risk 0.73, 95% CI 0.59–0.89), postoperative nausea at 24-hour (relative risk 0.41, 95% CI 0.22–0.76), and overall 24-hour postoperative nausea (relative risk 0.66, 95% CI 0.46–0.95). Liberal IV crystalloids also reduced overall 24-hour PONV (relative risk 0.48, 95% CI 0.29–0.79), late PONV (relative risk 0.27, 95% CI 0.13–0.54), and overall 24-hour PONV (relative risk 0.59, 95% CI 0.42–0.84), as well as the need for antiemetic rescue treatment (relative risk 0.56, 95% CI 0.45–0.68).[127]

ANTIEMETIC PROPHYLAXIS

Because the gynecologic patient population is at high risk for PONV, combination antiemetic therapy should be used for prophylaxis. Studies have consistently reported the superior antiemetic efficacy of combination therapy compared with single-agent antiemetic prophylaxis. The multimodal approach incorporates combination antiemetic therapy in addition to measures to reduce the baseline risk of PONV, as discussed earlier, and should be used in high-risk patients.[117] The most commonly investigated therapies include a combination of 5-HT$_3$ antagonists with either dexamethasone or droperidol, with both combinations having comparable antiemetic efficacy.[128,129] Longer-acting antiemetics might provide additional protection against delayed PONV and postdischarge nausea and vomiting. Those agents include palonosetron, transdermal scopolamine, and the neurokinin-1 receptor antagonist aprepitant, with the last one being significantly more effective than ondansetron in prophylaxis against vomiting in women undergoing major gynecologic surgery.[130]

FLUID MANAGEMENT FOR MAJOR GYNECOLOGIC SURGERY

In contrast to ambulatory surgeries, in which PONV may be the primary outcome of concern, for major nonvascular abdominal surgeries, goal-directed fluid management improves major outcomes, such as cardiopulmonary function, gastric motility, and wound healing, and reduces hospital length of stay.[124] However, studies investigating goal-directed therapy in gynecologic surgery are limited. **Table 6**[131–133] summarizes the studies in gynecologic surgery examining the impact of intraoperative fluid administration regimen on patients' outcomes. A meta-analysis of 32 trials by Cecconi and colleagues[134] reported that patients with the highest risk of surgical mortality benefited the most from goal-directed therapy, which seems to be supported by 1 prospective observational trial in patients undergoing laparotomies for gynecologic cancer.[132] RCTs are clearly lacking in the gynecologic surgery population with regards to whether goal-directed fluid therapy confers benefits in these patients.

OTHER ENHANCED RECOVERY AFTER SURGERY PRINCIPLES FOR MAJOR GYNECOLOGIC SURGERY

Other elements of ERAS for major gynecologic surgeries include the approach to preoperative preparation, bowel management, surgical approach, thromboprophylaxis, and postoperative planning. A summary of the literature regarding those elements in the gynecologic patient population is presented in **Table 7**.

Table 7
Summary of outcomes in major gynecologic surgery when comparing a traditional approach with ERAS interventions

Traditional Approach	ERAS Intervention	Study Outcomes
Lack of focus on preoperative nutrition	Improve nutritional status	No known effective strategies identified in patients with ovarian cancer [136]

Bowel preparations	No bowel preparations	Bowel preparations[137–139]
		Do not:
		  Prevent infection
		  Improve surgical visualization
		Do:
		  Reduce patient satisfaction

Routine NG tubes	No routine NG tubes	NG tubes[140]
		Do not:
		  Reduce postoperative ileus
		  Reduce aspiration
		Do:
		  Increase aspiration risk
		  Increase patient discomfort

Delayed feeding	Early feeding	Early feeding[141,142]
		Does:
		  Promote early return of bowel function
		  Shorten HLOS
		  Increase nausea

±Antibiotic prophylaxis	Appropriate antibiotic prophylaxis	Antibiotic prophylaxis[143,144]
		  Indicated: all open procedures
		  Unclear indication: some laparoscopic procedures
		  Not indicated: minor or intrauterine procedures

Open procedures	Minimally invasive procedures when feasible	Hysterectomies[1]
		VH vs AH: VH has less blood loss, fastest recovery, shortest HLOS, lowest infection rate
		VH vs LH: VH has less blood loss, lower infection rate
		Laparoscopic vs open for all gynecologic surgeries[1,145]
		Advantage:
		  Less pain
		  Less blood loss
		  Shorter HLOS
		Disadvantage:
		  Increased urinary tract injuries
		Robotic[146]:
		  No RCTs comparing robotic procedures with laparoscopic or open procedures

(continued on next page)

Traditional Approach	ERAS Intervention	Study Outcomes
Table 7 *(continued)*		
No routine thromboprophylaxis	Routine thromboprophylaxis	Patients with ovarian cancer[147]: Heparin SQ 3 times daily to prevent thromboembolism No increase in bleeding complications Laparoscopic procedures[148]: Unclear if needed in minor laparoscopic procedures More extensive surgeries increase the risk of thromboembolism, so prophylaxis warranted Hysterectomy[149]: Pharmaceutical prophylaxis highly effective Possible increased risk of postoperative bleeding
Drains, tubes, catheters placed	No drains, tubes, catheters	Early removal of urinary catheters reduces HLOS[142]
Discharge patient when they are ready	Preplanning discharge	Scant literature on this topic in gynecology literature[142]

Abbreviations: AH, abdominal hysterectomy; HLOS, hospital length of stay; LH, laparoscopic hysterectomy; NG, nasogastric; SQ, subcutaneous; VH, vaginal hysterectomy.

SUMMARY

- Studies on ERAS after gynecologic surgery are limited and mainly extrapolate several ERAS principles from colorectal surgery and apply them to gynecologic surgery to a variable extent. Similar outcome benefits, namely a reduction in hospital length of stay, have been reported in those studies.
- Despite recommendations for use of regional anesthesia for colorectal procedures, an ideal, standardized anesthetic technique has not been identified, and thus, it is important to evaluate the best evidence for regional techniques in gynecologic surgery when developing ERAS guidelines in this surgical population.
- Effective regional anesthetic techniques in gynecologic surgery include spinal anesthesia, epidural analgesia, TAP blocks, local anesthetic instillation catheters, and intraperitoneal local anesthetic instillation.
- Effective nonopioid analgesics include pregabalin, gabapentin, NSAIDs, COX-2 inhibitors, and paracetamol.
- Ketamine infusions may provide benefit for some patients after major gynecologic surgery but should not be used routinely. Lidocaine infusions, although effective in other abdominal surgeries, provide no benefit for gynecologic surgery.
- A multimodal antiemetic strategy must be used, including strategies to reduce the baseline risk of PONV in conjunction with combination antiemetic therapy.
- RCTs exploring fluid management strategies on ERAS outcomes in the major gynecologic surgery population are lacking.
- Anesthesiologists should be aware of all ERAS principles from colorectal surgery that are also beneficial in major gynecologic surgery, such as bowel management, goal-directed fluid management strategies, timely administration of appropriate antibiotics, and thromboprophylaxis, because many of these may become quality measures for anesthesiologists in the future.

REFERENCES

1. Nieboer TE, Johnson N, Lethaby A, et al. Surgical approach to hysterectomy for benign gynaecological disease. Cochrane Database Syst Rev 2009;(3):CD003677.
2. Fleming ND, Havrilesky LJ, Valea FA, et al. Analgesic and antiemetic needs following minimally invasive vs open staging for endometrial cancer. Am J Obstet Gynecol 2011;204:65.e1–6.
3. Zhuang CL, Ye XZ, Zhang XD, et al. Enhanced recovery after surgery programs versus traditional care for colorectal surgery: a meta-analysis of randomized controlled trials. Dis Colon Rectum 2013;56:667–78.
4. Spanjersberg WR, Reurings J, Keus F, et al. Fast track surgery versus conventional recovery strategies for colorectal surgery. Cochrane Database Syst Rev 2011;(2):CD007635.
5. Kehlet H, Wilmore DW. Multimodal strategies to improve surgical outcome. Am J Surg 2002;183:630–41.
6. Campesi I, Fois M, Franconi F. Sex and gender aspects in anesthetics and pain medication. Handb Exp Pharmacol 2012;(214):265–78.
7. Ottesen M, Sorensen M, Rasmussen Y, et al. Fast track vaginal surgery. Acta Obstet Gynecol Scand 2002;81:138–46.
8. Kroon UB, Radstrom M, Hjelthe C, et al. Fast-track hysterectomy: a randomised, controlled study. Eur J Obstet Gynecol Reprod Biol 2010;151:203–7.
9. Kalogera E, Bakkum-Gamez JN, Jankowski CJ, et al. Enhanced recovery in gynecologic surgery. Obstet Gynecol 2013;122:319–28.
10. Dickson E, Argenta PA, Reichert JA. Results of introducing a rapid recovery program for total abdominal hysterectomy. Gynecol Obstet Invest 2012;73:21–5.
11. Marx C, Rasmussen T, Jakobsen DH, et al. The effect of accelerated rehabilitation on recovery after surgery for ovarian malignancy. Acta Obstet Gynecol Scand 2006;85:488–92.
12. Sjetne IS, Krogstad U, Odegard S, et al. Improving quality by introducing enhanced recovery after surgery in a gynaecological department: consequences for ward nursing practice. Qual Saf Health Care 2009;18:236–40.
13. Yoong W, Sivashanmugarajan V, Relph S, et al. Can enhanced recovery pathways improve outcomes of vaginal hysterectomy? Cohort control study. J Minim Invasive Gynecol 2014;21:83–9.
14. Wijk L, Franzen K, Ljungqvist O, et al. Implementing a structured enhanced recovery after surgery (ERAS) protocol reduces length of stay after abdominal hysterectomy. Acta Obstet Gynecol Scand 2014;93:749–56.
15. Snyder GL, Greenberg S. Effect of anaesthetic technique and other perioperative factors on cancer recurrence. Br J Anaesth 2010;105:106–15.
16. Fletcher D, Martinez V. Opioid-induced hyperalgesia in patients after surgery: a systematic review and a meta-analysis. Br J Anaesth 2014;112:991–1004.
17. Kumar L, Barker C, Emmanuel A. Opioid-induced constipation: pathophysiology, clinical consequences, and management. Gastroenterol Res Pract 2014;2014: 141737.
18. Carli F, Kehlet H, Baldini G, et al. Evidence basis for regional anesthesia in multidisciplinary fast-track surgical care pathways. Reg Anesth Pain Med 2011;36: 63–72.
19. Beattie WS, Badner NH, Choi PT. Meta-analysis demonstrates statistically significant reduction in postoperative myocardial infarction with the use of thoracic epidural analgesia. Anesth Analg 2003;97:919–20.

20. Hahnenkamp K, Herroeder S, Hollmann MW. Regional anaesthesia, local anaesthetics and the surgical stress response. Best Pract Res Clin Anaesthesiol 2004; 18:509–27.

21. Hart SR, Bordes B, Hart J, et al. Unintended perioperative hypothermia. Ochsner J 2011;11:259–70.

22. Jorgensen H, Wetterslev J, Moiniche S, et al. Epidural local anaesthetics versus opioid-based analgesic regimens on postoperative gastrointestinal paralysis, PONV and pain after abdominal surgery. Cochrane Database Syst Rev 2000;(4):CD001893.

23. Kabon B, Fleischmann E, Treschan T, et al. Thoracic epidural anesthesia increases tissue oxygenation during major abdominal surgery. Anesth Analg 2003;97:1812–7.

24. Popping DM, Elia N, Marret E, et al. Protective effects of epidural analgesia on pulmonary complications after abdominal and thoracic surgery: a meta-analysis. Arch Surg 2008;143:990–9 [discussion: 1000].

25. Guay J. The benefits of adding epidural analgesia to general anesthesia: a metaanalysis. J Anesth 2006;20:335–40.

26. Block BM, Liu SS, Rowlingson AJ, et al. Efficacy of postoperative epidural analgesia: a meta-analysis. JAMA 2003;290:2455–63.

27. Andreae MH, Andreae DA. Local anaesthetics and regional anaesthesia for preventing chronic pain after surgery. Cochrane Database Syst Rev 2012;(10):CD007105.

28. Rodgers A, Walker N, Schug S, et al. Reduction of postoperative mortality and morbidity with epidural or spinal anaesthesia: results from overview of randomised trials. BMJ 2000;321:1493.

29. Sprung J, Sanders MS, Warner ME, et al. Pain relief and functional status after vaginal hysterectomy: intrathecal versus general anesthesia. Can J Anaesth 2006;53:690–700.

30. Catro-Alves LJ, De Azevedo VL, De Freitas Braga TF, et al. The effect of neuraxial versus general anesthesia techniques on postoperative quality of recovery and analgesia after abdominal hysterectomy: a prospective, randomized, controlled trial. Anesth Analg 2011;113:1480–6.

31. Borendal Wodlin N, Nilsson L, Carlsson P, et al. Cost-effectiveness of general anesthesia vs spinal anesthesia in fast-track abdominal benign hysterectomy. Am J Obstet Gynecol 2011;205(326):e1–7.

32. Massicotte L, Chalaoui KD, Beaulieu D, et al. Comparison of spinal anesthesia with general anesthesia on morphine requirement after abdominal hysterectomy. Acta Anaesthesiol Scand 2009;53:641–7.

33. Vaida SJ, Ben David B, Somri M, et al. The influence of preemptive spinal anesthesia on postoperative pain. J Clin Anesth 2000;12:374–7.

34. Ferguson SE, Malhotra T, Seshan VE, et al. A prospective randomized trial comparing patient-controlled epidural analgesia to patient-controlled intravenous analgesia on postoperative pain control and recovery after major open gynecologic cancer surgery. Gynecol Oncol 2009;114:111–6.

35. Katz J, Cohen L, Schmid R, et al. Postoperative morphine use and hyperalgesia are reduced by preoperative but not intraoperative epidural analgesia: implications for preemptive analgesia and the prevention of central sensitization. Anesthesiology 2003;98:1449–60.

36. Jorgensen H, Fomsgaard JS, Dirks J, et al. Effect of peri- and postoperative epidural anaesthesia on pain and gastrointestinal function after abdominal hysterectomy. Br J Anaesth 2001;87:577–83.

37. Chinachoti T, Niruthisard S, Tuntisirin O, et al. A double-blind, randomized study comparing postoperative pain management using epidural ropivacaine with intravenous ketorolac or intravenous ketorolac alone following transabdominal hysterectomy. J Med Assoc Thai 2002;85(Suppl 3):S837–47.
38. Wattwil M, Thoren T, Hennerdal S, et al. Epidural analgesia with bupivacaine reduces postoperative paralytic ileus after hysterectomy. Anesth Analg 1989; 68:353–8.
39. Thorn SE, Wattwil M, Kallander A. Effects of epidural morphine and epidural bupivacaine on gastroduodenal motility during the fasted state and after food intake. Acta Anaesthesiol Scand 1994;38:57–62.
40. Geddes SM, Thorburn J, Logan RW. Gastric emptying following caesarean section and the effect of epidural fentanyl. Anaesthesia 1991;46:1016–8.
41. Vallejo MC, Edwards RP, Shannon KT, et al. Improved bowel function after gynecological surgery with epidural bupivacaine-fentanyl than bupivacaine-morphine infusion. Can J Anaesth 2000;47:406–11.
42. Asantila R, Eklund P, Rosenberg PH. Continuous epidural infusion of bupivacaine and morphine for postoperative analgesia after hysterectomy. Acta Anaesthesiol Scand 1991;35:513–7.
43. Thoren T, Sundberg A, Wattwil M, et al. Effects of epidural bupivacaine and epidural morphine on bowel function and pain after hysterectomy. Acta Anaesthesiol Scand 1989;33:181–5.
44. Blythe JG, Hodel KA, Wahl TM, et al. Continuous postoperative epidural analgesia for gynecologic oncology patients. Gynecol Oncol 1990;37:307–10.
45. Rapp SE, Ready LB, Greer BE. Postoperative pain management in gynecology oncology patients utilizing epidural opiate analgesia and patient-controlled analgesia. Gynecol Oncol 1989;35:341–4.
46. de Leon-Casasola OA, Parker BM, Lema MJ, et al. Epidural analgesia versus intravenous patient-controlled analgesia. Differences in the postoperative course of cancer patients. Reg Anesth 1994;19:307–15.
47. Rivard C, Dickson EL, Vogel RI, et al. The effect of anesthesia choice on postoperative outcomes in women undergoing exploratory laparotomy for a suspected gynecologic malignancy. Gynecol Oncol 2014;133:278–82.
48. Chen LM, Weinberg VK, Chen C, et al. Perioperative outcomes comparing patient controlled epidural versus intravenous analgesia in gynecologic oncology surgery. Gynecol Oncol 2009;115:357–61.
49. Belavy D, Janda M, Baker J, et al. Epidural analgesia is associated with an increased incidence of postoperative complications in patients requiring an abdominal hysterectomy for early stage endometrial cancer. Gynecol Oncol 2013;131:423–9.
50. Lin L, Liu C, Tan H, et al. Anaesthetic technique may affect prognosis for ovarian serous adenocarcinoma: a retrospective analysis. Br J Anaesth 2011;106:814–22.
51. Capmas P, Billard V, Gouy S, et al. Impact of epidural analgesia on survival in patients undergoing complete cytoreductive surgery for ovarian cancer. Anticancer Res 2012;32:1537–42.
52. de Oliveira GS Jr, Ahmad S, Schink JC, et al. Intraoperative neuraxial anesthesia but not postoperative neuraxial analgesia is associated with increased relapse-free survival in ovarian cancer patients after primary cytoreductive surgery. Reg Anesth Pain Med 2011;36:271–7.
53. Lacassie HJ, Cartagena J, Branes J, et al. The relationship between neuraxial anesthesia and advanced ovarian cancer-related outcomes in the Chilean population. Anesth Analg 2013;117:653–60.

54. Tonnesen E, Wahlgreen C. Influence of extradural and general anaesthesia on natural killer cell activity and lymphocyte subpopulations in patients undergoing hysterectomy. Br J Anaesth 1988;60:500–7.
55. Hong JY, Lim KT. Effect of preemptive epidural analgesia on cytokine response and postoperative pain in laparoscopic radical hysterectomy for cervical cancer. Reg Anesth Pain Med 2008;33:44–51.
56. Champaneria R, Shah L, Geoghegan J, et al. Analgesic effectiveness of transversus abdominis plane blocks after hysterectomy: a meta-analysis. Eur J Obstet Gynecol Reprod Biol 2013;166:1–9.
57. De Oliveira GS Jr, Castro-Alves LJ, Nader A, et al. Transversus abdominis plane block to ameliorate postoperative pain outcomes after laparoscopic surgery: a meta-analysis of randomized controlled trials. Anesth Analg 2014;118:454–63.
58. De Oliveira GS Jr, Fitzgerald PC, Marcus RJ, et al. A dose-ranging study of the effect of transversus abdominis block on postoperative quality of recovery and analgesia after outpatient laparoscopy. Anesth Analg 2011;113:1218–25.
59. Kane SM, Garcia-Tomas V, Alejandro-Rodriguez M, et al. Randomized trial of transversus abdominis plane block at total laparoscopic hysterectomy: effect of regional analgesia on quality of recovery. Am J Obstet Gynecol 2012;207: 419.e1–5.
60. Favuzza J, Brady K, Delaney CP. Transversus abdominis plane blocks and enhanced recovery pathways: making the 23-h hospital stay a realistic goal after laparoscopic colorectal surgery. Surg Endosc 2013;27:2481–6.
61. Liu SS, Richman JM, Thirlby RC, et al. Efficacy of continuous wound catheters delivering local anesthetic for postoperative analgesia: a quantitative and qualitative systematic review of randomized controlled trials. J Am Coll Surg 2006; 203:914–32.
62. Zohar E, Fredman B, Phillipov A, et al. The analgesic efficacy of patient-controlled bupivacaine wound instillation after total abdominal hysterectomy with bilateral salpingo-oophorectomy. Anesth Analg 2001;93:482–7, 4th contents page.
63. Leong WM, Lo WK, Chiu JW. Analgesic efficacy of continuous delivery of bupivacaine by an elastomeric balloon infusor after abdominal hysterectomy: a prospective randomised controlled trial. Aust N Z J Obstet Gynaecol 2002;42: 515–8.
64. Kushner DM, LaGalbo R, Connor JP, et al. Use of a bupivacaine continuous wound infusion system in gynecologic oncology: a randomized trial. Obstet Gynecol 2005;106:227–33.
65. Gupta A, Perniola A, Axelsson K, et al. Postoperative pain after abdominal hysterectomy: a double-blind comparison between placebo and local anesthetic infused intraperitoneally. Anesth Analg 2004;99:1173–9 Table of contents.
66. Kristensen BB, Christensen DS, Ostergaard M, et al. Lack of postoperative pain relief after hysterectomy using preperitoneally administered bupivacaine. Reg Anesth Pain Med 1999;24:576–80.
67. Hafizoglu MC, Katircioglu K, Ozkalkanli MY, et al. Bupivacaine infusion above or below the fascia for postoperative pain treatment after abdominal hysterectomy. Anesth Analg 2008;107:2068–72.
68. Cobby TF, Reid MF. Wound infiltration with local anaesthetic after abdominal hysterectomy. Br J Anaesth 1997;78:431–2.
69. Klein JR, Heaton JP, Thompson JP, et al. Infiltration of the abdominal wall with local anaesthetic after total abdominal hysterectomy has no opioid-sparing effect. Br J Anaesth 2000;84:248–9.

70. Hannibal K, Galatius H, Hansen A, et al. Preoperative wound infiltration with bu-
    pivacaine reduces early and late opioid requirement after hysterectomy. Anesth
    Analg 1996;83:376–81.
71. Updike GM, Manolitsas TP, Cohn DE, et al. Pre-emptive analgesia in gyneco-
    logic surgical procedures: preoperative wound infiltration with ropivacaine in
    patients who undergo laparotomy through a midline vertical incision. Am J
    Obstet Gynecol 2003;188:901–5.
72. Fong SY, Pavy TJ, Yeo ST, et al. Assessment of wound infiltration with bupiva-
    caine in women undergoing day-case gynecological laparoscopy. Reg Anesth
    Pain Med 2001;26:131–6.
73. Segal JL, Owens G, Silva WA, et al. A randomized trial of local anesthesia with
    intravenous sedation vs general anesthesia for the vaginal correction of pelvic
    organ prolapse. Int Urogynecol J Pelvic Floor Dysfunct 2007;18:807–12.
74. Ng A, Swami A, Smith G, et al. The analgesic effects of intraperitoneal and inci-
    sional bupivacaine with epinephrine after total abdominal hysterectomy. Anesth
    Analg 2002;95:158–62 Table of contents.
75. Ali PB, Cotton BR, Williamson KM, et al. Intraperitoneal bupivacaine or lidocaine
    does not provide analgesia after total abdominal hysterectomy. Br J Anaesth
    1998;80:245–7.
76. Kahokehr A, Sammour T, Soop M, et al. Intraperitoneal local anaesthetic in
    abdominal surgery–a systematic review. ANZ J Surg 2011;81:237–45.
77. Gupta N, Dadhwal V, Mittal S. Combined intraperitoneal instillation and port site
    infiltration of local anaesthetic (bupivacaine) for postoperative analgesia in
    women undergoing daycare diagnostic gynaecological laparoscopy. Eur J
    Obstet Gynecol Reprod Biol 2012;161:109–10.
78. Perniola A, Fant F, Magnuson A, et al. Postoperative pain after abdominal hys-
    terectomy: a randomized, double-blind, controlled trial comparing continuous
    infusion vs patient-controlled intraperitoneal injection of local anaesthetic. Br J
    Anaesth 2014;112:328–36.
79. Perniola A, Magnuson A, Axelsson K, et al. Intraperitoneal local anesthetics
    have predominant local analgesic effect: a randomized, double-blind study.
    Anesthesiology 2014;121:352–61.
80. Yao Z, Shen C, Zhong Y. Perioperative pregabalin for acute pain after gyneco-
    logical surgery: a meta-analysis. Clin Ther 2014. [Epub ahead of print].
81. Mishriky BM, Waldron NH, Habib AS. Impact of pregabalin on acute and persis-
    tent postoperative pain: a systematic review and meta-analysis. Br J Anaesth
    2015;114:10–31.
82. Alayed N, Alghanaim N, Tan X, et al. Preemptive use of gabapentin in abdominal
    hysterectomy: a systematic review and meta-analysis. Obstet Gynecol 2014;
    123:1221–9.
83. Pandey CK, Navkar DV, Giri PJ, et al. Evaluation of the optimal preemptive dose of
    gabapentin for postoperative pain relief after lumbar diskectomy: a randomized,
    double-blind, placebo-controlled study. J Neurosurg Anesthesiol 2005;17:65–8.
84. Hayes EC, Rock JA. COX-2 inhibitors and their role in gynecology. Obstet
    Gynecol Surv 2002;57:768–80.
85. Maund E, McDaid C, Rice S, et al. Paracetamol and selective and non-selective
    non-steroidal anti-inflammatory drugs for the reduction in morphine-related side-
    effects after major surgery: a systematic review. Br J Anaesth 2011;106:292–7.
86. Ng A, Parker J, Toogood L, et al. Does the opioid-sparing effect of rectal diclo-
    fenac following total abdominal hysterectomy benefit the patient? Br J Anaesth
    2002;88:714–6.

87. Cobby TF, Crighton IM, Kyriakides K, et al. Rectal paracetamol has a significant morphine-sparing effect after hysterectomy. Br J Anaesth 1999;83:253–6.

88. Scott RM, Jennings PN. Rectal diclofenac analgesia after abdominal hysterectomy. Aust N Z J Obstet Gynaecol 1997;37:112–4.

89. Blackburn A, Stevens JD, Wheatley RG, et al. Balanced analgesia with intravenous ketorolac and patient-controlled morphine following lower abdominal surgery. J Clin Anesth 1995;7:103–8.

90. Balestrieri P, Simmons G, Hill D, et al. The effect of intravenous ketorolac given intraoperatively versus postoperatively on outcome from gynecologic abdominal surgery. J Clin Anesth 1997;9:358–64.

91. Rogers JE, Fleming BG, Macintosh KC, et al. Effect of timing of ketorolac administration on patient-controlled opioid use. Br J Anaesth 1995;75:15–8.

92. Ng A, Smith G, Davidson AC. Analgesic effects of parecoxib following total abdominal hysterectomy. Br J Anaesth 2003;90:746–9.

93. Nong L, Sun Y, Tian Y, et al. Effects of parecoxib on morphine analgesia after gynecology tumor operation: a randomized trial of parecoxib used in postsurgical pain management. J Surg Res 2013;183:821–6.

94. Barton SF, Langeland FF, Snabes MC, et al. Efficacy and safety of intravenous parecoxib sodium in relieving acute postoperative pain following gynecologic laparotomy surgery. Anesthesiology 2002;97:306–14.

95. Viscusi ER, Frenkl TL, Hartrick CT, et al. Perioperative use of etoricoxib reduces pain and opioid side-effects after total abdominal hysterectomy: a double-blind, randomized, placebo-controlled phase III study. Curr Med Res Opin 2012;28: 1323–35.

96. Chau-in W, Thienthong S, Pulnitiporn A, et al. Prevention of post operative pain after abdominal hysterectomy by single dose etoricoxib. J Med Assoc Thai 2008;91:68–73.

97. Gobble RM, Hoang HL, Kachniarz B, et al. Ketorolac does not increase perioperative bleeding: a meta-analysis of randomized controlled trials. Plast Reconstr Surg 2014;133:741–55.

98. McNicol ED, Tzortzopoulou A, Cepeda MS, et al. Single-dose intravenous paracetamol or propacetamol for prevention or treatment of postoperative pain: a systematic review and meta-analysis. Br J Anaesth 2011;106:764–75.

99. Arici S, Gurbet A, Turker G, et al. Preemptive analgesic effects of intravenous paracetamol in total abdominal hysterectomy. Agri 2009;21:54–61.

100. Olonisakin RP, Amanor-Boadu SD, Akinyemi AO. Morphine-sparing effect of intravenous paracetamol for post operative pain management following gynaecological surgery. Afr J Med Med Sci 2012;41:429–36.

101. Moon YE, Lee YK, Lee J, et al. The effects of preoperative intravenous acetaminophen in patients undergoing abdominal hysterectomy. Arch Gynecol Obstet 2011;284:1455–60.

102. Varrassi G, Marinangeli F, Agro F, et al. A double-blinded evaluation of propacetamol versus ketorolac in combination with patient-controlled analgesia morphine: analgesic efficacy and tolerability after gynecologic surgery. Anesth Analg 1999;88:611–6.

103. Montgomery JE, Sutherland CJ, Kestin IG, et al. Morphine consumption in patients receiving rectal paracetamol and diclofenac alone and in combination. Br J Anaesth 1996;77:445–7.

104. Apfel CC, Turan A, Souza K, et al. Intravenous acetaminophen reduces postoperative nausea and vomiting: a systematic review and meta-analysis. Pain 2013; 154:677–89.

105. Ong CK, Seymour RA, Lirk P, et al. Combining paracetamol (acetaminophen) with nonsteroidal antiinflammatory drugs: a qualitative systematic review of analgesic efficacy for acute postoperative pain. Anesth Analg 2010;110:1170–9.

106. McCarthy GC, Megalla SA, Habib AS. Impact of intravenous lidocaine infusion on postoperative analgesia and recovery from surgery: a systematic review of randomized controlled trials. Drugs 2010;70:1149–63.

107. Vigneault L, Turgeon AF, Cote D, et al. Perioperative intravenous lidocaine infusion for postoperative pain control: a meta-analysis of randomized controlled trials. Can J Anaesth 2011;58:22–37.

108. Grady MV, Mascha E, Sessler DI, et al. The effect of perioperative intravenous lidocaine and ketamine on recovery after abdominal hysterectomy. Anesth Analg 2012;115:1078–84.

109. Bryson GL, Charapov I, Krolczyk G, et al. Intravenous lidocaine does not reduce length of hospital stay following abdominal hysterectomy. Can J Anaesth 2010; 57:759–66.

110. Yardeni IZ, Beilin B, Mayburd E, et al. The effect of perioperative intravenous lidocaine on postoperative pain and immune function. Anesth Analg 2009; 109:1464–9.

111. Laskowski K, Stirling A, McKay WP, et al. A systematic review of intravenous ketamine for postoperative analgesia. Can J Anaesth 2011;58:911–23.

112. Sen H, Sizlan A, Yanarates O, et al. A comparison of gabapentin and ketamine in acute and chronic pain after hysterectomy. Anesth Analg 2009;109:1645–50.

113. Bilgin H, Ozcan B, Bilgin T, et al. The influence of timing of systemic ketamine administration on postoperative morphine consumption. J Clin Anesth 2005; 17:592–7.

114. Apfel CC, Laara E, Koivuranta M, et al. A simplified risk score for predicting postoperative nausea and vomiting: conclusions from cross-validations between two centers. Anesthesiology 1999;91:693–700.

115. Centers for Disease Control and Prevention. Current cigarette smoking among adults–United States, 2005–2012. MMWR Morb Mortal Wkly Rep 2014;63(2): 29–34.

116. Apfel CC, Heidrich FM, Jukar-Rao S, et al. Evidence-based analysis of risk factors for postoperative nausea and vomiting. Br J Anaesth 2012;109: 742–53.

117. Gan TJ, Diemunsch P, Habib AS, et al. Consensus guidelines for the management of postoperative nausea and vomiting. Anesth Analg 2014;118:85–113.

118. Sinclair DR, Chung F, Mezei G. Can postoperative nausea and vomiting be predicted? Anesthesiology 1999;91:109–18.

119. Callesen T, Schouenborg L, Nielsen D, et al. Combined epidural-spinal opioid-free anaesthesia and analgesia for hysterectomy. Br J Anaesth 1999;82:881–5.

120. Apfel CC, Kranke P, Katz MH, et al. Volatile anaesthetics may be the main cause of early but not delayed postoperative vomiting: a randomized controlled trial of factorial design. Br J Anaesth 2002;88:659–68.

121. Fernandez-Guisasola J, Gomez-Arnau JI, Cabrera Y, et al. Association between nitrous oxide and the incidence of postoperative nausea and vomiting in adults: a systematic review and meta-analysis. Anaesthesia 2010;65:379–87.

122. Tramer M, Moore A, McQuay H. Propofol anaesthesia and postoperative nausea and vomiting: quantitative systematic review of randomized controlled studies. Br J Anaesth 1997;78:247–55.

123. McDaid C, Maund E, Rice S, et al. Paracetamol and selective and non-selective non-steroidal anti-inflammatory drugs (NSAIDs) for the reduction

of morphine-related side effects after major surgery: a systematic review. Health Technol Assess 2010;14:1–153, iii–iv.

124. Holte K, Kehlet H. Fluid therapy and surgical outcomes in elective surgery: a need for reassessment in fast-track surgery. J Am Coll Surg 2006;202:971–89.

125. Maharaj CH, Kallam SR, Malik A, et al. Preoperative intravenous fluid therapy decreases postoperative nausea and pain in high risk patients. Anesth Analg 2005;100:675–82 Table of contents.

126. Ali SZ, Taguchi A, Holtmann B, et al. Effect of supplemental pre-operative fluid on postoperative nausea and vomiting. Anaesthesia 2003;58:780–4.

127. Apfel CC, Meyer A, Orhan-Sungur M, et al. Supplemental intravenous crystalloids for the prevention of postoperative nausea and vomiting: quantitative review. Br J Anaesth 2012;108:893–902.

128. Habib AS, El-Moalem HE, Gan TJ. The efficacy of the 5-HT3 receptor antagonists combined with droperidol for PONV prophylaxis is similar to their combination with dexamethasone. A meta-analysis of randomized controlled trials. Can J Anaesth 2004;51:311–9.

129. Apfel CC, Korttila K, Abdalla M, et al. A factorial trial of six interventions for the prevention of postoperative nausea and vomiting. N Engl J Med 2004;350:2441–51.

130. Gan TJ, Apfel CC, Kovac A, et al. A randomized, double-blind comparison of the NK1 antagonist, aprepitant, versus ondansetron for the prevention of postoperative nausea and vomiting. Anesth Analg 2007;104:1082–9 Tables of contents.

131. McKenny M, Conroy P, Wong A, et al. A randomised prospective trial of intraoperative oesophageal Doppler-guided fluid administration in major gynaecological surgery. Anaesthesia 2013;68:1224–31.

132. Chattopadhyay S, Mittal S, Christian S, et al. The role of intraoperative fluid optimization using the esophageal Doppler in advanced gynecological cancer: early postoperative recovery and fitness for discharge. Int J Gynecol Cancer 2013;23:199–207.

133. Gan TJ, Soppitt A, Maroof M, et al. Goal-directed intraoperative fluid administration reduces length of hospital stay after major surgery. Anesthesiology 2002;97:820–6.

134. Cecconi M, Corredor C, Arulkumaran N, et al. Clinical review: goal-directed therapy–what is the evidence in surgical patients? The effect on different risk groups. Crit Care 2013;17:209.

135. de Groot JJ, van Es LE, Maessen JM, et al. Diffusion of enhanced recovery principles in gynecologic oncology surgery: is active implementation still necessary? Gynecol Oncol 2014;134:570–5.

136. Billson HA, Holland C, Curwell J, et al. Perioperative nutrition interventions for women with ovarian cancer. Cochrane Database Syst Rev 2013;(9):CD009884.

137. Siedhoff MT, Clark LH, Hobbs KA, et al. Mechanical bowel preparation before laparoscopic hysterectomy: a randomized controlled trial. Obstet Gynecol 2014;123:562–7.

138. Lijoi D, Ferrero S, Mistrangelo E, et al. Bowel preparation before laparoscopic gynaecological surgery in benign conditions using a 1-week low fibre diet: a surgeon blind, randomized and controlled trial. Arch Gynecol Obstet 2009;280:713–8.

139. Ballard AC, Parker-Autry CY, Markland AD, et al. Bowel preparation before vaginal prolapse surgery: a randomized controlled trial. Obstet Gynecol 2014;123:232–8.

140. Nelson R, Edwards S, Tse B. Prophylactic nasogastric decompression after abdominal surgery. Cochrane Database Syst Rev 2007;(3):CD004929.
141. Charoenkwan K, Phillipson G, Vutyavanich T. Early versus delayed (traditional) oral fluids and food for reducing complications after major abdominal gynaeco-logic surgery. Cochrane Database Syst Rev 2007;(4):CD004508.
142. Murphy M, Olivera C, Wheeler T 2nd, et al. Postoperative management and restrictions for female pelvic surgery: a systematic review. Int Urogynecol J 2013;24:185–93.
143. Morrill MY, Schimpf MO, Abed H, et al. Antibiotic prophylaxis for selected gynecologic surgeries. Int J Gynaecol Obstet 2013;120:10–5.
144. Van Eyk N, van Schalkwyk J. Antibiotic prophylaxis in gynaecologic procedures. J Obstet Gynaecol Can 2012;34:382–91.
145. Lin YS. Preliminary results of laparoscopic modified radical hysterectomy in early invasive cervical cancer. J Am Assoc Gynecol Laparosc 2003;10:80–4.
146. Weinberg L, Rao S, Escobar PF. Robotic surgery in gynecology: an updated systematic review. Obstet Gynecol Int 2011;2011:852061.
147. Einstein MH, Kushner DM, Connor JP, et al. A protocol of dual prophylaxis for venous thromboembolism prevention in gynecologic cancer patients. Obstet Gynecol 2008;112:1091–7.
148. Bouchard-Fortier G, Geerts WH, Covens A, et al. Is venous thromboprophylaxis necessary in patients undergoing minimally invasive surgery for a gynecologic malignancy? Gynecol Oncol 2014;134:228–32.
149. Brummer TH, Heikkinen A, Jalkanen J, et al. Pharmaceutical thrombosis pro-phylaxis, bleeding complications and thromboembolism in a national cohort of hysterectomy for benign disease. Hum Reprod 2012;27:1628–36.

Anesthesia for Emergency Abdominal Surgery

Carol Peden, MB ChB, MD, FRCA, FFICM, MPH[a],*, Michael J. Scott, MB ChB, MRCP, FRCA, FFICM[b,c]

KEYWORDS

- Emergency surgery • Laparotomy • Sepsis • Surviving Sepsis • Enhanced recovery
- High mortality • ELPQuIC bundle

KEY POINTS

- Emergency laparotomy is a common procedure with high mortality and morbidity.
- There is a diverse range of causes and surgical treatment, with up to 40% of patients having sepsis at the time of presentation.
- Patients who are elderly often have multiple comorbidities and a mortality of up to 25%, and for those undergoing emergency colorectal resection their life expectancy at 1 year is around 50%.
- Patients presenting for surgery have deranged body homeostasis and gut dysfunction, and a high incidence of sepsis; they are effectively experiencing a complication before surgery.
- Little research has been done in this area; however, the introduction of standardized pathways of care expediting diagnosis, resuscitation, and sepsis management with urgent surgery followed by critical care admission may improve outcomes.

INTRODUCTION

This article reviews the epidemiology and pathophysiology of patients presenting for emergency intra-abdominal surgery (excluding vascular and trauma-related surgery), particularly the generic operation known as emergency laparotomy. This procedure is well known to every anesthesiologist who deals with emergency surgery; however, the common factor of a surgeon opening an abdomen to manage an intra-abdominal emergency can have multiple causes, and multiple different procedures are encompassed by the overarching term laparotomy. This article examines the organizational issues that may challenge health care teams trying to optimize care for this group of patients. It reviews the latest developments and evidence base for anesthesia and perioperative care pathways to optimize outcomes.

[a] Royal United Hospital, Combe Park, Bath BA1 3NG, UK; [b] Department of Anesthesia and Perioperative Medicine, Royal Surrey County Hospital NHS Foundation Trust, Surrey, Guildford GU1 7XX, UK; [c] Surrey Perioperative Anesthesia Critical Care Research Group (SPACeR), University of Surrey, Surrey, Guildford GU2 7XH, UK
* Corresponding author.
E-mail address: cpeden@nhs.net

Anesthesiology Clin 33 (2015) 209–221
http://dx.doi.org/10.1016/j.anclin.2014.11.012
anesthesiology.theclinics.com

EPIDEMIOLOGY

Patients undergoing emergency general surgery (EGS) have much higher mortality and morbidity than those patients undergoing elective or scheduled procedures. US outcomes, using data from the American College of Surgeons (ACS) National Surgical Quality Improvement Program (NSQIP), showed a mortality of 14% at 30 days for patients who had undergone emergency laparotomy.[1] Comparison of hospital performance in emergency versus elective general surgery, adjusted for patient-related and operation-related risk factors, showed that emergency status was a significant predictor for morbidity, serious morbidity, and mortality.[2] Outcomes from other countries are similarly poor, with a large UK database study showing an average mortality of 15.6%,[3] and a prospective study with data from 35 hospitals showing a mortality of 14.4% overall, with mortality in patients more than 80 years of age increasing to an average 24.4%.[4] Other countries also show high average mortality, with a Danish cohort study showing a mean mortality of 18.5% at 30 days.[5] Long-term outcomes are even worse, with only 49% of patients more than 80 years of age who had undergone nonelective colorectal resection alive at 1 year.[6]

The resource burden of emergency general surgery is high, with a 10-year analysis of the US Nationwide Inpatient sample (2001–2010) showing that 7.1% of all hospital admissions were related to EGS, with 29% of these patients requiring surgery; the population-adjusted case rate of 1290 admissions per 100,000 people was higher than the sum of all new cancer diagnoses, and has increased annually since 2001.[7]

Despite the volume of patient episodes, high mortality, and use of resources by this patient group there has been, until recently, little discussion about the management of these patients in the anesthetic or surgical literature. One of the reasons for this may be the number and diversity of causes of EGS, ranging from an incarcerated hernia to infarcted bowel, with an associated range of morbidity and mortality. Symons and colleagues[3] analyzed the hospital episode statistics (HES) database of the UK National Health Service system for EGS admissions with a greater than 5% 30-day mortality. From a total of 367,796 patients, the investigators defined 8 groups of high-risk diagnoses, with 30-day mortality ranging between 7.4% and 47.4%. Al-Temimi and colleagues[1] found that the commonest indications for EGS in the NSQIP database were intestinal obstruction (33.6%), perforation (19%), and exploratory laparotomy with or without wound debridement or abscess drainage (10%); the strongest predictors of mortality were a white blood cell count of less than 4500/mm^3 or greater than 20,000 mm^3, septic shock, an American Society of Anesthesiologists (ASA) class IV at the time of surgery, age 70 years or older, and a dependent functional status. Patients with all these risk factors present had a predicted 30-day mortality of 50%.

The studies showing poor outcomes from EGS also show significant variation between hospitals after risk adjustment, with clear high and low outlying hospitals.[1–4] Hospitals with low mortality from EGS had significantly more intensive care beds per 1000 hospital beds and made significantly greater use of computed tomography (CT) and ultrasonography.[3] Saunders and colleagues[4] showed that, despite the high mortality for patients undergoing EGS, and a Cochrane Review showing benefit for goal-directed fluid therapy in high-risk patients,[8] only 15% of patients undergoing emergency laparotomy received intraoperative goal-directed fluid therapy. Hospital outcomes for EGS are not consistent with performance as an elective provider (ie, a hospital with good outcomes for elective surgery may not provide good outcomes for EGS).[2]

Patient outcomes for emergency surgery are likely to be improved by prompt investigation, diagnosis, and management. The National Emergency Laparotomy Audit in the United Kingdom collected data on organizational facilities[9] from 191 English and Welsh hospitals performing EGS and compared them with agreed standards.[10,11] Most centers met key recommendations; however, there was substantial variation between hospitals in their ability to provide optimal care, with, for example, two-thirds of hospitals unable to provide 24-hour on-site interventional radiology. The aim of collecting and publishing this type of data, which is linked to a National Audit of Emergency Laparotomy outcomes,[12] is to identify organizational structures, processes, and practices that need improvement or that, more positively, may be linked to good outcomes and from which other centers may learn.

Pathophysiology of Patients Presenting for Emergency Abdominal Surgery

Symons and colleagues[3] analyzed 10 years of hospital data from the United Kingdom and categorized the types of presentation for emergency surgical patients into 6 main categories with a seventh to include other miscellaneous causes. When the pathophysiologic process of intra-abdominal disorder is mapped it can be seen that patients already have a significant physiologic insult, with the development of a stress response, gut dysfunction, insulin resistance, and a systemic inflammatory response syndrome (SIRS) response, with up to 40% of patients having a septic focus. The presence of hypotension secondary to sepsis has a particularly poor outcome and delay in antibiotic administration leads to increased mortality.[13] The derangement in pathophysiology in each case depends on the patient's physiologic, metabolic, and immune status, the type of disorder, and the duration of injury before presentation to hospital (**Table 1**).

Why are Outcomes so Poor for this Group of Patients and is there any Evidence that Improvement Could Occur?

There are several key reasons why this group of patients may have such a poor outcome.[14] First, they can present from several sources; elderly patients in particular may present with nonspecific abdominal pain and gut disturbance and may initially be

Table 1
Potential pathophysiologic processes that develop in emergency surgical patients

Diagnostic Group	No. of Patients	30-d Mortality (%)	Length of Stay (d)*	28-d Readmission (%)	Surgical Treatment (%)	
Liver and biliary conditions	49,611	7.4	8 (5–14)	14.8	5.1	—
Hernias with obstruction or gangrene	31,156	8.2	6 (3–12)	10.7	83.1	Fluid shifts/ Sepsis
Bowel obstruction	158,652	9.8	6 (3–13)	16.3	26.8	Fluid shifts
Gastrointestinal ulcers	26,050	21.5	9 (6–17)	8.5	80.9	Bleeding
Peritonitis	28,218	27.3	9 (4–16)	18.2	25.7	Sepsis
Miscellaneous diagnoses	27,843	28.0	11 (5–21)	16.3	39.9	Sepsis
Bowel ischemia	20,766	47.4	13 (7–23)	14.2	52.5	Sepsis/SIRS
Total	367,796	15.6	8 (4–15)	14.9	37.4	—

* Values are median (interquartile range).
    Data from Symons NR, Moorthy K, Almoudaris AM, et al. Mortality in high-risk emergency general surgical admissions. Br J Surg 2013;100:1318–25.

presumed to have an infective problem and be managed by physicians, delaying time to definitive surgical management. There is some evidence that mortality increases in this group of patients.[15] Second, the patients are often elderly with comorbidities and with additional condition-related insults of sepsis and dehydration. Ingraham and colleagues[2] found that 42.4% of patients for EGS presented with SIRS, sepsis, and septic shock, compared with 4.3% in elective general surgery group data, supported by another small study showing that 46% of patients requiring emergency colorectal surgery presented in septic shock.[16] Third, many hospitals organize their services around elective patients with emergency general surgical patients receiving low priority; there is considerable data to support this.[2,9]

Although the specialty of EGS is developing around the world,[17] it is still possible to have a complex colorectal procedure performed on a critically ill patient at night by a general surgeon whose main expertise is in breast surgery. There is evidence to show that availability of acute care surgeons improves outcomes in patients requiring emergent colon surgery.[16] Moore and colleagues[16] argue that a paradigm shift is needed for the management of patients having emergency surgery, with early evidence-based resuscitation using Surviving Sepsis, guidelines including volume resuscitation and early antibiotics, surgery within 6 hours of presentation, damage control laparotomy, and postoperative care in the intensive care unit (ICU) (**Fig. 1**).

The pathophysiologic insults to patients presenting for EGS are significant, as discussed earlier. It could be argued that the nature of the insult and the limited ability to influence preoperative optimization could explain the high levels of morbidity and mortality. However, case study reviews show multiple defects in the care of these high-risk patients. The 2011 UK National Confidential Enquiry into Patient Outcome and Death[18] examined the care of patients undergoing surgery, both elective and emergency, and found significant deficits; for example, only 26% of high-risk patients had an arterial line placed and only 14% had a central venous catheter. A review of high mortality in patients undergoing colorectal surgery in Veterans Affairs hospitals (63% of the cases were emergencies)[19] showed that delay in diagnosis occurred in 19% of cases, 22% had a delay to surgery, and 14% should have received less radical surgery;

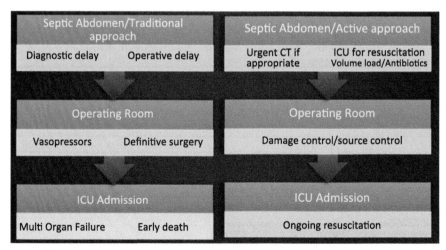

Fig. 1. Changing the way clinicians think: understanding urgency and risk. MOF, multi-organ failure. (*Adapted from* Moore LJ, Turner KL, Jones SL, et al. Availability of acute care surgeons improves outcomes in patients requiring emergent colon surgery. Am J Surg 2011;202(6):840; with permission.)

system issues were identified in 19% and practitioner-related issues in 20% of the cases of patients who died. These findings suggest that there is significant need for improvement in perioperative management in high-risk emergency cases.

CONDUCT OF ANESTHESIA

Anesthetists face many challenges with this group of patients. The emergency presentation means there is often minimal time to assess and optimize the patient before operation. However, a short time spent assessing and resuscitating patients before induction of anesthesia; ensuring that the patient has had broad-spectrum antibiotics, if appropriate; and that they are resuscitated with satisfactory intravascular volume, cardiac output, and oxygen delivery can lead to a more stable perioperative period. Depending on the institute, this can be done in the operating room, an anesthetic room, or on the ICU. Arterial line insertion and central venous line insertion can be performed to assess the patient. Although a central venous line is not a good predictor of fluid responsiveness, it is useful for delivering inotropes and to sample blood for venous extraction. Minimally invasive cardiac output monitoring may also be of benefit. Many anesthetists and intensivists are now becoming skilled at transthoracic echocardiography assessment and this can be used to assess cardiac structure and function, guide resuscitation, and identify perioperative issues such as valve stenosis and regurgitation and areas of myocardial dyskinesia.

Many patients in this group have a SIRS response or are septic and need vasopressors such as a noradrenaline infusion to maintain mean arterial pressure. Vasopressor infusions should ideally be commenced once intravascular volume is replete to avoid occult splanchnic hypovolemia and hypoperfusion; this may not be possible if the patient's condition is critical, but the anesthesiologist should be aware that gut perfusion may be compromised. In elective surgical patients the role of hemodynamic optimization and targeting oxygen delivery is still unclear. However, Surviving Sepsis supports early restoration and maintenance of intravascular volume and mean arterial pressure with crystalloid and noradrenaline infusions and ensuring adequate oxygen delivery using inotropes and blood transfusion as necessary.[20]

Induction and Maintenance of Anesthesia

Anesthetists should aim to induce anesthesia and rapidly secure the airway to avoid the risk of pulmonary aspiration. A rapid sequence induction is classically performed with a predetermined dose of induction agent, suxamethonium, and the addition of cricoid pressure to reduce this risk. Experienced anesthetists often modify the induction by using opioids and titration of induction agents to maintain better hemodynamic stability and use rocuronium to avoid the use of suxamethonium to enable rapid endotracheal intubation. Intubation aids such as a gum elastic bougie and fiberoptic laryngoscopes should be immediately available. An awake fiberoptic intubation can be performed if difficult intubation is predicted.

Anesthesia should be maintained using oxygen-enriched air with a short-acting anesthetic such as sevoflurane or desflurane. There is no evidence to support one anesthetic agent rather than another or to use propofol target-controlled infusions in this group. Short-acting opioids can be used, such as fentanyl of a remifentanil infusion. Muscle relaxation guided by a peripheral nerve stimulator should be maintained through the procedure to help the surgeon. Fluids and blood products should be warmed and forced-air warming used to maintain normothermia as appropriate throughout the procedure. Some patients may have sepsis or a SIRS response, and may have pyrexia, so nasopharyngeal temperature monitoring should be used to guide warming.

Ventilation should be done using a low tidal volume and high respiratory rate with optimal positive end-expiratory pressure to reduce the risk of acute lung injury.[21,22] In order to reduce the risk of microaspiration around the tracheal cuff, which can predispose to postoperative pneumonia, polyurethane cuffs and correctly sized endotracheal tubes should be used.

ANALGESIA

In elective midline laparotomy the use of thoracic epidural analgesia (TEA) offers many benefits in addition to analgesia, such as reduced use of opioids, reduced pulmonary complications, reduced thromboembolic risk, reduced incidence of ileus, and reduction of the stress response[23]; however, as an emergency procedure its use is more problematic. Patients can be too unstable to insert the epidural before surgery or may have contraindications such as sepsis or a coagulation disorder. There may be an opportunity to insert TEA on the ICU or to use an alternative such as rectus sheath catheters, wound catheters, and transversus abdominis plane blocks, so where possible consent should be taken for this before anesthesia.[24] Intravenous morphine is effective and efficacious but has the disadvantage of increasing postoperative nausea and vomiting, increasing the risk of ileus, and increasing somnolence and sleep disturbance.

SURGERY

There is evidence that, for this group of patients, the duration of surgery is critical.[25] Although patients may require a simple procedure, such as oversewing of a perforation to save their life, others require complex, difficult surgery. The concept of damage-control surgery was first developed to minimize surgical stress for patients following major trauma; however, the concept can equally be applied to those patients undergoing emergency surgery for nontrauma intra-abdominal disorders.[26] If the patient is septic, urgent source control of the sepsis is required. For many procedures encompassed by the term emergency laparotomy, the surgeon must consider whether a primary anastomosis and closure of the patient's abdomen are appropriate at the time of the initial surgery, or whether these procedures should be delayed until the patient's physiologic state has improved.[16,26,27]

POSTOPERATIVE CARE

Although in most elective surgical cases it is the intention of the anesthetist to wake and extubate the patient at the end of surgery, the physiologic processes in this group of patients may require a period of postoperative ventilatory support in the ICU to optimize outcome. Reasons for this include:

- Septic shock with an oxygen deficit and increased lactate level
- Hemodynamic instability or the need for large doses of vasopressors and inotropes
- Significant acidosis
- Massive bleeding with coagulopathy
- Requirement for renal support/continuous venovenous hemodialysis
- Abdominal distension that can cause significant reduction in functional residual capacity so that there would be respiratory compromise at extubation

Careful assessment should be made of patients before extubation. Depending on the length and nature of the intra-abdominal surgery, reassessment of the patient's predicted outcome using a scoring system taking into account blood loss, temperature, blood glucose, lactate, and surgical findings is likely to be justified.[28] Depending on the results of this assessment an informed decision can be made about whether or not the patient should be extubated, and what level of postoperative care is needed.

Evidence suggests that postoperative management is an area in which major improvements in care could be made for patients having EGS.[29] In an important article examining determinants of long-term survival after major surgery, the occurrence of a 30-day postoperative complication was more important than preoperative patient risk and intraoperative factors in determining survival after major surgery. The complications with the greatest impact, pneumonia and myocardial infarction occurring within 30 days of surgery, reduced survival up to 5 years after surgery. This article and others from the ACS NSQIP program also show that, when attention is paid to quality and process improvement in perioperative care, outcomes even for high-risk patients improve. Hall and colleagues[30] reported on 118 hospitals participating in the NSQIP programme; 66% of hospitals improved risk-adjusted mortality and 82% improved risk-adjusted complication rates. There was a correlation between initial observed/expected outcome ratios and the degree of improvement, initially worse-performing hospitals had more likelihood of improvement but hospitals that originally performed well also improved and the variation in outcome was reduced.

Preventing mortality and morbidity in patients undergoing EGS may require improved postoperative monitoring to detect and manage complications early. Ghaferi and colleagues[31] described high-mortality and low-mortality surgical hospitals, and these hospitals had similar rates of major complications and postoperative complications overall; what determined the different rates of death between low-mortality and high-mortality hospitals seemed to be the timely recognition and management of complications when they occurred, which may be best achieved by admission to a critical care bed. Although there are many scoring systems that can be used to assess operative risk,[32] there is little evidence that these are routinely used to enhance decision making about postoperative location for the emergency patient,[12] and triage may be required when bed availability is limited.[33] High-risk patients undergoing EGS may not always get optimal postoperative care and may be less likely to be admitted to critical care than patients undergoing major elective procedures with much lower mortality.[34–36] Most patients undergoing emergency laparotomy are likely to need critical care. The Emergency Laparotomy Network report found that patients who were more than 65 years of age and/or ASA III or more had a mortality of greater than 10%; these are criteria for ICU admission by most standards, but 33% of these patients were not admitted to a monitored bed postoperatively.[4] One of the suggested reasons for the high mortality (18.5% at 30 days and 24% at 90 days) of patients in the Danish cohort study[5] was that 84% of the patients did not receive any postoperative critical care.

Older patients (>65 years) are at substantially greater risk for adverse events following EGS procedures, with evidence of substantial variation in the quality of care delivered.[37,38] When variation exists it is likely that significant improvement is achievable through the reliable delivery of evidence-based processes, such as objective decision making about postoperative location.[38]

IMPROVING PERIOPERATIVE CARE

There are many options and areas to focus on to improve outcomes for high-risk surgical patients. A work plan can be visualized through the development of a driver diagram such as is shown in **Fig. 2**.

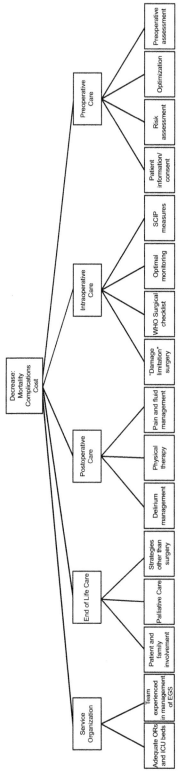

Fig. 2. Driver diagram. OR, operating room; SCIP, surgical care improvement project; WHO, World Health Organization. (*Adapted from* Peden CJ. Emergency surgery in the elderly patient: a quality improvement approach. Anaesthesia 2011;66:435–45; with permission.)

This list of areas that could have improvement projects attached is not comprehensive, but is a systematic approach to identifying areas on which to focus. Continued measurement for improvement of process and outcome data in each project area to understand how a service is performing will help to understand areas of practice to be worked on to drive better patient care and create the energy for improvement. Use of checklists to facilitate key components of care across surgical pathways has been shown to improve morbidity and mortality even in low-risk groups of patients.[39]

Improving outcomes for this complex patient group may be best achieved by standardization of the patient pathway and adherence to delivery of key components. The articles in this issue discuss the concept of fast track or enhanced recovery for patients undergoing elective procedures, but there is no reason why the principle should not be applied to emergency patients.[40] Simplification through protocolization of a high-risk hospital episode may enable delivery of essential components of care. An enhanced recovery programme is designed to deliver care that minimizes the patient's physiologic stress response to surgery with an evidence-based, patient-centered approach combining individual interventions, which, when used together consistently by a multidisciplinary team, are synergistic, with a greater impact on outcome than when used alone or in a haphazard way.[41–43] Although the preoperative components of such a programme may not be relevant to emergency patients, intraoperative management and postoperative care can be delivered in line with the principles of enhanced recovery.

Key elements for optimizing postoperative recovery following colorectal surgery:
1. Appropriate postoperative care location: ward/high dependency unit/ICU
2. Balanced analgesia
3. Appropriate monitoring during the initial postoperative period, when increased oxygen demand and fluid shifts demand individualized titration of fluids to maintain normovolemia, but avoid crystalloid excess
4. Early enteral nutrition
5. Early and structured postoperative mobilization
6. Venous thromboembolism prophylaxis
7. Patients should be involved in the process and motivated to reach predefined goals

A structured pathway for unscheduled adult general surgery is provided in "The Higher Risk General Surgical Patient" document from the Royal College of Surgeons England 2011,[10] which has 4 components: clinical assessment, diagnostics, intraoperative assessment, and postoperative care.

The principles of enhanced recovery and the pathway suggested earlier were tested in 4 hospitals. The hospitals developed a care bundle with 5 key components to be delivered to patients undergoing emergency laparotomy, termed the Emergency Laparotomy Quality Improvement Care (ELPQuIC) bundle.

The ELPQuIC bundle consists of:
1. Early assessment and resuscitation
2. Antibiotics administered to patients who show signs of sepsis
3. Prompt diagnosis and early surgery
4. Goal-directed fluid therapy in theaters and continued to ICU
5. Postoperative intensive care for all patients

The 4 participating hospitals measured their performance on these key metrics and several other process measures. No hospital achieved reliable delivery of all key processes, but all teams improved in delivery of all care bundle components from their baseline levels of performance. There was a significant reduction in risk-adjusted mortality across all 4 hospitals following implementation of the care bundle.[44] This study showed that it is possible to improve outcomes in the diverse group of patients undergoing emergency laparotomy using a quality-improvement approach to improve delivery of evidence-based components of a standardized care pathway.

The difficulty in undertaking randomized controlled trials in the diverse, sick patients who undergo emergency laparotomy may account for the paucity of research in this patient group to date. However, the increasing recognition that quality-improvement studies can lead to change, and are scientifically valid, is gaining traction. The British National Institute of Health Research has given major funding to the EPOCH (Enhanced Perioperative Care for High-risk patients) study to use quality-improvement methodology with the aim of reducing 90-day mortality in patients undergoing emergency mortality.[45] The EPOCH study draws its outcome data from participating hospitals' own submissions to the National Emergency Laparotomy Audit database.

Focus on the Elderly

Many of the patients presenting for EGS are elderly. Studies of older patients undergoing elective surgery have shown that proactive identification and management of problems such as nutrition and frailty can improve outcomes with a significant reduction in complications and length of stay[46]; this proactive approach is the same as that advocated by enhanced recovery programs. A small study in patients presenting for emergency surgery suggested that proactive referral to care of the elderly physicians, even if done at the time of surgery, may reduce length of stay.[47] The British Hip Fracture Database[48] shows that monitored delivery of key components of care, including perioperative management by orthogeriatric physicians, has led to a continued improvement in outcomes in elderly patients undergoing urgent surgery for fractured neck of femur. When outcomes of emergency intestinal surgery were compared with outcomes of similar procedures performed electively, elderly patients were much less likely to be discharged back to independent status, with 69% of elective patients discharged directly home compared with 6.5% of emergency surgical patients.[49] It is this type of outcome data that patients may value most when making decisions about undergoing high-risk EGS, but there are few data about long-term outcomes and quality of life following EGS, particularly in the elderly[50]; there is evidence of underappreciation of the impact of a hospital stay on functional performance of patients discharged to the community.[51] It may be that, for some patients, the risk of surgery is so high and the quality of survival so poor that a focus on pain relief and palliative care is in their best interests. However, more outcomes research is needed before clinicians can have truly informed discussions with their patients, particularly the elderly, before they undergo emergency laparotomy.[52]

SUMMARY AND FUTURE CONSIDERATIONS

Specific pathways of care may be needed to focus on patients having EGS who have different needs to those of patients undergoing elective general surgery. A focus on reliable delivery of key components of care, the early and optimal management of sepsis, preoperative resuscitation, and prevention of postoperative complications can lead to significantly improved outcomes for this high-risk group of surgical patients. Further research is needed into optimizing the perioperative care pathway, surgery, and rehabilitation after EGS.

REFERENCES

1. Al-Temimi MH, Griffee M, Enniss TM, et al. When is death inevitable after emergency laparotomy? Analysis of the American College of Surgeons National Surgical Quality Improvement Program Database. J Am Coll Surg 2012;215(4):503–11.

2. Ingraham AM, Cohen ME, Raval MV, et al. Comparison of hospital performance in emergency versus elective general surgery operations at 198 hospitals. J Am Coll Surg 2011;212:20–8.

3. Symons NR, Moorthy K, Almoudaris AM, et al. Mortality in high-risk emergency general surgical admissions. Br J Surg 2013;100:1318–25.

4. Saunders DI, Murray D, Pichel AC, et al. Variations in mortality after emergency laparotomy: the first report of the UK Emergency Laparotomy Network. Br J Anaesth 2012;109(3):368–75.

5. Vester-Andersen M, Lundstrøm LH, Møller MH, et al. Mortality and postoperative care pathways after emergency gastrointestinal surgery in 2904 patients: a population-based cohort study. Br J Anaesth 2014;112(5):860–70.

6. Mamidanna R, Eid-Arimoku L, Almoudaris AM, et al. Poor 1-year survival in elderly patients undergoing non-elective colorectal resection. Dis Colon Rectum 2012;55:788–96.

7. Gale SC, Shafi S, Dombrovskiy VY, et al. The public health burden of emergency general surgery in the United States: a 10-year analysis of the Nationwide Inpatient Sample–2001 to 2010. J Trauma Acute Care Surg 2014;77:202–8.

8. Grocott MP, Dushianthan A, Hamilton MA, et al. Perioperative increase in global blood flow to explicit defined goals and outcomes after surgery: a Cochrane Systematic Review. Br J Anaesth 2013;111(4):535–48. Available at: http://www.ncbi.nlm.nih.gov/pubmed/23661403.

9. NELA Project Team. First organisational report of the national emergency laparotomy audit. London: RCoA; 2014. Available at: http://www.hqip.org.uk/assets/NCAPOP-Library/NCAPOP-2014-15/National-Emergency-Laparotomy-Audit-Full-Report-May-2014.pdf. Accessed October 12, 2014.

10. The Royal College of Surgeons of England, Department of Health. The higher risk general surgical patient. 2011. Available at: http://www.rcseng.ac.uk/publications/docs/higher-risk-surgical-patient. Accessed October 12, 2014.

11. The Royal College of Surgeons of England. Emergency surgery: standards for unscheduled care. 2011. Available at: https://www.rcseng.ac.uk/publications/docs/emergency-surgery-standards-for-unscheduled-care. Accessed October 12, 2014.

12. The National Emergency Laparotomy audit NELA. Available at: http://www.nela.org.uk. Accessed October 12, 2014.

13. Kumar A, Roberts D, Wood KE, et al. Duration of hypotension before initiation of effective antimicrobial therapy is the critical determinant of survival in human septic shock. Crit Care Med 2006;34:1589–96.

14. Huddart S, Peden CJ, Quiney N. Emergency Major Abdominal Surgery – 'The times they are a changing'. Colorectal Dis 2013;5:645–9.

15. National Confidential Enquiry into Patient Outcome and Death 2010. An age old problem: a review of the care received by elderly patients undergoing surgery. Available at: http://www.ncepod.org.uk/2010report3/downloads/EESE_fullReport.pdf. Accessed October 12, 2014.

16. Moore LJ, Turner KL, Jones SL, et al. Availability of acute care surgeons improves outcomes in patients requiring emergent colon surgery. Am J Surg 2011;202(6):837–42. Available at: http://www.ncbi.nlm.nih.gov/pubmed/22014648.

17. Sorelli P, El-Masry N, Dawson P, et al. The dedicated emergency surgeon: towards consultant-based acute surgical admissions. Ann R Coll Surg Engl 2008;90:104–8. Available at: www.ncbi.nlm.nih.gov/pubmed/1832520.

18. National Confidential Enquiry into Patient Outcome and Death. Knowing the risk. A review of the peri-operative care of surgical patients. Published December

2011. Available at: http://www.ncepod.org.uk/2011poc.htm. Accessed January 11, 2013.

19. Kamal IM, Denwood R, Schifftener R, et al. Causes of high mortality in colorectal surgery. A review of episodes of care in Veterans Affairs Hospitals. Am J Surg 2007;19:639–45.

20. Dellinger RP, Levy MM, Rhodes A, et al. Surviving Sepsis campaign: international guidelines for management of severe sepsis and septic shock: 2012. Crit Care Med 2013;41(2):580–637. http://dx.doi.org/10.1097/CCM.0b013e31827e83af.

21. Futier E, Constatin JM, Paugam-Burtz C, et al. A trial of intraoperative low-tidal-volume ventilation in abdominal surgery. N Engl J Med 2013;369:428–37. http://dx.doi.org/10.1056/NEJMoa1301082.

22. Severgnini P, Selmo G, Lanza C, et al. Protective mechanical ventilation during general anesthesia for open abdominal surgery improves postoperative pulmonary function. Anesthesiology 2013;118:1307–21.

23. Nimmo SM, Harrington LS. What is the role of epidural analgesia in abdominal surgery? Contin Educ Anaesth Crit Care Pain 2014;14(5):224–9. Available at: http://ceaccp.oxfordjournals.org/content/early/2014/04/10/bjaceaccp.mkt062.

24. Ventham NT, Hughes M, O'Neill S, et al. Systematic review and meta-analysis of continuous local anaesthetic wound infiltration versus epidural analgesia for postoperative pain following abdominal surgery. Br J Surg 2013;100(10):1280–9.

25. Turrentine FE, Wang H, Simpson VB, et al. Surgical risk factors, morbidity and mortality in elderly patients. J Am Coll Surg 2006;203:865–77.

26. Weber DG, Bendinelli C, Balogh ZJ. Damage control surgery for abdominal emergencies. Br J Surg 2014;101(1):e109–18. Available at: http://www.ncbi.nlm.nih.gov/pubmed/24273018. Accessed August 10, 2014.

27. Godat L, Kobayashi L, Constantini T, et al. Abdominal damage control surgery and reconstruction: World Society of Emergency Surgery position paper. World J Emerg Surg 2013;8:53.

28. Hobson SA, Sutton CD, Garcea G, et al. Prospective comparison of POSSUM and P_POSSUM with clinical assessment of mortality following emergency surgery. Acta Anaesthesiol Scand 2007;51:94–100.

29. Khuri SF, Henderson WG, DePalma RG, et al, Participants in the VA National Surgical Quality Improvement Program. Determinants of long-term survival after major surgery and the adverse effect of postoperative complications. Ann Surg 2005;242:326–41.

30. Hall BL, Hamilton BH, Richards K, et al. Does surgical quality improve in the ACS NSQIP: an evaluation of all participating hospitals. Ann Surg 2009;250:363–76.

31. Ghaferi AA, Birkmeyer JD, Dimick JB. Variation in hospital mortality associated with inpatient surgery. N Engl J Med 2009;361:1368–75.

32. Moonesinghe SR, Mythen MG, Das P, et al. Risk stratification tools for predicting morbidity and mortality in adult patients undergoing major surgery: qualitative systematic review. Anesthesiology 2013;119:959–81.

33. Sobol JB, Wunsch H. Triage of high-risk surgical patients for intensive care. Crit Care 2011;15:217.

34. Pearse RM, Moreno RP, Bauer P, et al. Mortality after surgery in Europe: a 7 day cohort study. Lancet 2012;380:1059–65.

35. Pearse RM, Harrison DA, James P, et al. Identification and characterisation of the high-risk surgical population in the United Kingdom. Crit Care 2006;10:R81.

36. Jhanji S, Thomas B, Ely A, et al. Mortality and utilization of critical care resources amongst high-risk surgical patients in a large NHS trust. Anaesthesia 2008;63:695–700.

37. Ingraham AM, Cohen ME, Raval MV, et al. Variation in quality of care after emergency general surgery procedures in the elderly. J Am Coll Surg 2011;212: 1039–48.

38. Peden CJ. Emergency surgery in the elderly patient: a quality improvement approach. Anaesthesia 2011;66:435–45.

39. de Vries EN, Prins HA, Crolla RM, et al. Effect of a comprehensive surgical safety system on patient outcomes. N Engl J Med 2010;363:1928–37.

40. Gonenc M, Dural AC, Celik F, et al. Enhanced postoperative recovery pathways in emergency surgery: a randomised controlled clinical trial. Am J Surg 2014;207: 807–14. Available at: http://www.ncbi.nlm.nih.gov/pubmed/24119887. Accessed August 10, 2014.

41. Kehlet H. Fast track colorectal surgery. Lancet 2008;371:791–3.

42. Lassen K, Soop M, Nygren J, et al. Consensus review of optimal perioperative care in colorectal surgery: Enhanced Recovery After Surgery (ERAS) Group Recommendations. Arch Surg 2009;144(10):961–9.

43. Delivering enhanced recovery. Enhanced recovery partnership programme. Available at: http://webarchive.nationalarchives.gov.uk/20130107105354/http://www.dh.gov.uk/prod_consum_dh/groups/dh_digitalassets/@dh/@en/@ps/documents/digitalasset/dh_115156.pdf. Accessed December 14, 2014.

44. Huddart S, Peden CJ, Quiney N, et al. Use of the emergency laparotomy pathway quality improvement care bundle (ELPQuiC) to reduce mortality after emergency laparotomy. Br J Surg 2014. [Epub ahead of print].

45. Enhanced Peri-Operative Care for High-risk patients (EPOCH) trial. [Internet]. Available at: http://www.epochtrial.org/epoch.php. Accessed December 14, 2014.

46. Harari D, Hopper A, Dhesi J, et al. Proactive care of older people undergoing surgery ('POPS'): designing, embedding, evaluating and funding a comprehensive geriatric assessment service for older elective surgical patients. Age Ageing 2007;36:190–6.

47. Fitton L, Royds M, McNarry A, et al. Early multidisciplinary referral and length of stay of elderly emergency surgical patients. European J Anaesthesia 2010; 27:241.

48. National hip fracture database. National report 2013. Available at: www.nhfd.co.uk/20/hipfractureR.nsf/0/CA920122A244F2ED802579C900553993/$file/NHFD%20Report%202013.pdf. Accessed October 10, 2014.

49. Louis DJ, Hsu A, Brand MI, et al. Morbidity and mortality in octogenarians and older undergoing major intestinal surgery. Dis Colon Rectum 2009;52:59–63. http://dx.doi.org/10.1007/DCR.0b013e31819754d4.

50. Peden CJ, Grocott M. National research strategies: what outcomes are important in peri-operative elderly care? Anaesthesia 2014;69(Suppl 1):61–9. http://dx.doi.org/10.1111/anae.12491.

51. Krumholz HM. Post-hospital syndrome – an acquired transient condition of general risk. N Engl J Med 2013;368:100–2.

52. Kwok AC, Semel ME, Lipsitz SR, et al. The intensity and variation of surgical care at the end of life: a retrospective cohort study. Lancet 2011;378:1408–13.

Index

Note: Page numbers of article titles are in **boldface** type.

Anesthesiology Clin 33 (2015) 223–231
http://dx.doi.org/10.1016/S1932-2275(15)00009-9
anesthesiology.theclinics.com
1932-2275/15/$ – see front matter © 2015 Elsevier Inc. All rights reserved.

Printed and bound by CPI Group (UK) Ltd, Croydon, CR0 4YY

03/10/2024

01040487-0008